ANCA-associated Vasculitis

Guest Editors

BARRI J. FESSLER, MD
S. LOUIS BRIDGES JR, MD, PhD

RHEUMATIC DISEASE CLINICS OF NORTH AMERICA

www.rheumatic.theclinics.com

August 2010 • Volume 36 • Number 3

SAUNDERS an imprint of ELSEVIER, Inc.

W.B. SAUNDERS COMPANY

A Division of Elsevier Inc.

1600 John F. Kennedy Blvd., Suite 1800 • Philadelphia, PA 19103-2899

http://www.theclinics.com

**RHEUMATIC DISEASE CLINICS OF NORTH AMERICA Volume 36, Number 3
August 2010 ISSN 0889-857X, ISBN 13: 978-1-4377-2493-6**

Editor: Rachel Glover

Rheumatic Disease Clinics of North America (ISSN 0889-857X) is published quarterly by Elsevier Inc., 360 Park Avenue South, New York, NY 10010-1710. Months of issue are February, May, August, and November. Business and editorial offices: 1600 John F. Kennedy Boulevard, Suite 1800, Philadelphia, PA 19103-2899. Periodicals postage paid at New York, NY and additional mailing offices. Subscription prices are USD 264.00 per year for US individuals, USD 455.00 per year for US institutions, USD 132.00 per year for US students and residents, USD 311.00 per year for Canadian individuals, USD 563.00 per year for Canadian institutions, USD 369.00 per year for international individuals, USD 563.00 per year for international institutions, and USD 185.00 per year for Canadian and foreign students/residents. To receive student/resident rate, orders must be accompanied by name of affiliated institution, date of term, and the *signature* of program/residency coordinator on institution letterhead. Orders will be billed at individual rate until proof of status received. Foreign air speed delivery is included in all *Clinics* subscription prices. All prices are subject to change without notice. **POSTMASTER:** Send address changes to *Rheumatic Disease Clinics of North America,* Elsevier Health Sciences Division, Subscription Customer Service, 3251 Riverport Lane, Maryland Heights, MO 63043. **Customer Service: 1-800-654-2452 (US and Canada). From outside of the US and Canada: 314-453-7041. Fax: 314-453-5170. For print support, e-mail: JournalsCustomerService-usa@elsevier.com. For online support, e-mail: JournalsOnline Support-usa@elsevier.com.**

Reprints. For copies of 100 or more of articles in this publication, please contact the Commercial Reprints Department, Elsevier Inc., 360 Park Avenue South, New York, New York, 10010-1710; Tel.: (+1) 212-633-3813, Fax: (+1) 212-462-1935, and E-mail: reprints@elsevier.com.

Rheumatic Disease Clinics of North America is covered in *MEDLINE/PubMed (Index Medicus), Current Contents/Clinical Medicine, Science Citation Index, ISI/BIOMED,* and *EMBASE/Excerpta Medica.*

Printed and bound by CPI Group (UK) Ltd, Croydon, CR0 4YY
Transferred to Digital Print 2011

Contributors

GUEST EDITORS

BARRI J. FESSLER, MD
Associate Professor of Medicine, Division of Clinical Immunology and Rheumatology, University of Alabama at Birmingham, Birmingham, Alabama

S. LOUIS BRIDGES Jr, MD, PhD
Marguerite Jones Harbert-Gene V. Ball, MD Professor of Medicine; Director, Division of Clinical Immunology and Rheumatology, University of Alabama at Birmingham, Birmingham, Alabama

AUTHORS

CHIARA BALDINI, MD, PhD
Rheumatology Unit, Department of Internal Medicine, University of Pisa, Pisa, Italy

GENE V. BALL, MD
Professor Emeritus, Division of Clinical Immunology and Rheumatology, University of Alabama at Birmingham, Birmingham, Alabama

STEFANO BOMBARDIERI, MD
Professor of Rheumatology Unit, Department of Internal Medicine, University of Pisa, Pisa, Italy

SHARON A. CHUNG, MD, MAS
Assistant Professor of Medicine, Division of Rheumatology, Rosalind Russell Medical Research Center for Arthritis, University of California, San Francisco, California

JULIA FLINT, MBBS
Foundation Year 2 Doctor, Birmingham Children's Hospital NHS Foundation Trust; Renal Immunobiology, School of Immunity and Infection, College of Medical and Dental Sciences, University of Birmingham, Birmingham, United Kingdom

ANGELO L. GAFFO, MD, MSPH
Associate Professor of Medicine, Division of Clinical Immunology and Rheumatology, University of Alabama at Birmingham and Birmingham VA Medical Center, Birmingham, Alabama

WOLFGANG L. GROSS, MD, PhD
Professor of Medicine, Director, Department of Rheumatology and Clinical Immunology, Vasculitis Center, University Hospital Schleswig-Holstein, Bad Bramstedt, Germany

JULIA U. HOLLE, MD
Consultant Rheumatologist, Department of Rheumatology and Clinical Immunology, Vasculitis Center, University Hospital Schleswig-Holstein, Calikum Bad Bramstedt, Germany

CEES G.M. KALLENBERG, MD, PhD
Professor of Clinical Immunology, Department of Rheumatology and Clinical Immunology, University Medical Center Groningen, University of Groningen, Groningen, The Netherlands

ANUP A. KUBAL, MD
Instructor, Bascom Palmer Eye Institute, Miller School of Medicine, University of Miami, Miami, Florida

MARTIN LAUDIEN, MD
Consultant Otorhinolaryngologist, Department of Otorhinolaryngology, Head and Neck Surgery, University of Kiel, Kiel, Germany

RAASHID LUQMANI, DM, FRCP, FRCP(E)
Consultant Rheumatologist and Senior Lecturer, Department of Rheumatology, Nuffield Orthopaedic Centre, Oxford, United Kingdom

MATTHEW D. MORGAN, PhD, MRCP
Locum Senior Lecturer Renal Medicine, Renal Immunobiology, School of Immunity and Infection, College of Medical and Dental Sciences, University of Birmingham, Birmingham, United Kingdom

ELEANA NTATSAKI, MRCP
Specialist Registrar in Rheumatology, Ipswich Hospital NHS Trust, Ipswich, United Kingdom

VICTOR L. PEREZ, MD
Associate Professor of Opthalmology, Bascom Palmer Eye Institute, Miller School of Medicine, University of Miami, Miami, Florida

JOANNA ROBSON, MBBS, PhD, MRCP
Rheumatology Specialist Registrar, Department of Rheumatology, Nuffield Orthopaedic, Centre, Oxford, United Kingdom

ALESSANDRA DELLA ROSSA, MD, PhD
Rheumatology Unit, Department of Internal Medicine, University of Pisa, Pisa, Italy

ABRAHAM RUTGERS, MD, PhD
Assistant Professor of Clinical Immunology, Department of Rheumatology and Clinical Immunology, University Medical Center Groningen, University of Groningen, Groningen, The Netherlands

JAN S.F. SANDERS, MD, PhD
Assistant Professor, Department of Nephrology, University Medical Center Groningen, University of Groningen, Groningen, The Netherlands

CAROLINE O.S. SAVAGE, FRCP, FMedSci
Professor of Nephrology, Renal Immunobiology, School of Immunity and Infection, College of Medical and Dental Sciences, University of Birmingham, Birmingham, United Kingdom

DAVID G.I. SCOTT, MD, FRCP
Honorary Professor, School of Medicine, Health Policy and Practice, University of East Anglia; Consultant Rheumatologist, Norfolk and Norwich University Hospital NHS Foundation Trust, Norwich, United Kingdom

PHILIP SEO, MD
Assistant Professor of Medicine, Division of Rheumatology, Co-Director, The Johns Hopkins Vasculitis Center, Johns Hopkins University School of Medicine, Baltimore, Maryland

COEN A. STEGEMAN, MD, PhD
Associate Professor, Department of Nephrology, University Medical Center Groningen, University of Groningen, Groningen, The Netherlands

RAVI SUPPIAH, BHB, MBChB, PGDipSM
Rheumatology Fellow, Department of Rheumatology, Nuffield Orthopaedic Centre, Oxford, United Kingdom

ROSARIA TALARICO, MD, PhD
Rheumatology Unit, Department of Internal Medicine, University of Pisa, Pisa, Italy

RICHARD A. WATTS, DM, FRCP
Consultant Rheumatologist, Ipswich Hospital NHS Trust, Ipswich; Clinical Senior Lecturer, School of Medicine, Health Policy and Practice, University of East Anglia, Norwich, United Kingdom

STEFAN WIECZOREK, MD
Department of Human Genetics, Ruhr University, Bochum, Germany

ALLAN S. WIIK, MD, PhD
Emeritus Director, Department of Autoimmunology; Consultant, Department of Biochemistry and Immunology, Statens Serum Institut, Artillerivej, Copenhagen S, Denmark

Contents

An essential early step toward understanding vasculitis was recognition in 1948 of the differences between the small artery disease of polyarteritis, essentially sparing the glomerulus and lungs, and disease of glomerular vessels and small veins, often involving the lungs. By 1951, Churg and Strauss drew on their knowledge of vasculitis literature and renal pathology to provide an authoritative description of the syndrome bearing their names. One year later a paper from Australia described a syndrome of febrile systemic illness with myalgias, arthralgias, microscopic hematuria, and a serum antibody reacting with neutrophil cytoplasm antigens. Within 30 years, nephrologists and immunologists in northern Europe linked antineutrophil cytoplasm antibodies to a specific vasculitis, Wegener's granulomatosis. Falk and Jennette later determined that pANCA reacted with cytoplasmic myeloperoxidase, and that cANCA did not; the antigen with which cANCA reacted was soon identified as a novel serine proteinase. New and better treatments of AAV will follow progress in understanding their pathogenesis.

The epidemiology of the antineutrophil cytoplasm antibody (ANCA)-associated vasculitides (AAV), comprising Wegener's granulomatosis, microscopic polyangiitis, and Churg-Strauss syndrome, poses considerable challenges to epidemiologists. These challenges include the difficulty of defining a case with a lack of clear distinction between the different disorders, case capture, and case ascertainment. The AAV are rare and therefore a large population is required to determine the incidence and prevalence, and this poses questions of feasibility. Despite these difficulties a considerable body of data on the epidemiology of the AAV has been built in the past 20 years with an interesting age, geographic, and ethnic tropism gradually being revealed. Most of the data come from White populations of European descent, and the overall annual incidence is estimated at approximately 10–20/million with a peak age of onset in those aged 65 to 74 years.

Antineutrophil cytoplasm antibody (ANCA)-associated vasculitis (AAV) comprises a group of systemic inflammatory vasculitides associated with circulating autoantibodies directed against the neutrophil granule components proteinase 3 and myeloperoxidase. ANCA interact with their target antigens on cytokine primed neutrophils, causing neutrophil activation via several signaling pathways that culminates in endothelial interaction, degranulation, cytokine production, and endothelial and tissue damage. The presence of autoantibodies implies the assistance of autoreactive T-helper cells and B cells, and a failure of regulatory mechanisms. This article reviews the current evidence for the pathogenic mechanisms culminating in autoantibody production, the effects of ANCA-neutrophil and neutrophil-endothelial interactions, and the mechanisms of tissue damage.

Antineutrophil cytoplasmic autoantibody (ANCA)-associated vasculitides are systemic or more limited conditions characterized by necrotizing destruction of small and medium-sized vessels (eg, capillaries, venules, and arterioles). ANCAs are the most predominant autoantibodies in patients affected by vasculitis, but other autoantibodies may also occur, probably reflecting pathogenetic events in affected tissue. These autoantibodies are assumed to play a role in the intiation and propagation of chronic inflammation. ANCAs are valuable for clinical diagnosis, follow-up, and guidance in therapy.

Antineutrophil cytoplasmic antibody (ANCA)-associated vasculitides (AAV) include Wegener's granulomatosis, microscopic polyangiitis, and Churg-Strauss syndrome. Given their rarity, protean clinical manifestations, imperfect diagnostic tests, and wide differential diagnosis, they pose a diagnostic challenge even to experienced clinicians. This article describes diagnostic approaches for patients suspected of having one of the ANCA-associated vasculitides. The clinical findings at presentation, the role of laboratory and imaging tests, and the importance of tissue diagnosis are presented. In each section, issues relevant to the differential diagnosis of AAV are discussed.

Wegener's granulomatosis (WG) is characterized by granulomatous lesions and vasculitic disease manifestations. Granulomatous lesions are found in the upper and lower respiratory tract (eg, granulomatous sinusitis, orbital masses, and pulmonary granuloma), whereas vasculitic manifestations occur frequently in lung (alveolar hemorrhage) and kidney (glomerulonephritis). Vasculitis is typically associated with antineutrophil cytoplasmic antibodies (ANCA) directed against proteinase 3. WG has been traditionally associated with a poor outcome and increased mortality as documented by numerous studies; however, recent cohort studies report an improved outcome, probably a consequence of increased awareness leading to an earlier diagnosis, and to improved treatment strategies derived from evidence from controlled trials. Treatment regimens for WG, adapted to disease stage and activity, are reviewed and discussed in this article.

Chiara Baldini, Rosaria Talarico, Alessandra Della Rossa, and Stefano Bombardieri

Churg-Strauss syndrome (CSS) is a systemic necrotizing vasculitis affecting small to medium-sized vessels, and characterized by asthma, blood hypereosinophilia, and eosinophil-rich granulomatous inflammation of the respiratory tract. In the past few years the pathogenesis of the disease and its clinical manifestations have been clarified, fostering important advances in the treatment of CSS. Systemic corticosteroids are still considered the cornerstone of treatment. Many issues need to be addressed, such as how to maintain remission, prevent disease relapses, and treat refractory disease. This review provides a clinical overview of CSS and a summary of the current treatments and novel therapies.

Sharon A. Chung and Philip Seo

In 1923, Friedrich Wohlwill described two patients with a "microscopic form of periarteritis nodosa," which was distinct from the classical form. This disease, now known as microscopic polyangiitis (MPA), is a primary systemic vasculitis characterized by inflammation of the small-caliber blood vessels and the presence of circulating antineutrophil cytoplasmic antibodies. Typically, microscopic polyangiitis presents with glomerulonephritis and pulmonary capillaritis, although involvement of the skin, nerves, and gastrointestinal tract is not uncommon. Treatment of MPA generally requires use of a cytotoxic agent (such as cyclophosphamide) in addition to high-dose glucocorticoids. Recent research has focused on identifying alternate treatment strategies that minimize or eliminate exposure to cytotoxic agents. This article reviews the history, pathogenesis, clinical manifestations, and treatment of MPA.

Abraham Rutgers, Jan S.F. Sanders, Coen A. Stegeman, and Cees G.M. Kallenberg

Pauci-immune necrotizing glomerulonephritis is the most frequent cause of rapidly progressive glomerulonephritis and, in most cases, is associated with antineutrophil cytoplasmic antibodies (ANCA). It is either the renal manifestation of Wegener's granulomatosis, microscopic polyangiitis of Churg-Strauss syndrome, or a renal-limited vasculitis. In this review, the histopathologic changes seen in renal biopsies of patients with pauci-immune glomerulonephritis are described. The authors also describe why the disease is sometimes limited to the kidneys, the clinical course of renal disease, treatment issues, how to deal with disease relapses, and how to prevent them from occurring. Furthermore, the necessity of renal biopsy and rebiopsy, the usefulness of rapid ANCA detection at diagnosis, and serial measurement of ANCA during follow-up are discussed. The effect of dialysis on the disease process and the possibility of renal transplantation after disease remission are also debated.

The antineutrophil cytoplasmic antibody (ANCA)-associated vasculitides—Wegener's granulomatosis, microscopic polyangiitis, and Churg-Strauss syndrome—can present with various ophthalmic manifestations. In a subset of patients, these findings may be the earliest indicators of systemic disease. Orbital and anterior segment findings are most common, whereas posterior segment complications such as retinal vasculitis and optic neuropathy occur much less frequently. This article describes the distinguishing features of associated ophthalmic disease, focusing on the manifestations clinicians are most likely to encounter and those with the most significant ocular morbidity. Although the ANCA-associated vasculitides require systemic workup and treatment, this article discusses diagnostic and therapeutic modalities often used concurrently for ophthalmic disease.

The outcome in patients with antineutrophil cytoplasm antibody (ANCA)-associated vasculitis has considerably improved with the use of potent immunosuppression. In the most severe cases, mortality remains an important risk despite aggressive intervention. However, for most patients who survive, quality of survival is affected by morbidity due to low-grade disease activity, episodes of relapse, damage from the effects of disease and its treatment, development of associated comorbidity, and the social and psychological problems of chronic disease. A rational approach to management of patients with ANCA-associated vasculitis requires careful measurement of these different facets of disease, so that treatment is appropriate. This article reviews the development of assessment tools used to quantify disease in vasculitis, which have been extensively used in clinical trials and are also appropriate for use in individual patient care.

The introduction of cyclophosphamide for treatment and the detection of antineutrophil cytoplasmatic antibodies (ANCA) as a seromarker for ANCA-associated vasculitis (AAV) have been the most important milestones in the history of AAV. Nevertheless, there are still many issues to resolve to fully understand the pathogenesis of AAV and to improve patient outcomes. There is a need for diagnostic criteria; treatment strategies need further improvement to reduce the toxicity of conventional immunosuppressants such as cyclophosphamide. The elucidation of the genetic background in patients with AAV and the role of granulomatous lesions found in Wegener's granulomatosis are required to fully understand the pathophysiology of AAV.

FORTHCOMING ISSUES

November 2010
Rheumatic Manifestations of Endocrine Disease
Joseph Markenson, MD,
Guest Editor

February 2011
Complimentary and Alternative Medicine in Rheumatology
Sharon L. Kolasinski, MD,
Guest Editor

RECENT ISSUES

May 2010
New Insights into Rheumatoid Arthritis
David A. Fox, MD, *Guest Editor*

February 2010
Systemic Lupus Erythematosus
Ellen M. Ginzler, MD, MPH, *Guest Editor*

November 2009
Quantitative Assessment of Musculoskeletal Conditions in Standard Clinical Care
Theodore Pincus, MD and
Yusuf Yazici, MD, *Guest Editors*

THE CLINICS ARE NOW AVAILABLE ONLINE!

Access your subscription at:
www.theclinics.com

Preface

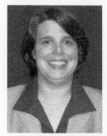 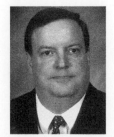

Barri J. Fessler, MD, MSPH   S. Louis Bridges Jr, MD, PhD
Guest Editors

This is the first issue of *Rheumatic Disease Clinics of North America* devoted entirely to antineutrophil cytoplasmic antibody (ANCA)-associated vasculitis. Because of their potentially life-threatening nature and the toxicity of the drugs used to treat them, ANCA-associated vasculitic syndromes are the subject of considerable immunologic and clinical research. Significant advances have emerged in the understanding of underlying immunologic mechanisms as well as the emergence of new therapeutic options. In this issue, we have called on leading international experts to provide updates on various aspects of these diseases. This issue includes a historical overview of ANCA-associated vasculitis, as well as articles describing advances in the understanding of the epidemiology, the role of autoantibodies, and the pathogenesis of these diseases. Pauci-immune renal disease and ophthalmologic manifestations are extensively discussed, as are outcome measures used to assess disease activity, damage, and effects of therapeutic agents. Separate articles focus on the overall diagnostic approach, as well as on clinical descriptions and treatment strategies for specific diseases, including Wegener's granulomatosis, Churg-Strauss syndrome, and microscopic polyangiitis. Finally, the future of research in ANCA-associated vasculitis is discussed.

We are grateful to the authors of these articles, who are busily engaged in patient care and research but have lent their time and expertise to make this issue up-to-date and useful to researchers and clinicians alike.

Barri J. Fessler, MD, MSPH
Division of Clinical Immunology and Rheumatology
University of Alabama at Birmingham
1813 6th Avenue South
MEB-609 Birmingham, AL 35294, USA

S. Louis Bridges Jr, MD, PhD
Division of Clinical Immunology and Rheumatology
University of Alabama Birmingham
1825 6th Avenue South, Birmingham, AL 35294, USA

E-mail addresses:
Barri.Fessler@ccc.uab.edu (B.J. Fessler)
Lou.Bridges@ccc.uab.edu (S.L. Bridges)

Rheum Dis Clin N Am 36 (2010) xiii
doi:10.1016/j.rdc.2010.06.001
0889-857X/10/$ – see front matter
rheumatic.theclinics.com

The History of ANCA-associated Vasculitis

Gene V. Ball, MD

KEYWORDS

• Antineutrophil cytoplasm antibodies • Vasculitis
• History • Polyarteritis

Until the discovery of antineutrophil cytoplasm antibodies (ANCA), it had been assumed that most vasculitis resulted from immune complex or antibasement membrane mediation. This article is based on the evidence that ANCA can directly activate neutrophils and monocytes[1] and lead to inflammation of small and medium-sized arteries, capillaries, and venules, hence ANCA-associated vasculitis (AAV). The detection of ANCA is not prima facie evidence of causation of vasculitis, but there is strong empiric evidence for the pathogenicity of MPO-ANCA, if not for PR3-ANCA, as is evident elsewhere in this issue. The reported frequencies of ANCA in the AAV depend on the population and methodology, but for Wegener's granulomatosis (WG), the frequencies range from 40% to 95% for PR3-ANCA and 5% to 60% for MPO-ANCA. For Churg-Strauss syndrome (CSS), the frequencies range from 30% to 70% for MPO-ANCA or PR3-ANCA, and as much as 75% for MPO-ANCA in microscopic polyangiitis (MPA). Other ANCA are directed against elastase, lactoferrin, azurocidin, lysozyme, H-lamp-2, and other antigens, and are of uncertain significance.

The disorders that are included in the AAV and polyarteritis nodosa spectrum can be difficult to differentiate in individuals. Clinical and objective laboratory and anatomic differences between MPA and classical polyarteritis nodosa (PAN), and MPA and WG are sometimes inconclusive. PAN is not included as an AAV because of its localization to arteries and the usual absence of ANCA. Incidentally, the term microscopic polyangiitis is preferred over microscopic polyarteritis because of the usual absence of arterial lesions in the former; however, both terms are used here to reflect their historical use.

Identification of the three primary ANCA-associated syndromes evolved from comparisons of their anatomic features with those of classical polyarteritis nodosa, which had been described in 1886[2] and 1908.[3] The kidney was the major focus for many relevant reports from the first half of the 20th century, exemplified by a comprehensive study entitled "The Kidney in Periarteritis Nodosa" by Davson, Ball, and Platt,

Division of Clinical Immunology and Rheumatology, University of Alabama at Birmingham, 510 20th Avenue South, Faculty Office Tower 827, Birmingham, AL 35294, USA
E-mail address: ballg@bellsouth.net

Rheum Dis Clin N Am 36 (2010) 439–446
doi:10.1016/j.rdc.2010.05.004
0889-857X/10/$ – see front matter © 2010 Elsevier Inc. All rights reserved.

rheumatic.theclinics.com

which established a precedent for separating renal lesions of periarteritis nodosa from those of malignant nephrosclerosis, and suggested the separation of classical periarteritis from microscopic polyarteritis.[4]

Fourteen autopsied cases were divided into two groups, the first with systemic arteritis without aneurysms but with lesions in the lungs and widespread necrotizing glomerulitis. The authors called this microscopic periarteritis and emphasized the necessity of considering this entity in patients with what might otherwise be considered focal embolic nephritis or type 1 nephritis. The second group had systemic arteritis without significant glomerular change or lung lesions and would correspond to today's PAN. In this, they anticipated the current distinction between PAN, which excludes glomerulonephritis or vasculitis in arterioles, capillaries or venules, and microscopic polyarteritis with vasculitis affecting small vessels including capillaries, venules, and arterioles. They also stressed that cases with renal failure or hypertension occurring in a pyrexial illness should be suspect for periarteritis. The first group appeared to be compatible with what is today called microscopic polyangiitis. Davson's view of the glomerulus as a specialized blood vessel was explicit in a later paper.[5] Zeek also suggested that there were two distinct types of periarteritis: hypersensitivity angiitis with glomerulonephritis and true periarteritis.[6,7]

In 1985, Savage and colleagues described the presentation, pathology, and prognosis of what they termed microscopic polyarteritis, based on studies of 34 patients. Their definition required clinical or histologic evidence of small vessel systemic vasculitis associated with focal segmental necrotizing glomerulonephritis for which there was no other explanation; this corresponds to the definition now in use for MPA. The predominating symptoms were fever, arthralgia, cutaneous purpura, hemoptysis or pulmonary hemorrhage, abdominal pain, mouth ulcers, and sensory neuropathy. Laboratory findings included anemia, elevated creatinine, and microscopic hematuria in all patients, and proteinuria in excess of 3 g in 41% of patients. Seven had definite alveolar hemorrhage, and it was suspected in three others. Visceral arteriograms, done in 12 patients to exclude PAN, were normal. Focal segmental necrotizing glomerulonephritis was found in all renal specimens from 32 patients, and crescents were found in 88% of patients. Of note, granular glomerular immunoglobulin deposits were found by direct immunofluorescence in only a few of 20 specimens. This is an example of pauci-immune glomerulonephritis, which is included often in the definition of the renal disease found in AAV. Small-vessel vasculitis with fibrinoid necrosis was found in five of nine skin biopsies. The patients were treated with varying regimens of glucocorticoids and immunosuppressive drugs, and the actuarial survival rate at 1 year was 70%. The authors compared microscopic polyarteritis with WG, PAN, and CSS, convincingly establishing its singularity.[8]

Fourteen years later and in the era of ANCA, Guillevin and other members of the French Vasculitis Study Group published an analysis of the clinical and laboratory features of 85 MPA patients, of whom 81 were biopsy-proven. They were similar to those of Savage, the dominant symptoms being weight loss, rash, fever, neuropathy, arthralgias, and myalgias. A large number (17.6%) had heart failure. Serum creatinine was elevated in 47 patients. Microaneurysms were seen by angiography in 4 of 30 patients who were examined. ANCA were found in 38 of 51 patients; in 33 this was pANCA and in 5, cANCA. Four patients had PR3-ANCA, and 31 had MPO-ANCA. The 5-year survival rate of 74% was better in patients treated with glucocorticoids and immunosuppressive drugs than those treated with glucocorticoids alone.[9]

Klinger, writing in 1931, is thought to have authored the first description of what is now termed WG.[10] Of Klinger's description, Wegener wrote that it depicted a man with a borderline form of polyarteritis nodosa and severe nasal changes. In the late 1930s, Wegener established the disease as a distinct entity thought to be most likely an allergic reaction to infection. A short paper entitled "On Generalized Septic Vessel Diseases," identified the major characteristics of the disease as a septic course, with extremely severe necrotizing granulomatous inflammation of the inner nose, pharynx, and larynx; localized glomerulonephritis; and generalized arteritis with the picture of periarteritis nodosa.[11] Godman and Churg described the features of WG more fully, and concluded that it and microscopic polyarteritis and CSS were related through a similar pathogenesis involving hypersensitivity.[12] In the same year, a major clinical study of WG was published, by which time 18 autopsied cases had been reported, to which six more were added, plus one patient still living after 19 months of cortisone or corticotropin (ACTH). The authors, Jacob Churg among them, confirmed the three characteristic anatomic features that Godman and Churg had identified:

1. Necrotizing granulomatous lesions in the upper or lower respiratory tract
2. Generalized focal necrotizing vasculitis involving both arteries and veins and almost always present in the lungs
3. Glomerulitis comprising necrosis and thrombosis of loops of the capillary tuft and evolution as a granulomatous lesion.

They acknowledged the similarity to what is now termed Churg-Strauss vasculitis, but felt that WG can be distinguished on the basis of marked predominance of necrotizing granulomatous lesions in the respiratory tract, the regular occurrence and severity of the renal lesions, and the usual absence of allergy or tissue eosinophilia.[13]

An influential paper by Fauci and Wolff reviewed the clinical and laboratory features of 18 patients with WG who had been studied during the 12 years before its publication in 1973. They built upon their earlier pioneering studies of cyclophosphamide in this disease,[14] and in so doing, further rationalized its use, thereby altering the prognosis from relentless morbidity and death to remission. Their guidelines for the use of glucocorticoids and cyclophosphamide still determine or influence the treatment of this disease and others.[15] Investigations of immunologic markers by Shillitoe and colleagues,[16] which included tests for autoantibodies to thyroid, gastric cells, adrenal, smooth muscle, DNA, mitochondria, and reticulin in 10 patients were negative, as were tests for rheumatoid factors and immune complexes, and they felt confident to dismiss circulating immune complexes as major players in the etiology of WG. Searches for infectious causes of WG have been considered fruitless, although it is thought that *Staphylococcus aureus* might be associated both with onset of disease and relapses.[17] A putative relationship between *S aureus* and other infectious agents has been reviewed recently,[18] and there is persisting interest in the use of trimethoprimsulfamethoxazole popularized by DeRemee and others for the prevention of relapse.[19,20] Unlike infections, drugs have been clearly implicated as causes of ANCA-positive vasculitis syndromes, including WG, which often subside after withdrawal of the drug.[21,22] Choi and colleagues described 30 patients with exposures to drugs including hydralazine and propythiouracil whose vasculitis was associated with anti-MPO titers more than 12 times the median of 250 patients.[23] Ninety-two patients in Japan with MPO-ANCA associated vasculitis who had taken methimazole or propylthiouracil were reported to a firm marketing antithyroid drugs. Forty-one of the 92 had single-organ failure; 32 had double-organ failure. Thirteen had triple-organ failure and in two, there was quadruple-organ failure. The median time of onset of symptoms after starting drug treatment was 42 months, with a range of 1 to 372 months. The severity or number of involved organs did not correlate with the MPO-ANCA titer, suggesting to the investigators a need for vigilance even among patients with low titers.[24]

The significance of a five-paragraph report from Australia entitled "Segmental Necrotising Glomerulonephritis with Antineutrophil Antibody: Possible Arbovirus Etiology?" was not recognized at the time of its publication in 1982. It described eight patients who had arthralgias and myalgias, anorexia, vomiting and diarrhea, and microscopic hematuria. Five had abnormal chest radiographs, and renal biopsies showed segmental necrotizing glomerulonephritis with frequent crescents. All patients had a factor in their serum that stained the cytoplasm of neutrophil leucocytes by indirect immunofluorescence; similar staining had not been seen in more than 5000 sera examined in the preceding 5 years. The glomerular lesions were morphologically identical to those of microscopic polyarteritis, referring to the criteria elaborated by Davson in the study mentioned earlier. Although the authors mused over the possibility that the illness was caused by Ross River virus, the patients had been treated by their clinicians with a regimen of prednisone and cyclophosphamide or azathioprine.[25]

Within 2 years, a different Australian group cited this report, and added four patients who had malaise, arthralgia, and pulmonary involvement; two had a rash due to vasculitis, and three had active urinary sediment and segmental necrotizing lesions on kidney biopsy. All four had cytoplasmic staining of neutrophils on immunofluorescence examination. The investigators thought this represented a homogenous illness "loosely labeled arteritis," for which treatment with steroids and cytotoxics was encouraged.[26]

In 1985, nephrologists and immunologists from the Netherlands and Denmark published the first of what would be many studies identifying ANCA in WG, and by extrapolation, other polyarteritis syndromes. The authors were seasoned investigators whose previous work had centered on glomerulonephritis and vasculitis, and the laboratory assessment of indicators of immunologic disease. They studied 41 patients with biopsy-proven WG, finding ACPA (an early designation for ANCA) by indirect immunofluorescence in 25 of 27 patients with active disease and 4 of 32 with inactive disease. They rather prematurely concluded that the autoantibody was specific for WG.[27] In this regard, it was fortuitous that ANCA were not found among their control patients, of whom 15 had tuberculosis (in which ANCA have been repeatedly identified) and 14 had "various forms of small-vessel vasculitis." Inasmuch as 33 of the controls were said to have classical polyarteritis, it is surprising that ANCA were not found among the 14 with small vessel disease, which they differentiated from polyarteritis.

Falk and Jennette studied sera from seven patients with WG and three with microscopic polyarteritis, and from 35 persons with idiopathic necrotizing and crescentic glomerulonephritis, 11 with lupus nephritis and 71 with other renal lesions. On indirect immunofluorescence (IIF) microscopy, they found two different staining patterns of ANCA: diffuse granular staining with accentuation near the center, and perinuclear to nuclear depending upon the method used for preparing the neutrophils. None of the 50 blood bank sera controls were positive for ANCA; however, positive reactions were found in significant titers in sera representing necrotizing and crescentic glomerulonephritis but not in lupus and other renal lesions. They concluded from the IIF and enzyme-linked immunosorbent assay (ELISA) that ANCA were found in patients with necrotizing and crescentic glomerulonephritis whose clinical disease ranged from kidney-limited to overt vasculitis including WG and polyarteritis. ANCA associated with the necrotizing and crescentic glomerulonephritis were specific for constituents of neutrophil primary granules, and there were at least two types of antibodies. Some produced perinuclear staining of alcohol-fixed neutrophils that reacted with myeloperoxidase (pANCA), and others produced diffuse cytoplasmic immunostaining

The History of ANCA-associated Vasculitis

not due to myeloperoxidase (cANCA).[28] These important discoveries have inspired much of the later ANCA research.

In the following year, in a study of sera producing cytoplasmic staining in 10 patients with WG, Niles and colleagues identified the antigen to which cANCA reacts as a novel serine proteinase. The antigen was distinct from neutral proteases elastase and cathepsin G, and they surmised that it might be proteinase 3.[29] Confirmation of this came from Ludemann, Utecht, and Gross, who identified the antigen as an elastinolytic enzyme.[30] Shortly thereafter they revised the antigen's nucleotide and amino acid sequence that they had published earlier.[31] Sera from 277 patients with WG and 1657 controls were analyzed for ACPA (ANCA) by IIF and ELISA in 1989. The specificity for WG among the sera was 99% by IIF and 98% by ELISA, and sensitivity depended on extent and activity of the disease. For example, it was 67% by IIF for patients with active but localized symptoms, and for patients in full remission, the sensitivity by IIF was 41%. The investigators concluded, as did others, that APCA could be used as a marker to follow disease activity.[32,33]

By 1990, the authors of the 1982 report that had first described ANCA in patients with vasculitis and glomerulonephritis had screened 7500 sera for ANCA by IIF, finding it in 17. Eleven of the patients with ANCA were diagnosed with microscopic polyarteritis based on small vessel disease with focal segmental glomerulonephritis without evidence of WG, and four patients with WG. Remissions were induced in all patients who were treated with prednisolone and cyclophosphamide, and tests for ANCA became negative except in three patients thought to have MPA. There were five relapses, with return of ANCA positivity in patients who had been ANCA negative. Anticipating questions about the relationship between ANCA and activity of vasculitis, the authors specifically noted that ANCA were a sensitive but not specific marker of disease relapse, but also that ANCA persisted in three patients even though there was no clinical evidence of disease activity. They also noted the absence of ANCA by IIF in 15 patients with active MPA or WG, but they did not relate its presence or absence to extent of disease, as others had.[34]

Boomsma and colleagues[35] studied 100 patients with WG from 1996 to 1998, and obtained serum samples for ANCA analysis every 2 months. During this time, relapses occurred in 37 patients; of these, 34 showed a rise in the level of ANCA preceding the relapse. The predictive value for relapse was greater for increases in cANCA determined by ELISA than by IIF. In 29% of patients, the rise in ANCA titers was not followed by a relapse during an extended observation, and only 39% had a relapse within 6 months. They therefore cautioned against starting or escalating immunosuppressive therapy based solely on ANCA levels.

Periarteritis was linked with asthma in a prescient 1939 account by Rackemann and Greene of eight persons with severe asthma, pain and numbness in the extremities, and eosinophilia. The index case was a 36-year-old woman, who for 3 years had nasal stuffiness, rhinitis, and for 6 months cough and mild attacks of wheezing. Her leukocyte count was about 18,000/mm³ with 30% to 40% eosinophils. Antemortem diagnoses were tuberculosis, lupus erythematosus and, finally, periarteritis nodosa. At autopsy, there was extensive pericarditis, enlargement of the heart, and "lesions of periarteritis nodosa" in many organs. "Tremendous eosinophilia" was "the important feature" in each of the eight cases. Including their own, 27 cases were reviewed; 19 had both asthma and periarteritis nodosa. Increased eosinophils were counted in 74%, and this triad was regarded as virtually diagnostic of a polyarteritis syndrome. Their next steps were to learn what periarteritis nodosa is and determine the functions of the eosinophil, still worthy goals.[36]

This description of the triad of asthma, periarteritis, and eosinophilia was acknowledged by Churg and Strauss in their monograph entitled "Allergic Granulomatosis, Allergic angiitis, and Periarteritis nodosa." In it, they reviewed the clinical histories of 13 patients with asthma, fever, and pneumonia; central and peripheral neuropathy; skin rashes including purpura and nodules; mild generalized lymphadenopathy; arthralgias; and mild hematuria and proteinuria. The anatomic changes they described so carefully and illustrated with clear photographs were widespread vascular lesions like those of periarteritis; "tissue alteration" comprising eosinophilic necrosis; fibrinoid collagen, and granulomatous proliferation of epithelioid and giant cells termed "allergic granuloma." The granuloma within vessel walls and connective tissue throughout the body differed from lesions of classical periarteritis, which they knew well. The most characteristic lesions were granulomatous nodules associated with inflammation within and near small vessel walls. Small dense aggregates of eosinophils were observed along with macrophages around a focus with the appearance and radial arrangement of epithelioid cells. Lesions in blood vessels in 9 of 10 autopsied cases were similar to those seen in periarteritis nodosa except for the granulomatous lesions, which distinguished them from periarteritis. All stages of arteritis were seen, including aneurysms, although healed fibrosed lesions predominated. The epicardium was the most common seat of granulomatous nodules, which were found in 6 of 10 autopsied cases. Branches of pulmonary arteries were involved, and lung lesions suggested pneumonia with eosinophils and giant cells. Focal glomerular lesions involved a few capillary loops. Cutaneous nodules were of great diagnostic importance.

They noted that their findings were in agreement with those of Wilson and Alexander, who in their review of 300 published cases of periarteritis nodosa found that high eosinophilia was present in 94% of the cases associated with asthma and in only 6% of those without a history of asthma.[37] Churg and Strauss concluded that there were valid clinical and anatomic reasons for defining their symptom complex as allergic angiitis and allergic granulomatosis. Its allergic etiology was clearly proved, at least as long as asthma is considered an allergic disease. The clinical manifestations of CSS were recognized as highly variable.[38]

An authoritative explication of the syndrome now bearing their names was possible because of their knowledge of the literature pertaining to vasculitis and their expertise in renal and vascular pathology. They were both pathologists at Mount Sinai Hospital in New York City, and two of a distinguished group that has been memorialized in that institution's Hall of Fame. Incidentally, six of them are remembered in eponymic syndromes. Dr Churg was especially expert in renal pathology as other vasculitis investigators have been, and he published more than 300 papers during his career at Mount Sinai. Dr Strauss was also a prolific investigator and author of about 100 scientific papers. She was interested in vascular and uterine diseases, and she is regarded as the founder of pediatric pathology. The rapidly evolving ANCA paradigm promises to explain certain phenomena of the immune systems, and to provide targeted treatment of AAV.

REFERENCES

1. Falk RJ, Terrell R, Huneycutt-Calder L, et al. Antineutrophil cytoplasmic autoantibodies (ANCA) stimulate neutrophil activation in vitro. Kidney Int 1989;35:346.
2. Kussmaul A, Maier R. Ueber eine bisher nicht beschriebene eigenthumliche Arterienerkrankung (Periarteritis nodosa), die mit morbus Brightii und rapid fortschreitender allgemeiner Muskellahmung einhergeht. Deutsches Archiv fur Klinische Medizin 1866;1:484–518 [in German].

3. Dickson WEC. Polyarteritis acuta nodosa and periarteritis nodosa. J Pathol Bacteriol 1908;12:32–57.
4. Davson J, Ball J, Platt R. The kidney in polyarteritis nodosa. Quart J Med New Series 1948;17:175–205.
5. Wainwright J, Davson J. The renal appearances in the microscopic form of periarteritis nodosa. J Pathol Bacteriol 1950;62:189–96.
6. Zeek PM, Smith CC, Weeter JC. Studies on periarteritis nodosa.111. The differentiation between the vascular lesions of periarteritis nodosa and of hypersensitivity. Am J Pathol 1948;24:889–917.
7. Zeek PM. Periarteritis nodosa: a critical review. Am J Clin Pathol 1952;22:777–90.
8. Savage COS, Winearls CG, Evans DJ. Microscopic polyarteritis: presentation, pathology and prognosis. Q J Med 1985;220:467–83.
9. Guillevin L, Durand-Gasselin B, Cevallos R, et al. Microscopic polyangiitis: clinical and laboratory findings in eighty-five patients. Arthritis Rheum 1999; 42(3):421–30.
10. Klinger H. Grenzformen der periarteritis nodosa. Frankfurt Pathol 1931;42:455 [in German].
11. Socias R, Poznia A. On generalised septic vessel diseases. Translation of a classic paper by Friedrich Wegener. Thorax 1987;42:918–9.
12. Godman G, Churg J. Wegener's granulomatosis. Pathology and review of the literature. Arch Pathol Lab Med 1954;58:533–53.
13. Fahey JL, Leonard E, Churg J, et al. Wegener's granulomatosis. Am J Med 1954;168–79.
14. Fauci AS, Wolff SM. Treatment of Wegener's granulomatosis with cyclophosphamide. J Clin Invest 1971;50:28a.
15. Fauci AS, Wolff SM. Wegener's granulomatosis: studies in eighteen patients and a review of the literature. Medicine 1976;52:536–56.
16. Shillitoe EJ, Lehner T, Lessof MH, et al. Immunological features of Wegener's granulomatosis. Lancet 1974;23:281–4.
17. Stegeman CA, Cohen Tervaert JW, Sluiter WJ, et al. Association of chronic nasal carriage of *Staphylococcus aureus* and higher relapse rates in Wegener's granulomatosis. Ann Intern Med 1994;120:12–7.
18. Csernak E, Lamprecht P, Gross WL. Clinical and immunological features of drug-induced and infection-induced proteinase 3-antineutrophil cytoplasmic antibodies. Curr Opin Rheumatol 2010;22:43–8.
19. DeRemee RA, McDonald TJ, Weiland LH. Wegener's granulomaatosis: observation on treatment with antimicrobial agents. Mayo Clin Proc 1985;60:27–32.
20. Stegeman CA, Cohen Tervaert JW, de Jong PE, et al. Trimethoprim-sulfamethoxazole (co-trimoxazole) for the prevention of relapses of Wegener's granulomatosis. N Engl J Med 1996;335:16–20.
21. Dolman KM, Gans RD, Verveat TJ, et al. Vasculitis and antineutrophil cytoplasmic autoantibodies associated with propylthiouracil therapy. Lancet 1993;342(8872): 651–2.
22. Pillinger M, Staud R. Wegener's granulomatosis in a patient receiving propylthiouracil for Grave's disease. Semin Arthritis Rheum 1996;28(2):124–9.
23. Choi HK, Merkel PA, Walker AM, et al. Drug-associated antineutrophil cytoplasmic antibody-positive vasculitis: relevance among patients with high titers of antimyeloperoxidase antibodies. Arthritis Rheum 2000;43:405–13.
24. Noh JY, Yasuda S, Sato S, et al. Clinical characteristics of myeloperoxidase antineutrophil cytoplasmic antibody-associated vasculitis caused by antithyroid drugs. J Clin Endocrinol Metab 2009;94(8):2806–11.

25. Davies DJ, Moran JE, Niall JF, et al. Segmental necrotising glomerulonephritis with antineutrophil antibody: possible arbovirus etiology? BMJ 1982;285:606.
26. Hall JB, Wadham BM, Wood CJ, et al. Vasculitis and glomerulonephritis: a subgroup with an antineutrophil antibody. Aust N Z J Med 1984;14:277–8.
27. van der Woude FJ, Rasmussen N, Lobatto S, et al. Autoantibodies against neutrophils and monocytes: tool for diagnosis and marker of disease activity in Wegener's granulomatosis. Lancet 1985;23:425–9.
28. Falk RJ, Jennette JC. Antineutrophil cytoplasmic autoantibodies with specificity for myeloperoxidase in patients with systemic vasculitis and idiopathic necrotizing and crescentic glomerulonephritis. N Engl J Med 1988;318:1651–7.
29. Niles JL, McCluskey RT, Ahmad MF, et al. Wegener's granulomatosis is a novel neutrophil serine protease. Blood 1989;74:1888–93.
30. Ludemann J, Utecht B, Gross WL. Antineutrophil cytoplasm antibodies in Wegener's granulomatosis recognize an elastinolytic enzyme. J Exp Med 1990;171:357–62.
31. Jenne DE, Tschopp J, Ludemann J, et al. Wegener's autoantigen decoded. Nature 1990;346:520.
32. Nolle B, Specks U, Ludemann J, et al. Anticytoplasmic autoantibodies: their immunodiagnostic value in Wegener's granulomatosis. Ann Intern Med 1989;111(1):28–40.
33. Cohen Tervaert JW, Stegeman CA, Kallenberg CGM. Serial ANCA testing is useful in monitoring disease activity of patients with ANCA-associated vasculitides. Sarcoidosis Vasc Diffuse Lung Dis 1996;13:241–5.
34. MacIsaac AI, Moran JE, Davies DJ, et al. Antineutrophil cytoplasmic antibody (ANCA)-associated vasculitis. Clin Nephrol 1990;34(1):5–8.
35. Boomsma MM, Stegeman CA, van der Leij MJ, et al. Prediction of relapses in Wegener's granulomatosis by measurement of antineutrophil cytoplasmic antibody levels. Arthritis Rheum 2000;43(9):2025–33.
36. Rackemann FM, Greene JE. Periarteritis nodosa and asthma. Trans Assoc Am Physicians 1939;113–8.
37. Wilson KS, Alexander HL. The relation of periarteritis nodosa to bronchial asthma and other forms of human hypersensitiveness. J Lab Clin Med 1945;30:195–203.
38. Churg J, Strauss L. Allergic granulomatosis, allergic angiitis, and periarteritis nodosa. Am J Pathol 1951;27:277–301.

Epidemiology of ANCA-associated Vasculitis

Eleana Ntatsaki, MRCP[a], Richard A. Watts, DM, FRCP[a,b,*],
David G.I. Scott, MD, FRCP[b,c]

KEYWORDS

• Epidemiology • Vasculitis • Wegener's granulomatosis
• Microscopic polyangiitis • Churg-Strauss syndrome
• Polyarteritis nodosa • ANCA-associated vasculitis

The antineutrophil cytoplasm antibody (ANCA)-associated vasculitides (AAV) comprise Wegener's granulomatosis (WG), microscopic polyangiitis (MPA), and Churg-Strauss syndrome (CSS). For historical reasons polyarteritis nodosa (PAN) is often considered with the AAV although the presence of ANCA is now not considered to be a feature of PAN.

The epidemiology of the AAV poses considerable challenges to epidemiologists. The first is the difficulty of defining a case with a lack of clear distinction between the different disorders. There are 2 main systems of case definition or classification in current use: the American College of Rheumatology (ACR) (1990) classification criteria[1] and the Chapel Hill Consensus Definitions (CHCC).[2] There are several problems with these when used for epidemiology purposes. MPA does not feature in the ACR system but does in the CHCC and neither system use ANCA as a criterion. The CHCC were intended as definitions only and not classification criteria. Hence there are no validated classification criteria for MPA. To overcome this many studies have used both in parallel, but this leads to considerable overlap between categories.[3] To improve the situation, an algorithm was devised by international consensus to incorporate both systems and this has been validated in 2 separate populations and shown to reliably classify patients with AAV into WG, MPA, CSS, and PAN with a minimum of unclassified patients.[4,5]

The second difficulty is case capture. The AAV are rare and therefore a large population is required to determine the incidence and prevalence, and this poses questions of feasibility. A large population increases the risk of incomplete case

[a] Ipswich Hospital NHS Trust, Heath Road, Ipswich, IP4 5PD, UK
[b] School of Medicine, Health Policy and Practice, University of East Anglia, Norwich, NR4 7TJ, UK
[c] Norfolk and Norwich University Hospital NHS Foundation Trust, Colney Lane, Norwich, NR4 7UY, UK
* Corresponding author. Ipswich Hospital NHS Trust, Heath Road, Ipswich, IP4 5PD, UK.
E-mail address: Richard.watts@ipswichhospital.nhs.uk

Rheum Dis Clin N Am 36 (2010) 447–461
doi:10.1016/j.rdc.2010.04.002
0889-857X/10/$ – see front matter © 2010 Elsevier Inc. All rights reserved.

detection but permits a reasonable number of cases to be collected in a practicable time frame; whereas a smaller population requires a much longer time frame to collect the necessary cases, which also may not be feasible. Statistical methods of capture-recapture analysis enable estimates to be made of the number of missing cases.

The third difficulty is case ascertainment. The AAV are rare potentially life-threatening conditions and therefore usually come to the attention of physicians. Ascertainment of cases can therefore be achieved by monitoring clinical facilities and hospital activity statistics. The AAV are multisystem and therefore surveillance of many different specialties is necessary. However, patients with fulminating disease may die before diagnosis and not be ascertained.

The rarity of the conditions makes prospective case-control studies difficult to conduct because the population size required to achieve statistical confidence is in excess of that readily available. Thus, much of the data on risk factors are derived from retrospective studies with inherent potential bias.

Despite these difficulties, a considerable body of data on the epidemiology of the AAV has been built in the past 20 years. However, much of the data comes from White populations of European descent. There are relatively few studies from non-White populations and none from Africa or the Indian Subcontinent.

AAV

There is a broad consensus that for primary, systemic, medium- and small-vessel vasculitis (including WG, CSS, PAN, and MPA) the overall annual incidence is approximately 10 to 20/million and the peak age of onset is 65 to 74 years (**Table 1**).[8,10,11]

WG

In 1936, Wegener first described a disease characterized by necrotizing granulomata of the upper and lower respiratory tract, focal glomerulonephritis, and necrotizing systemic vasculitis.[12] The annual incidence of WG in the past decade has been estimated to be 8 to 10/million. WG is slightly more common in men than women.

Age

WG is generally considered to be rare in childhood with an incidence of 0.3/million.[13] However, a recent Canadian study in the Southern Alberta childhood population reported that the average incidence of childhood WG during 1993 to 2008 was 2.75/million/y, which is comparable with the incidence observed in adults. This was driven primarily by a high incidence in the last 5 years of the study of 6.39/million/y.

Table 1
Incidence of AAV

Place	Period	Incidence (Per Million)	References
Australian Capital Territory, Australia	1995–1999	17.0	6
	2000–2004	16.2	6
Lugo, Spain	1988–1994	13.0	7
Norwich, UK	1988–2008	20.1	8
Crete, Greece[a]	1995–2003	19.5	9
Sweden	1997–2006	21.8	10

[a] Primary systemic vasculitides including Henoch-Schönlein purpura.

This could be a regional phenomenon and further studies in pediatric populations are needed to see if this is indeed a global trend.[14]

Many series report a peak age of onset of 64 to 75 years.[8,10,11] A recent Swedish study reported the peak age to be more than 75 years; this is probably because of increased recognition of vasculitis in the very elderly.[10]

Time Trends

The incidence of WG seems to have increased from the 1980s to 1990s. An increase in the annual incidence of WG from 0.7/million (1980–1986) to 2.8/million (1987–1989) was reported by Andrews and colleagues[15] in Leicester, United Kingdom. Studies conducted during the late 1990s and 2000s in the United Kingdom suggest a relatively stable incidence. No significant change was noted during the 20-year period of a study conducted in secondary care by the Norwich group in the United Kingdom.[8] There was an increase in the annual prevalence from 28.8/million in 1990 to 64.8/million in 2005 in a primary care population. This was felt to be to the result of improved outcome because of improved treatment regimens.[11]

Some Scandinavian studies suggest that the incidence of WG has increased in the last 2 decades with little change in clinical symptoms at presentation. In particular, a recent study from Finland reported an increase from 1.9/million in 1981 to 1985 to 9.3/million in 1996 to 2000[16] with a similar increase up to 1998 in Tromsø in northern Norway reported by Koldingsnes and Nossent.[17] In contrast, Swedish and German studies did not report such an increase.[10,18]

There are several possible explanations for these conflicting data. The earlier increase may be related to better case recognition after the introduction of ANCA testing in the 1980s and early 1990s, but this effect should have diminished by now. Since the 1990s the ACR classification criteria or CHCC definition have been used for most studies. The use of different criteria will result in different estimates of incidence. Some studies have used International Classification of Diseases (ICD) codes for case identification, assuming diagnostic validity based on previous studies.[19] In other studies, when assigned ICD codes for AAV in clinical registries were used to capture cases, only about 60% of identified cases fulfilled ACR criteria or were validated in accordance with the consensus algorithm.[10] These methodological differences may have resulted in a variation in the reported incidence rates. Overall it is likely that there has not been a significant increase in the 1980s and early 1990s.

Geographic Factors

Most of the studies have been conducted in Europe, United Sates, Australia, and Japan in a secondary care setting (**Tables 2** and **3**). The annual incidence of WG since 1986 in Europe is in the range of 2 to 10/million. The only study from a primary care setting suggests that the incidence is 8.4/million, indicating that the secondary care figures accurately reflect the occurrence in the community at large.

There are several studies on the incidence of WG from Europe. In Finland, the annual incidence of the population increased from 1.9/million in 1981 to 1985 to 9.3/million in 1996 to 2000. Only minor changes in the signs and symptoms at diagnosis were observed in this 20-year period.[16] In the population-based Swedish Inpatient Register during the period 1975 to 2001, the incidence of WG increased from 0.33/million in the period 1975 to 1985 to 0.77/million in 1986 to 1990, to 1.19/million in 1991 to 2001, resulting in a mean incidence of 0.78/million.[19] In southern Europe (Greece) the overall annual incidence of primary systemic vasculitides (PSV) was 19.5/million. The incidence of WG was 6.6/million and was more prevalent in younger patients (<65 years old).[9] In Spain the annual incidence of WG was estimated at 3/million.[27]

Table 2
Annual incidence of WG

Year	Place	Criteria	Incidence (Per Million)	References
1980–1986	Leicester, UK	Fauci[a]	0.7	[15]
1987–1989	Leicester, UK	Fauci	2.8	[15]
1988–2008	Norwich, UK	EMEA	10.8	[8]
1990–2005	UKGPRD, UK	ACR	8.4	[11]
1992–1996	Kristiansand, Norway	ACR	6.6	[20]
1984–1998	Tromso, Norway	ACR	8.0	[17]
1971–1993	Lund, Sweden	ACR	2.1	[21]
1975–2001	Sweden	ICD	0.78	[19]
1997–2006	South Sweden	ACR, CHCC	9.8	[10]
1980–1985	Finland	ACR	1.9	[16]
1996–2000	Finland	ACR	9.3	[16]
1998–2002	Schleswig-Holstein, Germany	CHCC	6–12	[18]
1995–2003	Crete, Greece	ACR	6.6	[9]
1988–1997	Lugo, Spain	ACR	4.8	[22]
1988–2001	Lugo, Spain	CHCC	2.95	[7]
1990–1999	Vilnius, Lithuania	ACR	2.1	[23]
1993–2004	Western Montana, USA	ACR	8.6	[24]
1985–2004	South Australia	ACR, ICD	11.2	[25]
1995–1999	Australian Capital Territory,	ACR	8.8	[6]
2000–2004	Australia	ACR	8.4	[6]
1990–2004	Lima, Peru	CHCC	0.5	[26]

Abbreviations: ACR, American College of Rheumatology criteria (1990); CHCC, Chapel Hill Consensus Conference definition; EMEA, European Medicines Agency Algorithm; ICD, International Classification of Diseases; UKGPRD, United Kingdom General Practice Research Database.
[a] Fauci et al 1983.

The prevalence of WG has now been estimated in several populations. In the United Kingdom, the point prevalence on 31 December 2008 was 130/million.[8] In Germany in 1994 the prevalence of WG in the north and south of the country was reported to be 58/million and 42/million, respectively.[28] The estimated prevalence of WG in the United States was 26/million in 1986 to 1990.[29] WG seems to be much less common in Japan than the United Kingdom. Although the overall occurrence of renal vasculitis is similar in Japan and the United Kingdom, the clinical phenotype is very different, with MPA predominating in Japan and WG being more common in the United Kingdom.[30]

Epidemiologic studies in the Southern Hemisphere regions, using modified ACR criteria allowing for ANCA positivity in the absence of granulomatous vasculitis, have shown a 5-year period prevalence for WG at 152/million.[31] The 5-year incidence of WG in South Australia is higher than that in the same latitudinal region in New Zealand. This geographic variation might be relevant to exposure to different environmental factors. O' Donnell and colleagues[32] in New Zealand described a positive north-south gradient in the incidence of WG. This supports a hypothesis of a latitude-dependent risk factor that can affect both global hemispheres. WG is more common

Table 3 Prevalence of WG				
Year	Classification	Place	Prevalence (Per Million)	References
2008[a]	EMEA	Norwich, UK	130	8
1990	ACR	UKGPRD, UK	28.8	11
2005	ACR	UKGPRD, UK	64.8	11
2000	ACR	Paris, France	23.7	35
1994	CHCC	Germany (north)	58	28
1994	CHCC	Germany (south)	42	28
1977–2001	ICD	Denmark	100	67
2003[b]	ACR/CHCC	Southern Sweden	160	68
1992–96	ACR	Norway	53.0	20
1999–2003	ACR[d]	Canterbury,	131	31
2003[c]	ACR[d]	New Zealand	93.5	31
1986–90	ACR	New York, USA	32.0	29
1986–90	ACR	USA	26.0	29
2004	ACR	Western Montana, USA	90	24

Abbreviations: ACR, American College of Rheumatology criteria (1990); CHCC, Chapel Hill Consensus Conference definition; EMEA, European Medicines Agency Algorithm; ICD, International Classification of Diseases; UKGPRD, United Kingdom General Practice Research Database.
[a] Point prevalence on 31 December, 2008.
[b] Point prevalence on 1 January, 2003.
[c] Point prevalence on 31 December, 2003.
[d] Using unmodified ACR criteria.

in southeastern Australia than in southern Europe, whereas the opposite occurs in MPA. There is a trend for higher incidence of WG in rural compared with urban areas.[6]

There are limited data from the Indian subcontinent; however, case series suggest that there is increasing recognition of WG.[33]

Ethnic Factors

Most studies have been based on White population data. Data from the French prevalence study suggested that WG is less common than MPA in non-Europeans.[34,35] The rate among Europeans was double that of New Zealander Maoris or Asians in New Zealand.[32] In Japan, WG is not as common as MPA although the incidence of overall primary vasculitides does not differ from that in Europe. pANCA-associated disease is more frequent than cANCA-associated disease in the Japanese population, which is not the case in European or US patients.[36] In China, WG also seems to be less common than MPA.[5]

Genetics

There are familial cases in WG, but they are rare. Familial heritability is similar to that seen in rheumatoid arthritis and it has been estimated at a relative risk of 1.56.[37] Clusters of WG occurring in families usually involve no more than 2 affected members and those most commonly affected are first-degree relatives. Distant relatives are less affected, which is suggestive of a more dominant role for environmental factors.

HLA associations have been reported; the strongest for the AAV is with HLA DPB1*0401.[38] Associations with polymorphisms in genes encoding key regulators of the immune response such as CTL4A and PTPN22 have been identified. Alpha 1-antitrypsine deficiency has been repeatedly reported as a genetic susceptibility factor.[34]

Environmental Factors

The notion of seasonality has been suggested by reports of a higher incidence rate of onset in winter (29.8%) than in summer (14.3%).[39] This has been variable and not consistent with studies in the United States.[29] Difficulty in establishing an accurate date of onset of the disease process, methodological discrepancies, and variation of triggering factors in different geographic areas may explain this inconsistency. Lane and collegaues[40] were unable to confirm the occurrence of seasonal onset for WG or any other AAV.

A north-south declining gradient in disease risk in the Northern Hemisphere[34] and the opposite in the Southern Hemisphere[31] suggest there is indeed a latitudinal variation in occurrence of WG and the other AAVs. This could be explained by ambient ultraviolet radiation, which was shown to have a protective immunomodulatory effect on the onset of WG.[41] Possible mechanisms consider the effect of vitamin D on the immune system. However, ultraviolet radiation is known to be associated with autoimmunity especially in conditions mediated by TH1 cells, such as multiple sclerosis, type 1 diabetes mellitus, and Crohn disease.[42]

Infection

Infection is closely related to vasculitis not only as a triggering factor but also as a consequence of intensive immunosuppression used for the treatment of primary vasculitides. De novo expression and relapse of vasculitis could be related to infection. The hypothesis that infection acts as a trigger for autoimmunity is not new. That could occur via direct microbial toxicity affecting the endothelium, either by invasion (eg, Rickettsiae, Bartonella, or cytomegalovirus) or the effect of microbial toxins. Humoral or cellular immune response to infections can lead to vasculitis via immune complex pathways (such as in hepatitis C and cryoglobulinemia).

For WG, the only clear microbial association is that with *Staphylococcus aureus* infection. *S aureus* is frequently isolated in cultures from the upper airways of patients with WG and nasal carriage has been linked with higher risk of relapse in WG. The relative risk for relapse is modulated by the presence and type of *S aureus* and was calculated at 3.2. The presence of toxic-shock-syndrome-toxin-1 increases the relative risk for relapse to 13.3.[43]

Drugs

No specific drug has been linked with WG. There have been several clinical observations of cocaine abuse followed by WG suggestive of an active induction of a proteinase 3 (PR3)-ANCA–positive vasculitis by cocaine. Detection of human leukocyte elastase (HLE)-ANCA in a patient with cocaine-induced midline destructive lesions mimicking the midfacial osteocartilagenous changes of WG may be a valuable diagnostic marker. It is rarely detected in primary WG or MPA, thus is suggestive of a drug-induced vasculitis. Drug-induced PR3-ANCA and myeloperoxidase (MPO)-ANCA may be associated with vasculitis mimicking AAV. The mechanisms involved in the break of tolerance and induction of ANCA (eg, superantigens, neutrophil extracellular traps, Th17 cells, protease-activated receptor-2) are likely to be shared in a degree between drug-induced or infection-induced and primary AAV.[44]

Occupational Factors

Several studies have investigated possible links between occupation and development of vasculitis. A hospital discharge case-control study in Sweden with 2288 cases and 10 controls per case did not find any association with 32 occupations.[45] Systemic vasculitis has been associated with exposure to particulate silica (eg, quartz, granite, sandstone, and grain dust). Pulmonary silicosis in individuals exposed to high levels of silica (eg, miners and quarrymen) has been shown to associate with systemic vasculitis.[46]

Nuyts and colleagues[47] found an odds ratio (OR) of 5.0 for silica exposure in 16 cases of WG compared with community controls. Lane and colleagues,[40] in a case-control study in Norfolk, UK, reported an OR of 3.0 in 75 cases of AAV (47 cases of WG). There was no significant association between MPA or WG and occupational silica exposure. Hogan and colleagues[48] found an OR of 4.6 for reported silica exposure in ANCA-positive patients (36 MPA, 21 WG, 8 necrotizing glomerulonephritis) compared with renal controls. In a population-based case-control study by Hogan and colleagues,[49] silica exposure was found in 78 (60%) of 129 case patients and in 49 (45%) of 109 control subjects. The results showed no increased risk for disease from low/medium exposure relative to no exposure (OR 1.0) but identified increased risk with high exposure (OR 1.9).

A case-control study performed at the US National Institutes of Health (NIH)[50] reported an association with inhaled fumes and particulates and pesticides with WG compared with healthy and rheumatic disease controls but not compared with respiratory disease controls. Nuyts and colleagues[47] reported significantly raised OR for exposure to various metals and welding fumes (OR 2.0) in a group of renal patients including WG and glomerulonephritis. The Norfolk case-control study did not observe an association with occupational metal exposure and primary systemic vasculitis.[40]

Links between occupational exposure to hydrocarbons such as paints and glues and systemic vasculitis have been studied by different groups with varying outcomes. Pai and colleagues[51] reported significantly higher hydrocarbon exposure in male MPA and WG patients compared with matched blood donors and nonsignificantly greater exposures in female patients with pulmonary hemorrhage. Lane and colleagues[40] estimated OR of 4.8 for exposure to occupational solvents compared with matched controls for PSV overall. Heavy metal exposure (mercury, lead) has been associated with WG.[52] However, the large Swedish study did not find any association with relevant occupations.[45]

Farming in the year before the onset of vasculitis has been associated with primary systemic vasculitis with an OR of 2.3 (WG 2.7 and MPA 6.3). The association appeared stronger in livestock than crops.[40] This was not demonstrated in studies by the NIH and Knight and colleagues, which did not find a significant association between WG and farming.[45,50]

MPA

The original description of periarteritis nodosa by Kussmaul and Maier was of a patient with inflammation and necrosis of medium-sized arteries leading to aneurysm formation and organ infarction. Davson and colleagues[53] described patients with segmental necrotizing glomerulonephritis who also had features of PAN with extrarenal small and medium artery involvement. The term microscopic polyarteritis was used to describe these patients in whom the dominant feature was rapidly progressive renal failure. The current term for these patients is MPA. The dominant feature of PAN is organ infarction (intestine, nerve) as a result of involvement of medium-sized arteries. This illness is now termed classic PAN. The literature on the epidemiology of PAN and MPA has to be carefully interpreted, because many older studies used the term polyarteritis nodosa as a generic term for any form of necrotizing vasculitis. The accurate classification of patients as MPA is also difficult as there are no validated classification criteria for MPA. The introduction of the European Medicines Agency Algorithm (EMEA) has helped to ensure consistency of classification across studies.

Geographic/Ethnic Factors

The etiopathogenesis of the AAV is unknown and it is therefore difficult to differentiate the effects of ethnicity from environmental factors when studying the occurrence of the AAV in different populations.

Most studies on the epidemiology of vasculitis have been conducted in White populations, and there is relatively little data from outside Europe, United States, Australia, and Japan. There are very few studies looking at the occurrence of MPA in different ethnic groups in the same geographic region. From the data that are available it is clear that there are major differences between populations. The only study of a multiethnic population was conducted in Paris and showed that the prevalence of AAV in persons of European ancestry was twice (104.7/million) the rate in non-Europeans (52.5/million).[35] MPA was more frequent than WG in non-Europeans. The non-European population was derived from the Maghreb, sub-Saharan Africa, Asia, and the Caribbean and comprised 28% of the study population (1.09/million).

The occurrence of MPA shows some striking variations in different populations. In Europe, the overall occurrence of AAV is roughly stable across populations; however, there is a north-south variation in the ratio of WG to MPA. In the northern European populations WG is more common than MPA; in southern European populations MPA is more common.[27] There is an even more striking difference in the occurrence of renal AAV between the United Kingdom and Japan, together with a variation in the clinical phenotype of AAV between European populations and Japan. The authors have recently shown that ANCA-associated renal vasculitis in Japan is almost entirely caused by MPA, whereas in Europe only 50% is associated with MPA, the remainder being associated with WG or CSS. Renal vasculitis in Japan was exclusively caused by pANCA-MPO, whereas in Europe 33.3% is associated with the presence of cANCA-PR3 (**Table 4**).[30] The clinical features of the patients with renal vasculitis also support the rarity of renal vasculitis in WG in Japan, as upper respiratory tract manifestations and ear, nose, and throat features were much less common.

The Peruvian population seems to be another population where MPA is 8 times more common than WG.[26] The highest incidence yet reported comes from Kuwait where the incidence of MPA was 24/million[54]; there is unfortunately no corresponding data on the occurrence of WG in Kuwait. In a large evaluation of classification criteria performed in China on 550 patients with systemic vasculitis the ratio of MPA to WG was 3:1 and 75% of patients were pANCA positive and 13% cANCA positive.[5] These data suggest that granulomatous vasculitis may be less common than MPA in non-White populations. Detailed epidemiologic data from the Indian subcontinent and Africa are lacking.

Time Trends

There are now several lengthy studies of the epidemiology of MPA. The earliest study to suggest an increase came from Leicester, UK, where the annual incidence of MPA between 1980 and 1986 was 0.5/million and between 1987 and 1989, 3.3/million (**Tables 5** and **6**).[15] This increase followed introduction of testing for ANCA and was possibly ascribed to increased physician awareness. A renal biopsy study in Stockholm reported a doubling of the annual incidence from 6.0 to 12.0/million between 1986 and 1992.[56] More recent studies suggest that the incidence was greater during the 1990s than the 1980s.[22,27] In the prospective Norwich study, there was no

Table 4
Epidemiology and clinical features of renal vasculitis in the United Kingdom and Japan

	Japan	UK	P
Male/female	24:32	13:14	
Mean age (y)	70.4	63.5	
Incidence total/million	14.8 (10.8–18.9)	12.2 (8.0–17.7)	
Incidence MPA/million	14.8 (10.8–18.9)	5.0 (2.4–8.8)	
Incidence WG/million	0	5.8 (3.4–10.6)	
Incidence CSS/million	0	1.4 (0.3–3.9)	
Ear, nose, and throat	1 (1.8)	18 (66.6)	<.001
Respiratory	23 (41.1)	11 (40.7)	ns
Nervous	3 (5.4%)	8 (29.8)	.02
Gastrointestinal	2 (3.6)	3 (11.0)	ns
pANCA-MPO	51 (91.1)	15 (55.5)[a]	<.001
cANCA-PR3	0 (0.0)	9 (33.3)[a]	<.001
Negative ANCA	5 (8.9)	2 (7.4)[a]	ns

Abbreviation: ns, not significant.
[a] In 3 cases ANCA data were available.
Data from Watts RA, Scott DG, Jayne DR et al. Renal vasculitis in Japan and the UK—are there differences in epidemiology and clinical phenotype? Nephrol Dial Transplant 2008;23(12):3928–31.

Table 5
Annual incidence of MPA

Year	Place	Criteria	Incidence (Per Million)	References
1980–1986	Leicester, UK	MPA	0.5	[15]
1987–1989	Leicester, UK	MPA	3.3	[15]
1988–2008	Norwich, UK	EMEA	5.1	[8]
1984–1989	Heidelberg, Germany	MPA[a]	1.5	[55]
1998–2002	Schleswig-Holstein, Germany	MPA	3	[18]
1971–1993	Lund, Sweden	CHCC	2.5	[21]
1997–2006	Southern Sweden	EMEA	10.1	[10]
1988–1998	Tromso, Norway	CHCC	2.7	[17]
1988–2001	Lugo, Spain	CHCC	7.9	[7]
1995–2003	Crete, Greece	CHCC	10.2	[9]
1990–1999	Vilnius, Lithuania	MPA	3.0	[23]
1993–1996	Kuwait	CHCC	24.0	[54]
2000–2004	Miyazaki, Japan	MPA[b]	14.8	[36]
1993–2004	Western Montana, USA	MPA	2.9	[24]
2000–2004	Australia	CHCC	5.0	[6]

Abbreviations: ACR, American College of Rheumatology criteria (1990); CHCC, Chapel Hill Consensus Conference definition; EMEA, European Medicines Agency Algorithm; ICD, International Classification of Diseases; UKGPRD, United Kingdom General Practice Research Database.
[a] Renal involvement only.
[b] Includes renal limited vasculitis.

Table 6 Prevalence of MPA				
Year	Place	Criteria	Prevalence (Per Million)	References
01/01/2003	Southern Sweden	EMEA	94	68
2000–2004	Australia	CHCC	39.1	6
31/12/2008	Norwich, UK	EMEA	47.9	8

Abbreviations: CHCC, Chapel Hill Consensus Conference definition; EMEA, European Medicines Agency Algorithm.

significant change in incidence during the period 1988 to 2008.[8] Tidman and colleagues[57] also did not observe an increase in incidence during 1986 to 1995. It is likely that earlier reported increases in MPA reflected increased awareness of the condition as physicians became better acquainted with the condition and its differences from WG or classic PAN following the publication of the CHCC definitions.

Environmental Factors

The environmental factors associated with development of MPA have been studied often in association with the other forms of AAV including WG and CSS. An association has been demonstrated with silica and AAV.[48,49] Following the Kobe earthquake in 1995 there was an increase in the occurrence of MPA.[58]

CSS

In 1951, Churg and Strauss described the post-mortem features of 13 patients who died following an illness characterized by asthma, eosinophilia, fever, systemic features, and granulomatous necrotizing vasculitis. Several studies have now included data on CSS; the incidence is generally reported to be in the range of 1.0 to 3.0/million (**Tables 7** and **8**). The highest figure was based on a single case seen during the period

Table 7 Annual incidence of CSS				
Year	Place	Criteria	Incidence (Per Million)	References
1988–2008	Norwich, UK	EMEA	3.0	8
1988–1997	Lugo, Spain	ACR	1.1	22
1988–2001	Lugo, Spain	CHCC & ACR	1.3	7
1995–2003	Crete, Greece	CHCC	0	9
1998–2008	Burgundy, France		1.2	59
1998–2002	Schleswig-Holstein, Germany	CHCC	1	18
1990–1999	Vilnius, Lithuania	ACR	1.3	23
1988–1998	Tromsø, Norway	ACR	0.5	27
1997–2006	Southern Sweden	EMEA	0.9	10
1976–1979	Olmsted, Minnesota		4.0	60
1995–2004	Australia	ACR	2.3	6
1990–2004	Lima, Peru	CHCC	0.14	26

Abbreviations: ACR, American College of Rheumatology criteria (1990); CHCC, Chapel Hill Consensus Conference definition; EMEA, European Medicines Agency Algorithm; ICD, International Classification of Diseases; UKGPRD, United Kingdom General Practice Research Database.

Table 8 Prevalence of CSS				
Year	Place	Criteria	Prevalence (Per Million)	References
31/12/08	Norwich, UK	EMEA	45.7	8
01/01/2003	Southern Sweden	EMEA	14.0	68
2000–2004	Australia	ACR	22.3	6

Abbreviations: ACR, American College of Rheumatology (1990) criteria; EMEA, European Medicines Agency Algorithm.

1976 to 1979 in Olmsted County, MN.[60] CSS is the least common of the AAV. It is more common in women than men and has peak age of onset at 65 to 75 years. In our 20-year study, the longest yet reported, the annual incidence of CSS as defined by the ACR criteria was 3.0/million, and there was no significant change in incidence during this period.[8]

There are very little data on ethnic differences in the occurrence of CSS, but the lowest incidence figure comes from Lima, Peru (0.14/million); whether this truly represents ethnic differences is uncertain.[26] The prevalence of CSS is in the range of 11.3/million to 45.7/million, again, much lower than that observed for either MPA or WG.

Environmental Factors

Most cases of CSS are idiopathic; inhaled antigens, vaccination, and desensitization have been reported as triggering factors.[61] Drugs, including sulfonamides, penicillin, anticonvulsants, and thiazides, have also been associated with the syndrome. The onset of CSS has been associated with use of leukotriene inhibitors and more recently with the anti-IgE monoclonal antibody omalizumab.[62] In a recent study looking at the US Food and Drug Administration Adverse Events Reporting System database, leukotriene inhibitor therapy was a suspect medication in most confirmed cases of CSS reported.[63] The incidence of CSS among patients with asthma has been estimated to be 34.6/million person-years[64]; the occurrence of CSS following leukotriene inhibitors and omalizumab may be the result of unmasking previous undiagnosed disease with reduction in the glucocorticoid use. The epidemiologic data may be confounded by the severity of the preceding asthma.[65,66]

SUMMARY

The epidemiology of the systemic vasculitides has been increasingly well documented in the past 20 years. There is an interesting age, geographic, and ethnic tropism that is gradually being revealed. Slow progress is being made on understanding the underlying causative factors but despite detailed and numerous studies no unequivocal environmental factors have emerged. The challenge still remains to the epidemiologist as improvements in classification methodology are promising a better opportunity to unfold the true picture of systemic vasculitides.

REFERENCES

1. Hunder GG, Bloch DA, Michel BA, et al. The American College of Rheumatology 1990 criteria for the classification of giant cell arteritis. Arthritis Rheum 1990; 33(8):1122–8.

2. Jennette JC, Falk RJ, Andrassy K, et al. Nomenclature of systemic vasculitides. Proposal of an international consensus conference. Arthritis Rheum 1994;37(2): 187–92.

3. Watts RA, Jolliffe VA, Carruthers DM, et al. Effect of classification on the incidence of polyarteritis nodosa and microscopic polyangiitis. Arthritis Rheum 1996;39(7): 1208–12.

4. Watts RA, Lane S, Hanslik T, et al. Development and validation of a consensus methodology for the classification of the ANCA-associated vasculitides and poly-arteritis nodosa for epidemiological studies. Ann Rheum Dis 2007;66(2):222–7.

5. Liu LJ, Chen M, Yu F, et al. Evaluation of a new algorithm in classification of systemic vasculitis. Rheumatology (Oxford) 2008;47(5):708–12.

6. Ormerod AS, Cook MC. Epidemiology of primary systemic vasculitis in the Australian Capital Territory and south-eastern New South Wales. Intern Med J 2008;38(11):816–23.

7. Gonzalez-Gay MA, Garcia-Porrua C, Guerrero J, et al. The epidemiology of the primary systemic vasculitides in northwest Spain: implications of the Chapel Hill Consensus Conference definitions. Arthritis Rheum 2003;49(3):388–93.

8. Watts RA, Mooney J, Scott DGI, et al. A twenty year study of the epidemiology of ANCA associated vasculitis in UK [abstract]. APMIS Suppl 2009;117(Suppl 127): 159.

9. Panagiotakis SH, Perysinakis GS, Kritikos H, et al. The epidemiology of primary systemic vasculitides involving small vessels in Crete (southern Greece): a comparison of older versus younger adult patients. Clin Exp Rheumatol 2009;27(3):409–15.

10. Mohammad AJ, Jacobsson LT, Westman KW, et al. Incidence and survival rates in Wegener's granulomatosis, microscopic polyangiitis, Churg Strauss syndrome and polyarteritis nodosa. Rheumatology (Oxford) 2009;48(12):1560–5.

11. Watts RA, Al-Taiar A, Scott DG, et al. Prevalence and incidence of Wegener's granulomatosis in the UK general practice research database. Arthritis Rheum 2009;61(10):1412–6.

12. Godman GC, Churg J. Wegener's granulomatosis: pathology and review of the literature. AMA Arch Pathol 1954;58(6):533–53.

13. Gardner-Medwin JM, Dolezalova P, Cummins C, et al. Incidence of Henoch Schönlein purpura, Kawasaki disease, and rare vasculitides in children of different ethnic origins. Lancet 2002;360(9341):1197–202.

14. Grisaru S, Yuen GW, Miettunen PV, et al. Incidence of Wegener's granulomatosis in children. J Rheumatol 2010;37(2):440–2.

15. Andrews M, Edmunds M, Campbell A, et al. Systemic vasculitis in the 1980's – is there an increasing incidence of Wegener's granulomatosis and microscopic pol-yarteritis? J R Coll Physicians Lond 1990;24(4):284–8.

16. Takala JH, Kautiainen H, Malmberg H, et al. Incidence of Wegener's granuloma-tosis in Finland 1981–2000. Clin Exp Rheumatol 2008;26(3 Suppl 49):S81–5.

17. Koldingsnes W, Nossent JC. Epidemiology of Wegener's granulomatosis in northern Norway. Arthritis Rheum 2000;43(11):2481–7.

18. Reinhold-Keller E, Herlyn K, Wagner-Bastmeyer R, et al. Stable incidence of primary systemic vasculitides over five years: results from the German vasculitis register. Arthritis Rheum 2005;53(1):93–9.

19. Knight A, Ekbom A, Brandt L, et al. Increasing incidence of Wegener's granulo-matosis in Sweden, 1975–2001. J Rheumatol 2006;33(10):2060–3.

20. Haugeberg G, Bie R, Bendvold A, et al. Primary vasculitis in a Norwegian community hospital: a retrospective study. Clin Rheumatol 1998;17(5):364–8.

21. Westman KW, Bygren PG, Olsson H, et al. Relapse rate, renal survival, and cancer morbidity in patients with Wegener's granulomatosis or microscopic polyangiitis with renal involvement. J Am Soc Nephrol 1998;9(5):842–52.
22. González-Gay MA, García-Porrúa C. Systemic vasculitis in adults in northwestern Spain 1988–97. Clinical and epidemiological aspects. Medicine (Baltimore) 1999; 78(5):292–308.
23. Dadoniene J, Kirdaite G, Mackiewicz Z, et al. Incidence of primary systemic vasculitis in Vilnius: a university hospital population based study. Ann Rheum Dis 2005;64(2):335–6.
24. Zeft A, Schlesinger M, Weiss N, et al. Case control study of ANCA associated vasculitis in western Montana [abstract]. Arthritis Rheum 2005;52(Suppl):S648.
25. Hissaria P, Cai FZ, Ahern M, et al. Wegener's granulomatosis: epidemiological and clinical features in a South Australian study. Intern Med J 2008;38(10):776–80.
26. Sanchez AA, Acevedo EM, Sanchez CG, et al. Evaluation of epidemiology of the primary systemic vasculitides in a Latin-American well-defined population [abstract]. Arthritis Rheum 2006;54(Suppl):S757.
27. Watts RA, Gonzalez-Gay M, Garcia-Porrua C, et al. Geoepidemiology of systemic vasculitis. Ann Rheum Dis 2001;60(2):170–2.
28. Reinhold-Keller E, Zeidler A, Gutfleisch J, et al. Giant cell arteritis is more prevalent in urban than rural populations: results of an epidemiological study of primary systemic vasculitides in Germany. Rheumatology (Oxford) 2000;39(12): 1396–402.
29. Cotch MF, Hoffman GS, Yerg DE, et al. The epidemiology of Wegener's granulomatosis: estimates of the five year period prevalence, annual mortality and geographic disease distribution from population based data sources. Arthritis Rheum 1996;39(1):87–92.
30. Watts RA, Scott DG, Jayne DR, et al. Renal vasculitis in Japan and the UK—are there differences in epidemiology and clinical phenotype? Nephrol Dial Transplant 2008;23(12):3928–31.
31. Gibson A, Stamp LK, Chapman PT, et al. The epidemiology of Wegener's granulomatosis and microscopic polyangiitis in a Southern Hemisphere region. Rheumatology (Oxford) 2006;45(5):624–8.
32. O'Donnell JL, Stevanovic VR, Frampton C, et al. Wegener's granulomatosis in New Zealand: evidence for a latitude-dependent incidence gradient. Intern Med J 2007;37(4):242–6.
33. Malaviya AN, Kumar A, Singh YN, et al. Wegener's granulomatosis in India: not so rare. Br J Rheumatol 1990;29(6):499–500.
34. Mahr AD, Neogi T, Merkel PA. Epidemiology of Wegener's granulomatosis: lessons from descriptive studies and analyses of genetic and environmental risk determinants. Clin Exp Rheumatol 2006;24(2 Suppl 41):S82–91.
35. Mahr A, Guillevin L, Poissonnet M, et al. Prevalences of polyarteritis nodosa, microscopic polyangiitis, Wegener's granulomatosis, and Churg-Strauss syndrome in a French urban multiethnic population in 2000: a capture-recapture estimate. Arthritis Rheum 2004;51(1):92–9.
36. Fujimoto S, Uezono S, Hisanaga S, et al. Incidence of ANCA-associated primary renal vasculitis in the Miyazaki prefecture: the first population-based, retrospective, epidemiologic survey in Japan. Clin J Am Soc Nephrol 2006;1(5):1016–22.
37. Knight A, Sandin S, Askling J. Risks and relative risks of Wegener's granulomatosis among close relatives of patients with the disease. Arthritis Rheum 2008; 58(1):302–7.

38. Heckmann M, Holle JU, Arnig L, et al. The Wegener's granulomatosis quantitive trait locus on chromosome 6p21.3 as characterized by tagSNP genotyping. Ann Rheum Dis 2008;67(7):972–9.

39. Raynauld JP, Bloch DA, Fries JF. Seasonal variation in the onset of Wegener's granulomatosis, polyarteritis nodosa and giant cell arteritis. J Rheumatol 1993; 20(9):1524–6.

40. Lane SE, Watts RA, Bentham G, et al. Are environmental factors important in primary systemic vasculitis? A case control study. Arthritis Rheum 2003;48(3): 814–23.

41. Gatenby PA, Lucas RM, Engelsen O, et al. Antineutrophil cytoplasmic antibody-associated vasculitides: could geographic patterns be explained by ambient ultraviolet radiation? Arthritis Rheum 2009;61(10):1417–24.

42. Staples JA, Ponsonby AL, Lim L, et al. Ecologic analysis of some immune related disorders, including type I diabetes, in Australia: latitude, regional ultraviolet radiation, and disease prevalence. Environ Health Perspect 2003;111(4):518–23.

43. Popa ER, Stegeman CA, Abdulahad WH, et al. Staphylococcal toxic-shock-syndrome-toxin-1 as a risk factor for disease relapse in Wegener's granulomatosis. Rheumatology (Oxford) 2007;46(6):1029–33.

44. Csernok E, Lamprecht P, Gross WL. Clinical and immunological features of drug-induced and infection-induced proteinase 3-antineutrophil cytoplasmic antibodies and myeloperoxidase-antineutrophil cytoplasmic antibodies and vasculitis. Curr Opin Rheumatol 2010;22(1):43–8.

45. Knight A, Sandin S, Askling J. Occupational risk factors for Wegener's granulomatosis – a case control study. Ann Rheum Dis 2010;69(4):737–40.

46. Tervaert JW, Stegeman CA, Kallenberg CG. Silicon exposure and vasculitis. Curr Opin Rheumatol 1998;10(1):12–7.

47. Nuyts GD, van Vlem E, de Vos A, et al. Wegener's granulomatosis is associated with exposure to silicon compounds: a case control study. Nephrol Dial Transplant 1995;10(7):1162–5.

48. Hogan SL, Satterly KK, Dooley MA, et al. Silica exposure in anti-neutrophil cytoplasmic autoantibody-associated glomerulonephritis and lupus nephritis. J Am Soc Nephrol 2001;12(1):134–42.

49. Hogan SL, Cooper GS, Savitz DA, et al. Association of silica exposure with anti-neutrophil cytoplasmic autoantibody small-vessel vasculitis: a population-based, case-control study. Clin J Am Soc Nephrol 2007;2(2):290–9.

50. Duna GF, Cotch MF, Galperin C, et al. Wegener's granulomatosis: role of environmental exposures. Clin Exp Rheumatol 1998;16(6):669–74.

51. Pai P, Bone JM, Bell GM. Hydrocarbon exposure and glomerulonephritis due to systemic vasculitis. Nephrol Dial Transplant 1998;13(5):1321–3.

52. Albert D, Clarkin C, Komoroski J, et al. Wegener's granulomatosis: possible role of environmental agents in its pathogenesis. Arthritis Rheum 2004;51(4):656–64.

53. Davson J, Ball J, Platt R. The kidney in periarteritis nodosa. Q J Med 1948;17(67): 175–202.

54. El-Reshaid K, Kapoor M, El-Reshaid W, et al. The spectrum of renal disease associated with microscopic polyangiitis and classical polyarteritis nodosa in Kuwait. Nephrol Dial Transplant 1997;12(9):1874–82.

55. Andrassy K, Erb A, Koderisch J, et al. Wegener's granulomatosis with renal involvement: patient survival and correlations between initial renal function, renal histology, therapy and renal outcome. Clin Nephrol 1991;35(4):139–47.

56. Pettersson EE, Sundelin B, Heigl Z. Incidence and outcome of pauci-immune necrotising glomerulonephritis in adults. Clin Nephrol 1995;43(3):141–9.

57. Tidman M, Olander R, Svalander C, et al. Patients hospitalised because of small vessel vasculitides with renal involvement in the period 1975–95: organ involvement, anti-neutrophil cytoplasmic antibodies patterns, seasonal attack rates and fluctuation of annual frequencies. J Intern Med 1998;244(2): 133–41.
58. Yashiro M, Muso E, Itoh-Ihara T, et al. Significantly high regional morbidity of MPO-ANCA-related angitis and/or nephritis with respiratory tract involvement after the 1995 great earthquake in Kobe (Japan). Am J Kidney Dis 2000;35(5): 889–95.
59. Vinit J, Muller G, Bielefeld P, et al. Churg-Strauss syndrome: retrospective study in Burgundian population in France in past 10 years. Rheumatol Int 2009. [Epub ahead of print]. PMID: 20039171.
60. Kurland LT, Chuang TY, Hunder GG. The epidemiology of systemic arteritis. In: Lawrence RC, Shulman LE, editors. The epidemiology of the rheumatic diseases. New York: Gower Publishing; 1984. p. 196–205.
61. Guillevin L. Virus-associated vasculitides. Rheumatology (Oxford) 1999;38(7): 588–90.
62. Wechsler M, Wong D, Miller MK, et al. Churg Strauss syndrome in patients treated with omalizumab. Chest 2009;136(2):507–18.
63. Bibby S, Healy B, Steele R, et al. Association between leukotriene receptor antagonist therapy and Churg-Strauss syndrome: an analysis of the FDA AERS database. Thorax 2010;65(2):132–8.
64. Harrold LR, Andrade SE, Go AS, et al. Incidence of Churg Strauss Syndrome in asthma drug users: a population based perspective. J Rheumatol 2005;32(6): 1076–80.
65. Harrold LR, Patterson MK, Andrade SE, et al. Asthma drug use and the development of Churg-Strauss syndrome (CSS). Pharmacoepidemiol Drug Saf 2007; 16(6):620–6.
66. Hauser T, Mahr A, Metzler C, et al. The leucotriene receptor antagonist montelukast and the risk of Churg-Strauss syndrome: a case-crossover study. Thorax 2008;63(8):677–82.
67. Eaton WW, Rose NR, Kalaydjian A, et al. Epidemiology of autoimmune diseases in Denmark. J Autoimmun 2007;29(1):1–9.
68. Mohammad AJ, Jacobsson LT, Mahr AD, et al. Prevalence of Wegener's granulomatosis, microscopic polyangiitis, polyarteritis nodosa and Churg-Strauss syndrome within a defined population in southern Sweden. Rheumatology (Oxford) 2007;46(8):1329–37.

Pathogenesis of ANCA-associated Vasculitis

Julia Flint, MBBS[a,b], Matthew D. Morgan, MRCP, PhD[b,*], Caroline O.S. Savage, FRCP, FMedSci[b]

KEYWORDS

- Antineutrophil cytoplasm antibody • Vasculitis
- Wegener's granulomatosis • Microscopic polyangiitis
- T cell • Neutrophil • Endothelium

Wegener's granulomatosis (WG), microscopic polyangiitis (MPA), and Churg-Strauss syndrome are rare small-vessel vasculitides characterized by necrotizing inflammation of blood vessel walls. Classification criteria for the 3 diseases were agreed on at the Chapel Hill Consensus Conference.[1] The diseases are associated with circulating autoantibodies directed against the neutrophil granule components myeloperoxidase (MPO) and proteinase 3 (PR3). The presence of antineutrophil cytoplasm antibodies (ANCA) and shared pathologic and clinical features have led to MPA and WG often being termed ANCA-associated vasculitis (AAV). This review focuses mainly on WG and MPA.

AAV may cause localized or systemic disease, the commonest organ systems involved being the kidneys and the upper and lower respiratory tract. The clinical presentation is highly variable, but the disease may eventually lead to renal or respiratory failure or failure of other organ systems. Left untreated the disease has high mortality, and current treatment regimens have improved 5-year survival to between 49% and 90%. Current treatments with corticosteroids and cyclophosphamide, while effective, are associated with significant morbidity and mortality.

Much of the research and debate around the pathogenesis of AAV has centered on the role of ANCA in the disease, and this is reviewed herein. The presence of

---

Disclosure: C.O.S.S. is currently undertaking a sabbatical for GlaxoSmithKline. M.D.M. and J.F. have nothing to declare.

[a] Birmingham Children's Hospital NHS Foundation Trust, Steelhouse Lane, Birmingham B4 6NH, UK

[b] Renal Immunobiology, School of Immunity and Infection, College of Medical and Dental Sciences, University of Birmingham, Birmingham B15 2TT, UK

* Corresponding author.

E-mail address: m.d.morgan@bham.ac.uk

Rheum Dis Clin N Am 36 (2010) 463–477

doi:10.1016/j.rdc.2010.05.006

rheumatic.theclinics.com

autoantibodies also implies a loss of self tolerance and a role for T-helper cells and B cells in their production, as well as a defect in regulatory T-cell function.

ROLE OF ANCA IN ANCA-ASSOCIATED VASCULITIS

One of the most hotly debated topics in AAV research has been the pathogenic significance of ANCA. There is now a substantial body of evidence supporting a pathogenic role for ANCA in AAV. This evidence consists of in vitro experiments demonstrating that ANCA activate cytokine primed neutrophils, animal models of vasculitis that mimic some of the features of human disease and the transplacental transfer of anti-MPO ANCA, leading to neonatal disease.

IN VITRO ACTIVATION OF NEUTROPHILS BY ANCA

The potential involvement of these antibodies in the disease process was suggested in 1990 when Falk and colleagues[2] proposed a pathogenic mechanism whereby ANCA could lead to vascular damage. In vitro experiments demonstrated that neutrophils express the antigens for ANCA on the cell surface. Following cytokine priming, ANCA can activate neutrophils resulting in adhesion to endothelium, superoxide generation, degranulation, and the production of proinflammatory cytokines.[3,4]

Several cytokines, such as tumor necrosis factor α (TNF-α), interleukin (IL)-18, and granulocyte macrophage colony stimulating factor can prime neutrophils for ANCA activation. The cytokine priming may increase surface expression of ANCA antigens, mobilize components of the NADPH oxidase complex, and perform other functions necessary for subsequent neutrophil activation by ANCA.[5–8]

Studies of the intracellular signaling cascades of neutrophils following ANCA activation have demonstrated a role for multiple signaling pathways.[9] ANCA IgG Fc binding to the Fcγ receptors appears to activate tyrosine kinases,[10,11] whereas the F(ab′)2 portion of ANCA activates a separate G-protein pathway, including activation of phosphatidylinositol-3 kinase-γ, and an increased guanosine triphosphatase (GTPase) activity.[12] These distinct pathways appear to converge on a GTPase, p21^{ras}. p21^{ras} plays a central role in many cellular processes in the neutrophil, including the respiratory burst. ANCA F(ab′)2 binding and intact ANCA IgG binding activate only 1 of the 2 isoforms of p21^{ras} present in the neutrophil, with little effect on the other isoform.[9] Karussis and colleagues[13] have successfully used an inhibitor of p21^{ras}, farnesylthiosalicylic acid, in an animal model of autoimmune encephalitis to selectively inhibit active cells without affecting other immune functions. It is therefore theoretically possible that this particular p21^{ras} isoform could be inhibited to specifically inhibit the ANCA-activated signaling via p21^{ras} without affecting other p21^{ras} functions.[9] The effect of ANCA binding to neutrophils on gene transcription has also been investigated. It has been shown that changes in gene expression can reflect disease activity in vivo. Of note, binding of both intact ANCA and F(ab′)2 portions was found to be capable of inducing gene expression in the neutrophil.[14]

EFFECT OF ANCA ON NEUTROPHIL-ENDOTHELIAL ADHESION

Neutrophil-mediated damage of endothelial cells plays a key role in the pathogenesis of AAV, as the histologic features of AAV include fibrinoid necrosis of the endothelium. The earliest changes involve swelling, necrosis, and dehiscence of the vascular endothelial cells.[15] This process exposes the basement membrane, leading to platelet adherence, thrombosis, and vessel occlusion. Upregulation of adhesion molecules and the release of chemoattractant proteins by endothelial cells are likely to promote adhesion and transmigration of leukocytes, contributing to the endothelial damage.

In vitro studies have demonstrated that neutrophils exposed to ANCA adhere to TNF-α activated human umbilical vein endothelial cells (HUVEC).[16–18] ANCA induce adhesion of neutrophils to endothelial cells in vitro via the upregulation and conformational change of adhesion molecules such as CD11b.[19,20] The key steps involved in the model of ANCA-stimulated neutrophil-endothelial cell interaction are summarized in **Fig. 1**.

This process has been investigated using a flow model whereby neutrophils are perfused over monolayers of endothelial cells replicating the shear stresses found in capillaries. Pretreatment of the neutrophils with ANCA was shown to increase the stability of the adhesion of neutrophils, as well as significantly increasing neutrophil transmigration.[21] This adhesion of neutrophils to endothelium was shown to be dependent on activation of β2 integrins and CXCR2.[20] Of note, a recent study has

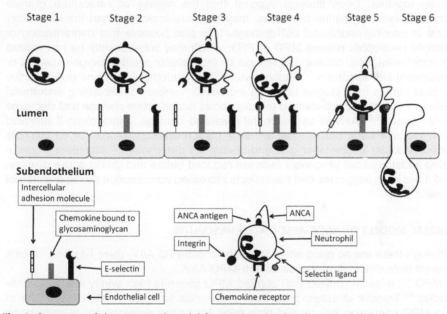

Fig. 1. Summary of the proposed model for ANCA-stimulated neutrophil-endothelial interaction. Stage 1: Unprimed neutrophils are present in the circulation and the endothelial cells are not activated. Stage 2: Cytokine priming leads to increased surface expression of ANCA antigens (MPO and PR3), integrins, chemokine receptors, and selectin ligands on the neutrophil cell surface. Cytokine activation of endothelial cells leads to increased expression of intercellular adhesion molecules (CAMs), E-selectin, and chemokines. Stage 3: ANCA interacts with its antigens on the neutrophil surface and cross-links the Fc gamma receptors, leading to conformation change in integrins. Stage 4: Rolling adhesion of the neutrophil on the endothelial surface is mediated by the interaction of CAMs and their ligands on the neutrophil (integrins). There may be some differences between various microvascular circulations; in the glomerulus it may be that neutrophils do not undergo rolling adhesion prior to firm adhesion and arrest. Stage 5: Firm adhesion and arrest is mediated by interaction between E-selectin and its ligands and glycosaminoglycan-bound chemokines on endothelial cells and chemokine receptors on the neutrophil. Stage 6: Neutrophils transmigrate the endothelial cell monolayer, undergo respiratory burst and degranulation with release of toxic products, leading to endothelial damage.

demonstrated that anti-PR3 ANCA, interacting with adherent cytokine primed neutrophils, increase membrane PR3 expression, providing a positive feedback loop that may amplify anti-PR3 ANCA–induced responses in the small vessels where adhesion occurs.[22]

ANCA have also been shown to induce F-actin polymerization in neutrophils, decreasing neutrophil deformability. This process may lead to impaired passage of neutrophils through capillary beds, such as in the glomerulus, promoting interaction with the endothelium and endothelial damage.[23]

ANCA may play a role in neutrophil-mediated cytotoxicity of endothelial cells.[24,25] It is known that ANCA can stimulate cytokine primed neutrophils to release both reactive oxygen species and proteases. These factors have been proposed as potential instigators of endothelial cell damage. However, it has recently been shown that endothelial cells inhibit the production of superoxide by neutrophils, and that the release of von Willebrand factor (vWF) by endothelial cells (a well-recognized marker of endothelial cell damage) was more dependent on serine proteases released from neutrophils.[26] Taken together, these findings suggest that the release of intracellular granule contents, including serine proteases, may be more important than the respiratory burst in causing endothelial cell damage. It is also possible that degranulating or necrotic neutrophils release MPO or PR3, which may subsequently be internalized by endothelial cells, causing the release of intracellular reactive oxygen species or endothelial cell apoptosis.[27] Further evidence of endothelial damage during active disease comes from studies reporting increased numbers of circulating endothelial cells and endothelial cell–derived microparticles during active disease that decrease in remission.[28,29] As well as neutrophil-mediated damage, angiopoietin-2 released from Weibel-Palade bodies may act in a paracrine/autocrine manner to promote further vascular inflammation and endothelial cell detachment.[28] Numbers of circulating endothelial cell progenitor cells are reduced before and during active disease, and it has been suggested that this reflects increased consumption during endothelial repair.[30–32]

ANIMAL MODELS OF ANCA-ASSOCIATED VASCULITIS

Although there are no good animal models of anti-PR3 AAV, there has been recent interest in murine and rat models of anti-MPO AAV.

MPO$^{-/-}$ mice immunized with purified MPO generate high avidity anti-MPO antibodies.[33] Transfer of splenocytes from these mice to Rag2$^{-/-}$ mice or transfer of anti-MPO containing IgG to wild-type mice led to the development of necrotizing and crescentic glomerulonephritis, granulomatous inflammation, and systemic necrotizing vasculitis. The addition of lipopolysaccharide (LPS) enhanced renal injury and increased levels of TNF-α. This effect was ameliorated by anti–TNF-α antibodies, demonstrating the importance of cytokines in this pathogenic process.[33] The model has also confirmed the central role of neutrophils in the pathogenesis of AAV. Neutrophil and macrophage infiltration was prominent at the sites of glomerular injury, and neutrophil-depleted mice did not develop crescentic glomerulonephritis.[34]

Intravital microscopy studies of the cremaster muscle of wild-type mice (pretreated with cytokines), showed that anti-MPO IgG enhances leukocyte adhesion and transmigration. This effect was shown to be dependent on Fcγ receptors and β2 integrins (CD18), as there was no increase in adherence or transmigration in Fc receptor γ chain$^{-/-}$ mice, or following coadministration of anti-CD18 antibodies.[35] Others have found that the mechanisms involved in anti-MPO–induced neutrophil adhesion is dose dependent; low-dose anti-MPO in the presence of LPS induced endothelial adhesion in a β2-integrin dependent manner whereas high-dose anti-MPO in the absence of LPS induced adhesion in a β4-integrin dependent manner.[36]

Other studies of ANCA activation of neutrophils in mice and humans have suggested a role for complement in the development of inflammation and glomerular damage, with immune complex deposition in renal biopsies demonstrated by electron microscopy.[37] In vitro studies demonstrate ANCA activation of cytokine-primed neutrophils results in activation of the alternative complement pathway and that C5a acting via the neutrophil C5a receptor further primes neutrophils for ANCA activation.[38,39] C5a-deficient mice were resistant to induction of glomerulonephritis following transfer of murine anti-MPO antibodies. Recent studies in human renal biopsy tissue have demonstrated the presence of the membrane attack complex, C3d, and factors B and P in the glomeruli and microvasculature,[40] and that complement deposition was associated with more severe renal disease.[41]

A recent rat model of anti-MPO ANCA vasculitis, termed experimental autoimmune vasculitis (EAV), has shown interesting results.[42] Wistar-Kyoto rats immunized with purified human MPO in adjuvant develop anti-MPO antibodies as well as pauci-immune crescentic glomerulonephritis and lung hemorrhage. In this model intravital microscopy demonstrated increased leukocyte adhesion and transmigration in response to a rat homologue of IL-8 (CXC Ligand-1, a chemokine that acts on neutrophils), as well as in naïve rats after passive transfer of anti-MPO IgG from animals with EAV.[43]

In humans, the most direct evidence for the pathogenicity of ANCA comes from a case study in which an infant was born to a mother with active MPA.[44] The infant developed pulmonary-renal syndrome 48 hours after delivery and was found to have serum MPO-ANCA titers similar to the mother. It is hypothesized that the neonate's disease developed due to transplacental transfer of pathogenic ANCA (and possibly cytokines). The neonate was treated with steroids and plasma exchange, and recovered.

EFFECT OF ANCA ON NEUTROPHIL APOPTOSIS

Neutrophil activation usually ends in cell death by apoptosis, which should not trigger an inflammatory response or expose the internal components of the cell to the immune system. It has been shown that when primed neutrophils interact with ANCA, the neutrophils undergo dysregulated and accelerated apoptosis,[45] which can lead to secondary necrosis and the release of toxic intracellular contents. Opsonization of neutrophils by ANCA may lead to enhanced macrophage uptake, and the release of proinflammatory cytokines such as IL-1 and IL-8 to perpetuate inflammation.[46] Furthermore, apoptosis of nonprimed neutrophils leads to translocation of granule contents to the cell surface, which may thus provide an additional mechanism whereby ANCA can interact with the intracellular granule contents PR3 and MPO.[47]

OTHER FUNCTIONS OF THE ANCA ANTIGENS

The membrane expression of PR3 (mPR3) is bimodal, with an mPR3-positive neutrophil subset distinguishable from a membrane PR3-negative neutrophil subset within a given individual. Although the proportion of mPR3-expressing neutrophils appears to be relatively stable within an individual, there is a wide variation between individuals (0%–100%). This variation has been shown to be genetically determined,[48] perhaps related to the major histocompatibility complex HLA region.[49] High levels of mPR3 expression have been associated with susceptibility to vasculitis and disease relapse in WG.[50,51] It has also been demonstrated that patients with AAV show increased transcription of PR3 and MPO compared with healthy controls. During the normal process of neutrophil maturation, the transcription of granule constituents (including MPO and PR3) is terminated by the time the neutrophil leaves the bone marrow. In patients with AAV, mRNA transcripts for PR3 and MPO were found in mature circulating monocytes and neutrophils.

The role of ANCA target antigens may extend beyond cross-linking of ANCA on the surface of neutrophils. The serum levels of PR3 have also been shown to be elevated in AAV in both active disease and remission, and in MPO-ANCA and PR3-ANCA vasculitis.[52,53] Circulating serum PR3 may contribute to the pathogenesis of disease by interaction with endothelial cells,[54] leading to IL-8 and MCP-1 production, recruiting neutrophils and macrophages,[55] or causing endothelial cell apoptosis.[27] PR3 may also increase the activity of multiple inflammatory cytokines.[56,57]

Anti-MPO ANCA have also been shown to interact with MPO directly, leading to generation of hypochlorous acid, which was strongly cytolytic in culture.[58]

α-1 Antitrypsin is the main physiologic inhibitor of PR3, and anti-PR3 ANCA has been shown to inhibit the inactivation of PR3 by α-1 antitrypsin.[59,60] In one study, this inhibitory effect of anti-PR3 ANCA correlated more closely with disease activity than the serum levels of ANCA.[61] However, the main evidence that the inhibition of PR3 by α-1 antitrypsin is important in the pathogenesis of AAV stems from the observation that deficiency of α-1 antitrypsin is associated with AAV. The z allele (which leads to reduced α-1 antitrypsin activity) for α-1 antitrypsin is more common in patients with WG, especially in those with more severe disease.[62,63]

The mechanisms by which the interaction of ANCA and neutrophils may contribute to microvascular inflammation are varied, and may include inappropriate degranulation at the endothelial surface, altered interaction with endothelial cells (with increased transmigration across the vessel wall and endothelial cell damage), and altered apoptosis and necrosis of neutrophils, leading to the release of proinflammatory cytokines.

LYSOSOMAL MEMBRANE PROTEIN 2

Antibodies against lysosomal membrane protein 2 (LAMP-2) have recently been reported in AAV. LAMP-2 ANCA are capable of damaging human microvascular endothelium and inducing focal necrotizing glomerulonephritis in rats. Of note, LAMP-2 antibodies recognize an epitope that has homology with a bacterial adhesion molecule, "Fim H." It is postulated that bacteria expressing the Fim H antigen could act as a molecular mimic to LAMP-2, thus triggering the production of LAMP-2 ANCA alongside anti-Fim H antibodies.[64]

ANTIENDOTHELIAL CELL ANTIBODIES

ANCA are the autoantibodies most closely associated with WG and MPA, but other autoantibodies have been reported in patients with these diseases, including antibodies against endothelial cell components. Some in vivo evidence of a pathogenic role for antiendothelial cell antibodies (AECA) exists, whereby mice were immunized with purified IgG AECA (from a patient with WG) and subsequently developed perivascular lymphocytic infiltrate of venules and arterioles but no glomerulonephritis.[65] AECA are prevalent in systemic vasculitis in humans as well as other inflammatory conditions, and levels may fluctuate with disease activity.[66] AECA also demonstrate some organ specificity: AECA specific to human nasal, kidney, and lung endothelial cells are found more frequently than AECA specific to HUVEC in patients with WG.[67] Mechanisms for a pathogenic role for AECA have been proposed. It is suggested that AECA may up-regulate endothelial surface adhesion molecules and secretion of inflammatory cytokines, promoting adhesion of activated neutrophils and monocytes as well as cytotoxicity.[67–69] It is conceivable that some of the pathogenic activity of AECA is due to anti–LAMP-2 antibodies.

THE ROLE OF LYMPHOCYTES CELLS IN ANCA-ASSOCIATED VASCULITIS
T Cells

The role of lymphocytes in AAV is less well defined than the role of ANCA in activating neutrophils. T cells are a predominant infiltrating cell in the interstitium of the kidney with crescentic glomerulonephritis,[70] and are found in other sites of inflammation.[71,72] ANCA are class switched high-affinity autoantibodies implying a role for T-cell help in their production, the presence of autoreactive T cells, and a failure of regulatory T-cell function.[73,74] In addition, patients with resistant disease have been reported to respond to T-cell–depleting treatment with antithymocyte globulin.[75] Similarly, depleting CD4+ T cells in a mouse model of anti-MPO vasculitis attenuated the glomerular crescent formation, despite the MPO ANCA titer being unaffected.[76]

Following activation T-helper cells differentiate into 1 of 4 distinct lineages depending on, amongst other things, the cytokine environment. Each lineage is characterized by the presence of specific transcription factors and patterns of cytokine.

Both Th1 and Th2 cell populations have been described in the tissues in AAV. High levels of interferon-γ production following nonspecific stimulation of these T cells suggest a predominantly Th1-driven response.[77–79] However, this conclusion is challenged by other studies reporting a predominantly Th2 response in WG.[80,81] MPO- and PR3-specific T cells have been reported in patients with AAV,[80] with proliferative responses to MPO or PR3 in culture and strong production of IL-6 and IL-10. At the time it was suggested that this may represent a Th2 response; however, in light of better understanding of Th17 cells (whose differentiation depends on IL-6 among other cytokines) and Treg cells, it may be possible to interpret these data differently. Recently a population of PR3-specific Th17 cells has been described in ANCA-positive patients.[82] IL-17 may be involved in neutrophil migration[83,84] and stimulate the generation of other proinflammatory cytokines.[85,86]

The role of regulatory T cells has also been studied.[87] The number and function of CD4+ CD25+ Treg cells has been shown to be reduced in AAV, especially in active disease,[88] and reduced numbers of Treg correspond to slower times to remission and increased relapse rates.

Peripheral blood T cells in patients with AAV have an abnormal phenotype and appear to be persistently activated, during periods of both active disease and remission.[89–91] Overall, there appears to be a peripheral lymphopenia, with low levels of CD4+ T-helper cells but a relative increase in the subset of CD4+ memory cells.[89] It is not understood how these differences in T-cell phenotype between healthy individuals and AAV patients relate to disease pathogenesis. Many previous studies were done before Th17 cells were recognized as a separate lineage and before human Treg cells were characterized. Many of the apparent inconsistencies in previous studies (the different reporting of Th1 and Th2 associations) and apparent persistent activation (such as high CD25 expression) may become more comprehensible as our understanding of T-cell biology improves.

B Cells

The importance of B cells in AAV is evident, due to their role in the production of ANCA. Histologically B cells are found in affected tissues in WG, such as nasal lesions and the renal interstitial infiltrate of those with renal involvement.[70,92] The proportion of active circulating B cells is also increased in active WG compared with disease in remission or healthy controls.[91]

The presence of autoreactive B cells implies a breakdown of normal mechanisms that ensure tolerance to self antigens. CD19 is a B-cell coreceptor that enhances B-cell receptor signal transduction, and surface expression of this coreceptor has been shown to be approximately 20% lower in AAV than in healthy controls.[93] It is possible that autoreactive B cells with low surface expression of CD19 may escape normal tolerance mechanisms due to the reduced strength of signaling achieved via the B-cell receptor.[93]

Granuloma formation is a feature of WG often found in the lungs and upper airways,[94] and may be a feature of early or "localized" disease.[95] Histologic examination of granulomatous inflammation in WG demonstrated B-cell clusters in close proximity to numerous PR3-positive cells. An analysis of the functional immunoglobulins from WG tissue was supportive of an antigen-driven selection process.[92] It is therefore possible that this early granulomatous inflammation provides a site for the selection and maturation of anti-PR3 ANCA producing B cells, contributing to progression to systemic vasculitis.

Recently there has been interest in the role of the anti-CD20 antibody rituximab in the treatment of autoimmune diseases, including AAV. CD20 is expressed on mature B cells but not plasma cells, yet there are several case series now describing rapid remission induction and reduction in ANCA titers following peripheral B-cell depletion with rituximab treatment.[96,97] A recently completed randomized controlled trial comparing cyclophosphamide with rituximab suggests that rituximab is as effective as cyclophosphamide (in conjunction with corticosteroids) at inducing disease remission.

ETIOLOGY THEORIES

Although the evidence for the pathogenicity of ANCA in AAV is substantial, it remains difficult to understand what triggers the breakdown in immune tolerance and initial generation of ANCA. It is recognized that drugs and infectious agents may trigger the generation of ANCA as well as a clinical picture of secondary vasculitis, which may bear strong clinical resemblance to primary vasculitis.[98] However, infectious agents have also long been suspected to have a role in the pathogenesis of primary AAV. For example, Staphylococcus aureus has been shown to be a strong independent risk factor for relapse in WG, leading some clinicians to advocate the use of long-term prophylactic cotrimoxazole.[99] Several case-control studies have also demonstrated an association of AAV with environmental silica exposure.[100]

It is conceivable that exposure to an infectious antigen may promote the development of an antibody with cross-reactivity to PR3 and MPO. The discovery of another ANCA target molecule, LAMP-2, which has structural homology with a bacterial adhesion molecule, Fim H, provides some support for this hypothesis.[64]

However, no molecular mimics of PR3 have been reliably demonstrated. The answer may lie in the recently proposed theory of antigen complementarity. Investigation of individuals with PR3 ANCA in some cases revealed antibodies not only to the PR3 peptide but also to a peptide derived from the complementary, or antisense, strand of the DNA coding for PR3.[101] It is postulated that antigens expressed on infectious agents may act as a complementary antigen (cPR3), triggering the production of complementary antibodies (anti-cPR3). Following a secondary immune response, anti-idiotype antibodies are generated against the initial complementary antibodies.

These anti-idiotype antibodies (anti-anti-cPR3) recognize the autoantigen PR3. More recently the same group has reported the presence of cPR3-specific T cells in patients with anti-cPR3 antibodies.[102] The anti-cPR3 antibodies have also been reported to have specificity for plasminogen and to be functional in that they delayed the dissolution of fibrin clots.[103] Several patients with these antibodies had a history of thrombosis.

SUMMARY

There is now a substantial body of evidence supporting a pathogenic role for ANCA in the development of organ damage and inflammation of AAV. What is still not understood is how ANCA develop in the first place, although studies of T and B cells in AAV and their regulatory mechanisms should continue to improve our understanding of this process. The recently described anti–LAMP-2 antibodies and anti-cPR3 antibodies provide interesting suggestions as to how molecular mimicry may lead to the subverting of regulatory mechanisms and the development of autoantibodies.

The development of animal models of AAV that recapitulate human disease more accurately allows us to investigate pathogenic mechanisms and interventions that may lead to improved treatment.

REFERENCES

1. Jennette J, Falk R, Andrassy K, et al. Nomenclature of systemic vasculitides. Proposal of an international consensus conference. Arthritis Rheum 1994;37: 187–92.
2. Falk R, Terrell R, Charles L, et al. Anti-neutrophil cytoplasmic autoantibodies induce neutrophils to degranulate and produce oxygen radicals in vitro. Proc Natl Acad Sci U S A 1990;87:4115–9.
3. Harper L, Savage C. Pathogenesis of ANCA-associated systemic vasculitis. J Pathol 2000;190:349–59.
4. Cockwell P, Brooks C, Adu D, et al. Interleukin-8: a pathogenetic role in antineutrophil cytoplasmic autoantibody-associated glomerulonephritis. Kidney Int 1999;55:1125–7.
5. Kettritz R, Jennette J, Falk R. Crosslinking of ANCA-antigens stimulates superoxide release by human neutrophils. J Am Soc Nephrol 1997;8:386–94.
6. Hewins P, Morgan M, Holden N, et al. IL-18 is up-regulated in the kidney and primes neutrophil responsiveness in ANCA-associated vasculitis. Kidney Int 2006;69:605–15.
7. Mulder AH, Heeringa P, Brouwer E, et al. Activation of granulocytes by anti-neutrophil cytoplasmic antibodies (ANCA): a Fc gamma RII-dependent process. Clin Exp Immunol 1994;98:270–8.
8. Kocher M, Edberg JC, Fleit HB, et al. Antineutrophil cytoplasmic antibodies preferentially engage Fc gammaRIIIb on human neutrophils. J Immunol 1998; 161:6909–14.
9. Williams JM, Savage CO. Characterization of the regulation and functional consequences of p21ras activation in neutrophils by antineutrophil cytoplasm antibodies. J Am Soc Nephrol 2005;16:90–6.
10. Hewins P, Williams JM, Wakelam MJ, et al. Activation of Syk in neutrophils by antineutrophil cytoplasm antibodies occurs via Fcgamma receptors and CD18. J Am Soc Nephrol 2004;15:796–808.
11. Ben-Smith A, Dove SK, Martin A, et al. Antineutrophil cytoplasm autoantibodies from patients with systemic vasculitis activate neutrophils through distinct

signaling cascades: comparison with conventional Fc{gamma} receptor ligation. Blood 2001;98:1448–55.

12. Kettritz R, Choi M, Butt W, et al. Phosphatidylinositol 3-kinase controls antineutrophil cytoplasmic antibodies-induced respiratory burst in human neutrophils. J Am Soc Nephrol 2002;13:1740–9.

13. Katzav A, Kloog Y, Korczyn AD, et al. Treatment of MRL/lpr mice, a genetic autoimmune model, with the Ras inhibitor, farnesylthiosalicylate (FTS). Clin Exp Immunol 2001;126:570–7.

14. Yang JJ, Preston GA, Alcorta DA, et al. Expression profile of leukocyte genes activated by anti-neutrophil cytoplasmic autoantibodies (ANCA). Kidney Int 2002;62:1638–49.

15. Donald KJ, Edwards RL, McEvoy JD. An ultrastructural study of the pathogenesis of tissue injury in limited Wegener's granulomatosis. Pathology 1976;8:161–9.

16. Ewert BH, Becker ME, Jennette JC, et al. Antimyeloperoxidase antibodies induce neutrophil adherence to cultured human endothelial cells. Ren Fail 1995;17:125–33.

17. Keogan MT, Rifkin I, Ronda N, et al. Anti-neutrophil cytoplasm antibodies (ANCA) increase neutrophil adhesion to cultured human endothelium. Adv Exp Med Biol 1993;336:115–9.

18. Mayet WJ, Meyer zum Buschenfelde KH. Antibodies to proteinase 3 increase adhesion of neutrophils to human endothelial cells. Clin Exp Immunol 1993; 94:440–6.

19. Johnson PA, Alexander HD, McMillan SA, et al. Up-regulation of the granulocyte adhesion molecule Mac-1 by autoantibodies in autoimmune vasculitis. Clin Exp Immunol 1997;107:513–9.

20. Calderwood JW, Williams JM, Morgan MD, et al. ANCA induces {beta}2 integrin and CXC chemokine-dependent neutrophil-endothelial cell interactions that mimic those of highly cytokine-activated endothelium. J Leukoc Biol 2005;77: 33–43.

21. Radford DJ, Luu NT, Hewins P, et al. Antineutrophil cytoplasmic antibodies stabilize adhesion and promote migration of flowing neutrophils on endothelial cells. Arthritis Rheum 2001;44:2851–61.

22. Brachemi S, Mambole A, Fakhouri F, et al. Increased membrane expression of proteinase 3 during neutrophil adhesion in the presence of anti proteinase 3 antibodies. J Am Soc Nephrol 2007;18:2330–9.

23. Tse W, Nash G, Hewins P, et al. ANCA-induced neutrophil F-actin polymerization: implications for microvascular inflammation. Kidney Int 2005;67:130–9.

24. Ewert BH, Jennette JC, Falk RJ. Anti-myeloperoxidase antibodies stimulate neutrophils to damage human endothelial cells. Kidney Int 1992;41:375–83.

25. Savage CO, Pottinger BE, Gaskin G, et al. Autoantibodies developing to myeloperoxidase and proteinase 3 in systemic vasculitis stimulate neutrophil cytotoxicity toward cultured endothelial cells. Am J Pathol 1992;141:335–42.

26. Lu X, Garfield A, Rainger GE, et al. Mediation of endothelial cell damage by serine proteases, but not superoxide, released from antineutrophil cytoplasmic antibody-stimulated neutrophils. Arthritis Rheum 2006;54:1619–28.

27. Yang JJ, Preston GA, Pendergraft WF, et al. Internalization of proteinase 3 is concomitant with endothelial cell apoptosis and internalization of myeloperoxidase with generation of intracellular oxidants. Am J Pathol 2001;158:581–92.

28. Kumpers P, Hellpap J, David S, et al. Circulating angiopoietin-2 is a marker and potential mediator of endothelial cell detachment in ANCA-associated vasculitis with renal involvement. Nephrol Dial Transplant 2009;24:1845–50.

29. Erdbruegger U, Grossheim M, Hertel B, et al. Diagnostic role of endothelial microparticles in vasculitis. Rheumatology (Oxford) 2008;47:1820–5.
30. de Groot K, Goldberg C, Bahlmann FH, et al. Vascular endothelial damage and repair in antineutrophil cytoplasmic antibody-associated vasculitis. Arthritis Rheum 2007;56:3847–53.
31. Zavada J, Kideryova L, Pytlik R, et al. Reduced number of endothelial progenitor cells is predictive of early relapse in anti-neutrophil cytoplasmic antibody-associated vasculitis. Rheumatology (Oxford) 2009;48:1197–201.
32. Zavada J, Kideryova L, Pytlik R, et al. Circulating endothelial progenitor cells in patients with ANCA-associated vasculitis. Kidney Blood Press Res 2008;31: 247–54.
33. Xiao H, Heeringa P, Hu P, et al. Antineutrophil cytoplasmic autoantibodies specific for myeloperoxidase cause glomerulonephritis and vasculitis in mice. J Clin Invest 2002;110:955–63.
34. Xiao H, Heeringa P, Liu Z, et al. The role of neutrophils in the induction of glomerulonephritis by anti-myeloperoxidase antibodies. Am J Pathol 2005; 167:39–45.
35. Nolan SL, Kalia N, Nash GB, et al. Mechanisms of ANCA-mediated leukocyte-endothelial cell interactions in vivo. J Am Soc Nephrol 2008;19:973–84.
36. Kuligowski MP, Kwan RY, Lo C, et al. Antimyeloperoxidase antibodies rapidly induce alpha-4-integrin-dependent glomerular neutrophil adhesion. Blood 2009;113:6485–94.
37. Haas M, Eustace JA. Immune complex deposits in ANCA-associated crescentic glomerulonephritis: a study of 126 cases. Kidney Int 2004;65:2145–52.
38. Schreiber A, Xiao H, Jennette JC, et al. C5a receptor mediates neutrophil activation and ANCA-induced glomerulonephritis. J Am Soc Nephrol 2009;20: 289–98.
39. Xiao H, Schreiber A, Heeringa P, et al. Alternative complement pathway in the pathogenesis of disease mediated by anti-neutrophil cytoplasmic autoantibodies. Am J Pathol 2007;170:52–64.
40. Xing GQ, Chen M, Liu G, et al. Complement activation is involved in renal damage in human antineutrophil cytoplasmic autoantibody associated pauci-immune vasculitis. J Clin Immunol 2009;29:282–91.
41. Chen M, Xing GQ, Yu F, et al. Complement deposition in renal histopathology of patients with ANCA-associated pauci-immune glomerulonephritis. Nephrol Dial Transplant 2009;24:1247–52.
42. Little MA, Smyth L, Salama AD, et al. Experimental autoimmune vasculitis: an animal model of anti-neutrophil cytoplasmic autoantibody-associated systemic vasculitis. Am J Pathol 2009;174:1212–20.
43. Little MA, Smyth CL, Yadav R, et al. Antineutrophil cytoplasm antibodies directed against myeloperoxidase augment leukocyte-microvascular interactions in vivo. Blood 2005;106:2050–8.
44. Schlieben DJ, Korbet SM, Kimura RE, et al. Pulmonary-renal syndrome in a newborn with placental transmission of ANCAs. Am J Kidney Dis 2005;45: 758–61.
45. Harper L, Ren Y, Savill J, et al. Antineutrophil cytoplasmic antibodies induce reactive oxygen-dependent dysregulation of primed neutrophil apoptosis and clearance by macrophages. Am J Pathol 2000;157:211–20.
46. Harper L, Cockwell P, Adu D, et al. Neutrophil priming and apoptosis in anti-neutrophil cytoplasmic autoantibody-associated vasculitis. Kidney Int 2001;59: 1729–38.

47. Gilligan HM, Bredy B, Brady HR, et al. Antineutrophil cytoplasmic autoantibodies interact with primary granule constituents on the surface of apoptotic neutrophils in the absence of neutrophil priming. J Exp Med 1996;184: 2231–41.

48. Schreiber A, Busjahn A, Luft FC, et al. Membrane expression of proteinase 3 Is genetically determined. J Am Soc Nephrol 2003;14:68–75.

49. von Vietinghoff S, Busjahn A, Schonemann C, et al. Major histocompatibility complex HLA region largely explains the genetic variance exercised on neutrophil membrane proteinase 3 expression. J Am Soc Nephrol 2006;17: 3185–91.

50. Witko-Sarsat V, Lesavre P, Lopez S, et al. A large subset of neutrophils expressing membrane proteinase 3 is a risk factor for vasculitis and rheumatoid arthritis. J Am Soc Nephrol 1999;10:1224–33.

51. Rarok AA, Stegeman CA, Limburg PC, et al. Neutrophil membrane expression of proteinase 3 (PR3) Is related to relapse in PR3-ANCA-associated vasculitis. J Am Soc Nephrol 2002;13:2232–8.

52. Henshaw TJ, Malone CC, Gabay JE, et al. Elevations of neutrophil proteinase 3 in serum of patients with Wegener's granulomatosis and polyarteritis nodosa. Arthritis Rheum 1994;37:104–12.

53. Ohlsson S, Wieslander J, Segelmark M. Increased circulating levels of proteinase 3 in patients with anti-neutrophilic cytoplasmic autoantibodies-associated systemic vasculitis in remission. Clin Exp Immunol 2003;131: 528–35.

54. Taekema-Roelvink ME, Van Kooten C, Heemskerk E, et al. Proteinase 3 interacts with a 111-kD membrane molecule of human umbilical vein endothelial cells. J Am Soc Nephrol 2000;11:640–8.

55. Taekema-Roelvink ME, Kooten C, Kooij SV, et al. Proteinase 3 enhances endothelial monocyte chemoattractant protein-1 production and induces increased adhesion of neutrophils to endothelial cells by upregulating intercellular cell adhesion molecule-1. J Am Soc Nephrol 2001;12:932–40.

56. Bank U, Ansorge S. More than destructive: neutrophil-derived serine proteases in cytokine bioactivity control. J Leukoc Biol 2001;69:197–206.

57. Novick D, Rubinstein M, Azam T, et al. Proteinase 3 is an IL-32 binding protein. Proc Natl Acad Sci U S A 2006;103:3316–21.

58. Guilpain P, Servettaz A, Goulvestre C, et al. Pathogenic effects of antimyeloperoxidase antibodies in patients with microscopic polyangiitis. Arthritis Rheum 2007;56:2455–63.

59. Dolman KM, van de Wiel BA, Kam CM, et al. Proteinase 3: substrate specificity and possible pathogenetic effect of Wegener's granulomatosis autoantibodies (c-ANCA) by dysregulation of the enzyme. Adv Exp Med Biol 1993; 336:55–60.

60. Griffith ME, Coulthart A, Pemberton S, et al. Anti-neutrophil cytoplasmic antibodies (ANCA) from patients with systemic vasculitis recognize restricted epitopes of proteinase 3 involving the catalytic site. Clin Exp Immunol 2001; 123:170–7.

61. Daouk GH, Palsson R, Arnaout MA. Inhibition of proteinase 3 by ANCA and its correlation with disease activity in Wegener's granulomatosis. Kidney Int 1995; 47:1528–36.

62. Savige JA, Chang L, Cook L, et al. Alpha 1-antitrypsin deficiency and anti-proteinase 3 antibodies in anti-neutrophil cytoplasmic antibody (ANCA)-associated systemic vasculitis. Clin Exp Immunol 1995;100:194–7.

63. Segelmark M, Elzouki AN, Wieslander J, et al. The PiZ gene of alpha 1-antitrypsin as a determinant of outcome in PR3-ANCA-positive vasculitis. Kidney Int 1995;48:844–50.
64. Kain R, Exner M, Brandes R, et al. Molecular mimicry in pauci-immune focal necrotizing glomerulonephritis. Nat Med 2008;14:1088–96.
65. Damianovich M, Gilburd B, George J, et al. Pathogenic role of anti-endothelial cell antibodies in vasculitis. An idiotypic experimental model. J Immunol 1996; 156:4946–51.
66. Chan TM, Frampton G, Jayne DR, et al. Clinical significance of anti-endothelial cell antibodies in systemic vasculitis: a longitudinal study comparing anti-endothelial cell antibodies and anti-neutrophil cytoplasm antibodies. Am J Kidney Dis 1993;22:387–92.
67. Holmen C, Christensson M, Pettersson E, et al. Wegener's granulomatosis is associated with organ-specific antiendothelial cell antibodies. Kidney Int 2004;66:1049–60.
68. Del Papa N, Conforti G, Gambini D, et al. Characterization of the endothelial surface proteins recognized by anti-endothelial antibodies in primary and secondary autoimmune vasculitis. Clin Immunol Immunopathol 1994;70:211–6.
69. Matsumoto T, Kaneko T, Seto M, et al. The membrane proteinase 3 expression on neutrophils was downregulated after treatment with infliximab in patients with rheumatoid arthritis. Clin Appl Thromb Hemost 2008;14:186–92.
70. Chow FY, Hooke D, Kerr PG. Severe intestinal involvement in Wegener's granulomatosis. J Gastroenterol Hepatol 2003;18:749–50.
71. Rasmussen N, Petersen J. Cellular immune responses and pathogenesis in c-ANCA positive vasculitides. J Autoimmun 1993;6:227–36.
72. Brouwer E, Cohen Tervaert JW, Weening JJ. Immunohistology of renal biopsies in Wegener's granulomatosis (WG):clues to its pathogenesis. Kidney Int 1991; 39:1055.
73. Mellbye OJ, Mollnes TE, Steen LS. IgG subclass distribution and complement activation ability of autoantibodies to neutrophil cytoplasmic antigens (ANCA). Clin Immunol Immunopathol 1994;70:32–9.
74. Berden AE, Kallenberg CG, Savage CO, et al. Cellular immunity in Wegener's granulomatosis: characterizing T lymphocytes. Arthritis Rheum 2009;60: 1578–87.
75. Schmitt W, Hagen E, Neumann I, et al. Treatment of refractory Wegener's granulomatosis with antithymocyte globulin (ATG): an open study in 15 patients. Kidney Int 2004;65:1440–8.
76. Filer AD, Gardner-Medwin JM, Thambyrajah J, et al. Diffuse endothelial dysfunction is common to ANCA associated systemic vasculitis and polyarteritis nodosa. Ann Rheum Dis 2003;62:162–7.
77. Giscombe R, Nityanand S, Lewin N, et al. Expanded T cell populations in patients with Wegener's granulomatosis: characteristics and correlates with disease activity. J Clin Immunol 1998;18:404–13.
78. Csernok E, Trabandt A, Muller A, et al. Cytokine profiles in Wegener's granulomatosis: predominance of type 1 (Th1) in the granulomatous inflammation. Arthritis Rheum 1999;42:742–50.
79. Ludviksson BR. Active Wegener's granulomatosis is associated with HLA-DR+CD4+ T-cells exhibiting an unbalanced Th1-type T-cell cytokine pattern: reversal with IL-10. J Immunol 1998;160:3602–9.
80. Popa ER, Franssen CF, Limburg PC, et al. In vitro cytokine production and proliferation of T cells from patients with anti-proteinase 3- and

antimyeloperoxidase-associated vasculitis, in response to proteinase 3 and myeloperoxidase. Arthritis Rheum 2002;46:1894–904.

81. Abdulahad WH, van der Geld YM, Stegeman CA, et al. Persistent expansion of CD4+ effector memory T cells in Wegener's granulomatosis. Kidney Int 2006;70: 938–47.

82. Abdulahad WH, Stegeman CA, Limburg PC, et al. Skewed distribution of Th17 lymphocytes in patients with Wegener's granulomatosis in remission. Arthritis Rheum 2008;58:2196–205.

83. Forlow SB, Schurr JR, Kolls JK, et al. Increased granulopoiesis through interleukin-17 and granulocyte colony-stimulating factor in leukocyte adhesion molecule-deficient mice. Blood 2001;98:3309–14.

84. Laan M, Cui ZH, Hoshino H, et al. Neutrophil recruitment by human IL-17 via C-X-C chemokine release in the airways. J Immunol 1999;162:2347–52.

85. Van Kooten C, Boonstra JG, Paape ME, et al. Interleukin-17 activates human renal epithelial cells in vitro and is expressed during renal allograft rejection. J Am Soc Nephrol 1998;9:1526–34.

86. Jovanovic DV, Di Battista JA, Martel-Pelletier J, et al. IL-17 stimulates the production and expression of proinflammatory cytokines, IL-beta and TNF-alpha, by human macrophages. J Immunol 1998;160:3513–21.

87. Abdulahad WH, Stegeman CA, van der Geld YM, et al. Functional defect of circulating regulatory CD4+ T cells in patients with Wegener's granulomatosis in remission. Arthritis Rheum 2007;56:2080–91.

88. Morgan MD, Day CJ, Piper KP, et al. Patients with Wegener's granulomatosis demonstrate a relative deficiency and functional impairment of T-regulatory cells. Immunology 2010;130(1):64–73.

89. Marinaki S, Neumann I, Kalsch AI, et al. Abnormalities of CD4 T cell subpopulations in ANCA-associated vasculitis. Clin Exp Immunol 2005;140:181–91.

90. Giscombe R, Wang XB, Kakoulidou M, et al. Characterization of the expanded T-cell populations in patients with Wegener's granulomatosis. J Intern Med 2006; 260:224–30.

91. Popa ER, Stegeman CA, Bos NA, et al. Differential B- and T-cell activation in Wegener's granulomatosis. J Allergy Clin Immunol 1999;103:885–94.

92. Voswinkel J, Mueller A, Kraemer JA, et al. B lymphocyte maturation in Wegener's granulomatosis: a comparative analysis of VH genes from endonasal lesions. Ann Rheum Dis 2006;65:859–64.

93. Culton DA, Nicholas MW, Bunch DO, et al. Similar CD19 dysregulation in two autoantibody-associated autoimmune diseases suggests a shared mechanism of B-cell tolerance loss. J Clin Immunol 2007;27:53–68.

94. Bajema IM, Hagen EC, van der Woude FJ, et al. Wegener's granulomatosis: a meta-analysis of 349 literary case reports. J Lab Clin Med 1997;129: 17–22.

95. Mueller A, Holl-Ulrich K, Feller AC, et al. Immune phenomena in localized and generalized Wegener's granulomatosis. Clin Exp Rheumatol 2003;21:S49–54.

96. Eriksson P. Nine patients with anti-neutrophil cytoplasmic antibody-positive vasculitis successfully treated with rituximab. J Intern Med 2005;257:540–8.

97. Ferraro AJ, Day CJ, Drayson MT, et al. Effective therapeutic use of rituximab in refractory Wegener's granulomatosis. Nephrol Dial Transplant 2005;20:622–5.

98. Csernok E, Lamprecht P, Gross WL. Clinical and immunological features of drug-induced and infection-induced proteinase 3-antineutrophil cytoplasmic antibodies and myeloperoxidase-antineutrophil cytoplasmic antibodies and vasculitis. Curr Opin Rheumatol 2010;22:43–8.

99. Stegeman CA, Cohen Tervaert JW, de Jong PE, et al. Trimethoprim-sulfamethox-azole (co-trimoxazole) for the prevention of relapses of Wegener's granulomato-sis. N Engl J Med 1996;335:16–20.
100. Hogan SL, Cooper GS, Savitz DA, et al. Association of silica exposure with anti-neutrophil cytoplasmic autoantibody small-vessel vasculitis: a population-based, case-control study. Clin J Am Soc Nephrol 2007;2:290–9.
101. Pendergraft WF 3rd, Preston GA, Shah RR, et al. Autoimmunity is triggered by cPR-3(105-201), a protein complementary to human autoantigen proteinase-3. Nat Med 2004;10:72–9.
102. Yang J, Bautz DJ, Lionaki S, et al. ANCA patients have T cells responsive to complementary PR-3 antigen. Kidney Int 2008;74:1159–69.
103. Bautz DJ, Preston GA, Lionaki S, et al. Antibodies with dual reactivity to plasmin-ogen and complementary PR3 in PR3-ANCA vasculitis. J Am Soc Nephrol 2008; 19:2421–9.

Autoantibodies in ANCA-associated Vasculitis

Allan S. Wiik, MD, PhD[a,b,*]

KEYWORDS

- Necrotizing vasculitis • ANCA • Autoantibodies
- Pathophysiology

Antineutrophil cytoplasmic autoantibodies (ANCAs) are frequently associated with diseases characterized by the presence of vasculitis, affecting small and medium-sized vessels (eg, arterioles, capillaries, and venules).[1,2] Although this association was realized already in the mid-1980s, ANCAs were not immediately included in the classification criteria for this type of vasculitis, and no agreed diagnostic criteria for the diagnosis of these conditions exist as yet. Presence of autoantibodies such as ANCAs most likely reflects pathobiologic events in the affected tissue, in this case neutrophils and monocytes attacking the vascular endothelium of small vessels, causing autoantigen release from these cells and presentation to the immune system.

Because endothelial cells (ECs) become activated and damaged by the attack, autoantibodies to EC constituents (anti–endothelial cell antibodies [AECAs]) are also commonly produced in ANCA-associated vasculitis (AAV).[3] During this inflammatory attack on the vessel walls, the basal membrane of some vessels can also be damaged and autoantibodies to the basement membrane α_3 domain of type IV collagen of glomeruli and pulmonary vessels are produced.[3]

The primary events leading to the onset of these necrotizing vasculitides are not known. However, several hypotheses have proposed that infectious agents can trigger and perhaps perpetuate events[4–6] that, if left untreated, will lead to irreversible tissue damage and organ function failure.[7,8]

Patients suffering from ANCA-associated small vessel necrotizing vasculitides, such as Wegener's granulomatosis (WG), microscopic polyangiitis (MPA), and Churg-Strauss syndrome (CSS), may produce autoantibodies to several different autoantigens and structures that are involved in the pathology of these diseases.[3]

Disclosures: The author has no conflicts of interest or financial disclosures.
[a] Department of Autoimmunology, Statens Serum Institut, Artillerivej 5, DK-2300 Copenhagen S, Denmark
[b] Department of Biochemistry and Immunology, Statens Serum Institut, Artillerivej 5, DK-2300 Copenhagen S, Denmark
* Digesmuttevej 10, DK-2970 Hoersholm, Denmark.
E-mail address: asw@dadlnet.dk

Although ANCAs have thus lent name to the group of diseases collectively called AAV, they may not be the only interesting autoantibodies in terms of pathophysiology or classification.

NEUTROPHIL-SPECIFIC AUTOANTIBODIES

Neutrophil-specific autoantibodies (NSAs) have been known to exist since 1959, when their presence was first described in patients with leukopenia[9] and later in those with ulcerative colitis.[10]

Using indirect immunofluorescence (IIF) technique, the autoantibodies found in leukopenia and ulcerative colitis decorated the nuclei of neutrophils, and therefore later work on NSAs in patients with rheumatoid arthritis and Felty syndrome called them granulocyte-specific antinuclear antibodies.[11] Similar NSAs have been described in chronic active hepatitis, sclerosing cholangitis, Sweet syndrome, and other conditions in which chronic recruitment of neutrophils is an essential part of the inflammatory process.[2,12] However, most of the NSAs are not directed to the classic cytoplasmic ANCA antigens proteinase 3 (PR3), myeloperoxidase (MPO), or human leukocyte elastase (HLE) but rather to components found in all compartments of neutrophils and monocytes,[13] probably just showing an immune response caused by chronic neutrophil cell death.

When autoantibodies to neutrophils were described in patients with WG, they were termed anticytoplasmic antibodies because of their preferential staining of granular material in the cytoplasm,[14] but this indistinct term was changed to ANCA during the Second International Workshop on ANCA in Noordwijkerhout, The Netherlands.[15] The main reason for this change was the identification of the 2 most important neutrophil granule antigens, PR3 and MPO, as the dominant targets in patients not only with WG but also in patients with MPA and CSS and their limited forms.[16]

ANCA

In 1982, Davies and colleagues[17] first recognized autoantibodies that were specific for neutrophils in small vessel necrotizing glomerulonephritis. It was initially proposed that the antibodies were produced in response to an arbovirus (Ross River virus) infection, although this was never substantiated. Morphologically similar antibodies giving rise to a coarse granular staining of neutrophil cytoplasm (**Fig. 1**) were subsequently reported in patients with WG,[14] preferentially in those having active disease. This particular pattern of reactivity with neutrophils was then called the classic cytoplasmic ANCA (C-ANCA).[15] In 1988, soon after the first International Workshop on ANCA in Copenhagen, Denmark, the C-ANCA antigen was reported to be directed to the proteolytic enzyme PR3 in azurophilic granules of neutrophils.[18–20]

ANCAs that caused staining of neutrophil nuclei and their close vicinity were called perinuclear ANCAs (P-ANCAs) (**Fig. 2**)[15]; this reactivity is caused by cationic granule antigens, for example, MPO and HLE, that have migrated to the oppositely charged nuclei and was first described for ANCAs directed to MPO.[21] P-ANCAs with specificity for MPO are commonly produced in AAV with kidney or lung manifestations.

Proteinase 3

The conformation of PR3 is essential for its reactivity with PR3-ANCA.[22] PR3 is a linear polypeptide containing 228 amino acids. In 1994, linear epitopes of PR3 were found, and these seemed to occur in regions close to the active site of the enzyme[23] where 4 of 5 epitopes are assumed to be located.[24] The crystal structure of PR3 was resolved in 1996.[25] PR3 is progressively more strongly expressed from the stage of early

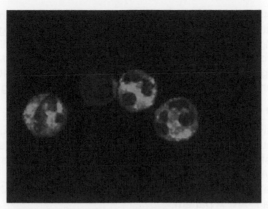

Fig. 1. Granular cytoplasmic staining of neutrophil granulocytes by IIF using serum from a patient with WG and an IgG-specific conjugate.

myelocyte maturation to the fully developed neutrophil.[26] The gene encoding PR3 is located close to the HLE site on chromosome 19.[27]

Myeloperoxidase

MPO is the main antigen for the P-ANCA reactivity in patients with AAV. The enzyme catalyzes the hydrogen peroxide–mediated peroxidation of chloride ions to hypochlorite, and the hypochlorous acid is effective in killing phagocytized bacteria and viruses. However, the hypochlorous acid can also inactivate proteinase inhibitors in blood and tissues, thus indirectly influencing inflammation through induction of highly reactive oxygen radical species among other mechanisms.[28] MPO is a hydrophilic and positively charged molecule located in azurophilic and primary granules. Thus, after fixation of neutrophils and monocytes by ethanol for use as substrate in IIF, the positively charged molecule migrates toward the nucleus and the ensuing staining pattern becomes perinuclear as shown in **Fig. 2.**[21]

MPO consists of 2 polypeptides of 467 and 113 amino acids, called the α and β chains, respectively. After glycosylation and final processing, the polypeptides form a 59-kDa α chain and a 13.5-kDa β chain that are linked together in

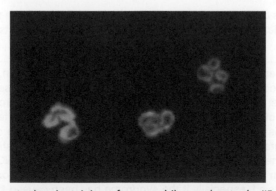

Fig. 2. Perinuclear cytoplasmic staining of neutrophil granulocytes by IIF using serum from a patient with MPA and an IgG-specific conjugate.

a heterodimeric 140-kDa molecule, in which each half has one α chain and one β chain. The crystal structure has been resolved,[29] and the gene encoding MPO has been found on the long arm of chromosome 17.[30] Reactivity with MPO-ANCA highly depends on conformational preservation of the structure.[31] The MPO molecule is very sensitive to light exposure, whereby it cleaves at position Met 409 of the α chain, a fact that is important for its stability during purification and coating on solid phases.

Human Leukocyte Elastase

HLE is a frequently targeted autoantigen in patients with drug-induced vasculitis or drug-induced lupus and in those with cocaine-induced nasal destruction, which may mimic late-stage WG.[32] HLE-ANCAs are rarely found alone and are mostly accompanied by ANCAs toward other neutrophil antigens.

HLE-ANCAs are rare in idiopathic AAV. If HLE-ANCA is the only ANCA contained in a serum, it gives a P-ANCA pattern.

Human Lysosomal Membrane Protein 2

Autoantibodies to a human lysosomal membrane protein (H-lamp-2) were first described in 78 of 84 individuals with ANCA-associated focal necrotizing glomerulo-nephritis (FNGN).[33] Kain and colleagues[33] reported that the H-lamp-2 protein is expressed in the plasma membrane of several human cells, such as neutrophils and ECs, but the protein is also integrated into membranes of neutrophil intracellular vesicles. A recent study from the same research group has suggested that the emergence of autoimmunity to H-lamp-2 is caused by molecular mimicry through reactivity with a H-lamp-2 peptide (P41–49) that shows 100% homology to a bacterial adhesin peptide (amino acids 72–80) found on mature FimH protein located on type 1 fimbriae of gram-negative bacteria.[34] Xenogeneic antibodies to H-lamp-2 were found to bind to fixed neutrophils in a C-ANCA–like reaction pattern by IIF as a result of reactivity with the intracellular vesicle membranes mentioned earlier.[34] These autoantibodies are thus not neutrophil-specific because they react with a variety of human cells, most importantly ECs, and it can be discussed whether it is justified to call them ANCA.

The H-lamp-2 protein is assumed to have physiologic roles in cell adhesion, auto-phagocytosis, and antigen presentation. Autoantibodies to H-lamp-2, however, may be able to induce pauci-immune FNGN per se because a monoclonal antibody to H-lamp-2 was found to induce apoptosis of microvascular endothelium when injected into rats. In addition, rats injected with rabbit antibodies to H-lamp-2 subsequently developed FNGN.[34]

Further studies on the prevalence and levels of anti–H-lamp-2 are needed to judge the potential clinical utility of this autoantibody in monitoring patients with AAV.

Other Antigens

Lactoferrin, bactericidal permeability-increasing protein, azurocidin, and lysozyme, which are also localized in neutrophil granules, may in some cases be targets of NSAs; however, such reactivity is rare in idiopathic small vessel necrotizing vasculitis. In contrast, any of these antigens may be a target in patients suffering from drug-induced vasculitis or drug-induced lupus-like syndromes. In these cases, there are often multiple granule protein targets, a finding so characteristic that a drug-induced syndrome should be suspected whenever multispecific ANCAs are found in serum. Sera from such patients can additionally harbor autoantibodies to histones and β_2-glycoprotein I, especially if the syndrome has been caused by an antithyroid drug.[35]

ANCA SCREENING AND QUANTIFICATION

Screening for ANCA is mostly done by IIF technique using human buffy coat leukocytes as substrate.[2,36] In cases in which either a C-ANCA or P-ANCA is found by IIF technique, specific methods for detection and quantification of PR3-ANCA and MPO-ANCA must be performed to reveal the specificity and quantity of the antibody. Most laboratories examine the specificity of ANCAs by enzyme-linked immunosorbent assay (ELISA) techniques using directly or indirectly coupled PR3 or MPO or such antigens coated on beads or chips.[2,36] The most important factor in such techniques is the use of strictly purified native antigens that are conformationally well preserved or recombinant antigens that can replace these native antigens without loss of reactivity with ANCAs. Further details of ANCA testing are available in the vast existing literature.[2]

PREVALENCE OF PR3-ANCA AND MPO-ANCA IN AAV

Reports from Europe and the United States on ANCA in different forms of AAV vary considerably (**Table 1**). Thus PR3-ANCA has been reported to be present in around 40% to 95% of patients with WG and in 9% to 30% of patients with CSS.[3] The reason for these discrepancies may rely on the selected cohorts studied, disease extent and activity at the time of serum sampling, the criteria used for setting the diagnoses, and the way positive cutoff values for the assays used have been set. This question has often not been addressed by producers of commercial ELISAs or by immunology laboratories using such kits. To be useful for clinicians who have to decide about differential diagnosis, a positive cutoff value for ANCA higher than that found not only in healthy blood donors but also in most patients with inflammatory conditions that mimic systemic vasculitis must be set.[37] This cutoff value is obtained in practice by setting up receiver operating characteristics (ROC) curves encompassing all values found in the vasculitis and nonvasculitis patient sera and then by choosing the level of diagnostic specificity required by clinicians to discriminate vasculitis from inflammatory controls, for example, 98% specificity of PR3-ANCA for patients with WG. Then the diagnostic sensitivity can be seen on the x-axis where the specificity line crosses the ROC curve. This method was found very useful in the European ANCA Assay Standardization Study in the 1990s.[38] Because intermediate levels of MPO-ANCA were found in inflammatory nonvasculitis patient sera, the positive cutoff had to be set high in this study. When ANCA values are to be compared among several laboratories, the same cohort of vasculitis and inflammatory disease control sera must be studied.

The exercise described earlier is necessary if quantitative ANCA levels are used clinically. By this approach, the number of borderline values can be kept to a minimum. In

Table 1		
Frequencies of PR3-ANCA and MPO-ANCA in ANCA-associated necrotizing vasculitic diseases		
Vasculitis	PR3-ANCA (%)	MPO-ANCA (%)
Wegener's Granulomatosis	40–95	5–60[a]
Microscopic Polyangiitis	25–30	50–70
Churg-Strauss Syndrome	9–30	30–40
Renal-limited Vasculitis	25–30	50–70
Drug-induced Vasculitis[b]	10–15	80–90

[a] As reported in studies from China; Chinese WG patients mostly produce MPO-ANCA.
[b] Several other ANCA specificities can be found in drug-induced vasculitis/drug-induced lupus.

principle, there is no difference in the nature of the quantitative assays used (eg, direct ELISA, capture ELISA, ligand ELISA, microbeads, chips) because all assays can be set to detect only those values that satisfy differential diagnostics. It is hoped that more extensive postmarketing surveillance studies meeting the standards described earlier will be performed in the future through collaboration between clinicians and commercial vendors of assay kits.[39]

CLINICAL USE OF ANCA TESTING FOR DIAGNOSIS, PROGNOSIS, AND FOLLOW-UP

The main indication for ordering ANCA tests is evidence of small vessel vasculitis or at least a clear suspicion of vasculitis. In practical terms, most clinicians base suspicion on symptoms and signs that have been set up by the Chapel Hill definitions and classification criteria in 1992[1] because there are still no agreed diagnostic criteria for these vasculitides. The classification criteria nevertheless have permitted a patient to be placed in a diagnostic subgroup of importance for clinical decision making and prognostication.[40] Presence of ANCA has not yet been proposed as a formal criterion for any of the 3 AAVs mentioned in the original proposal,[1] but there is strong agreement that ANCAs ought to be part of future diagnostic criteria for WG, MPA, and CSS.

Most experts on vasculitis agree that the level of PR3-ANCA and MPO-ANCA is higher in active and/or extensive phase of the disease than during remission phases and in cases of limited disease extent. However, there is still much controversy about the role of serial ANCA levels in monitoring disease activity and predicting relapses of AAV. Some investigators who prospectively planned frequent visits to the clinic and frequent blood sampling found a significant increase in PR3-ANCA level a short time preceding a relapse of disease activity.[41,42] A recent report described a strong association between increases in serum MPO-ANCA levels and clinical relapses of AAV.[43] The reason for some of the discrepancies seen in studies is likely to be a lack of prospective study design, lack of a clearly defined methodology, and a lack of carefully chosen patients with vasculitis.[44] If frequent visits and blood sampling are not part of follow-up, it is generally assumed that monitoring ANCA level has no value.

It seems that PR3-ANCA and MPO-ANCA have some influence on, or are reflective of, the development of clinical features in small vessel vasculitides.[45] Renal and respiratory involvement in vasculitis are common in patients positive for PR3-ANCA, whereas considerably fewer patients harboring MPO-ANCA exhibit this combination. Vasculitis limited to renal involvement is much more often seen in patients positive for MPO-ANCA. All patients positive for PR3-ANCA were found to fit the diagnosis of WG or, less often, MPA; however, granuloma formation in biopsy samples were found only in those with WG. Patients positive for PR3-ANCA suffered more frequent relapses than those positive for MPO-ANCA. This information may be useful in planning follow-ups in very early cases of AAV.

OTHER AUTOANTIBODIES THAT CAN BE PRESENT IN AAV

Although the vasculitides mentioned earlier often carry the term ANCA-associated vasculitis, these antibodies are not the only ones that can be encountered in AAV.[3] Some of the reported autoantibodies in AAV are shown in **Box 1**. Although ANCAs have been considered to possess pathogenic effects on cells in and around small affected vessels,[8,37] these antibodies cannot be assumed to be the only ones initiating, driving, or participating in the pathophysiology of AAV.[37] Although increased levels of the neutrophil-derived proteins neutrophil gelatinase-associated lipocalin and lactoferrin were described in the sera of ANCA-positive and ANCA-negative

---

Box 1
Autoantibodies that can co-occur in AAV

Anti–endothelial cell antibodies

Anti–glomerular basement membrane (collagen type IV) antibodies

Antibasal membrane laminin antibodies

Antiphospholipid antibodies (anti–β_2-glycoprotein I antibodies, lupus anticoagulant)

---

vasculitic patients with pauci-immune necrotizing glomerulonephritis, the findings indirectly suggest that neutrophil degranulation takes place in both types of vasculitis.[46] More convincing is that clinical features, prognosis, and histopathologic findings are similar.[47] The different autoantibodies are likely to reflect mechanisms operating in the inflammatory events and may even be part of an orchestrated attack on the endothelium and basement membrane.

AECAs

Antibodies to constituents of the endothelium have been described by several investigators.[48] Such antibodies are generally directed to small vessel ECs and thus reflect the typical distribution of such cells in the lungs, nose, and kidneys.[49] An increase in AECA levels has been described in patients with increasing vasculitis activity in idiopathic AAV and in drug-induced vasculitis.[48,50] An increase in AECA levels has been observed in ANCA-negative and ANCA-positive patients who encounter relapse of disease activity.[48] AECA found in sera from patients with MPA target several EC antigens,[51] but no predominant pattern of antigen-specific activity has been detected.

In vitro studies have shown that IgG class AECA from patients with WG can bind to human ECs, where they induce adhesion molecule expression and increased cytokine secretion.[52] Levels of ANCA and AECA fluctuate independently, and the autoantibodies do not cross-react with their target antigens.[53]

Antibodies to Glomerular Basement Membrane

It is well known that autoantibodies to the α_3 domain of type IV collagen are present in patients with anti–glomerular basement membrane (GBM) disease (formerly termed Goodpasture syndrome).[54] Several groups have found anti-GBM antibodies co-occurring with ANCAs in patients with idiopathic AAV.[55,56] The most common specificity of ANCAs in these patients is anti-MPO. In patients with pulmonary renal syndrome, it is essential to look for both types of autoantibodies because the clinical features are often not distinguishable but the follow-up and therapy may be different.[55,56] The co-occurrence of anti-GBM antibodies and ANCAs may influence outcome because more severe kidney disease often leads to end-stage renal disease, and fewer patients survive.[57]

Other Anti-GBM Antibodies

Although antibodies to basement membrane laminin have been described in AAV, there is uncertainty about the clinical value of detecting this antibody.[58]

Antiphospholipid Autoantibodies

Although rare, the presence of antiphospholipid antibodies, anti–β_2-glycoprotein 1, anticardiolipin, or the lupus anticoagulant, may have some importance in idiopathic AAV.[59] Scattered abstracts indicate that patients harboring both autoantibodies get more extensive and more severe disease. In drug-induced vasculitis, however, antiphospholipid antibodies of the IgM class are more frequently seen, as described earlier.[35] If antihistone antibodies and ANCAs directed to more than one ANCA antigen are found together, a drug-induced condition should be suspected.[32]

SUMMARY

Autoantibody responses against many different autoantigens can occur in AAV, probably reflecting details in the pathologic events occurring in the affected organs. Thus, there is interesting potential in studying the co-occurrence of such antibodies to glean more insight into pathophysiologic mechanisms in AAV. Perhaps a better understanding of the role of the various autoantibodies in vasculitis pathophysiology may lead to new and more targeted therapeutic options in individual patients. It is likely that certain autoantibodies, for example, AECAs and anti-GBM antibodies, may synergize with ANCAs in orchestrating damaging effects on cells and tissues in AAV.

REFERENCES

1. Jennette JC, Falk RJ, Andrassy K, et al. Nomenclature of systemic vasculitides: proposal of an international consensus conference. Arthritis Rheum 1994;37(2): 187–92.
2. Wiik A. Antineutrophil cytoplasm antibodies (ANCAs) and strategy for diagnosing ANCA-associated vasculitides. In: Detrick B, Hamilton RG, Folds JD, editors. Manual of molecular and clinical laboratory immunology. Washington, DC: ASM Press; 2006. p. 1053–8.
3. Wiik A. Autoantibodies in vasculitis. In: Hall G, Bridges L, editors. Vasculitis. 2nd edition. Oxford (UK): Oxford University Press; 2008. p. 53–65.
4. Brons RH, Bakker HI, van Wijk RT, et al. Staphylococcal acid phosphatase binds to endothelial cells via charge interaction; a pathogenic role in Wegener's granulomatosis? Clin Exp Immunol 2000;119(3):566–73.
5. Pendergraft WF 3rd, Preston GA, Shah RR, et al. Autoimmunity is triggered by cPR-3 (105-201), a protein complementary to human autoantigen proteinase-3. Nat Med 2004;10(1):72–9.
6. Salama AD, Pusey CD. Shining a LAMP on pauci-immune focal segmental glomerulonephritis. Kidney Int 2009;76(1):15–7.
7. Jennette JC, Falk RN. Antineutrophil cytoplasmic autoantibodies and associated diseases: a review. Am J Kidney Dis 1990;15(6):517–29.
8. Kallenberg CGM, Brouwer E, Mulder E, et al. ANCA - pathophysiology revisited. Clin Exp Immunol 1995;100(1):1–3.
9. Calabresi P, Edwards EA, Schilling RF. Fluorescent anti-globulin studies in leukopenic and related disorders. J Clin Invest 1959;38:2091–100.
10. Calabresi P, Thayer WR, Spiro HM. Demonstration of circulating antinuclear globulins in ulcerative colitis. J Clin Invest 1961;40:2126–33.
11. Wiik A. Granulocyte-specific antinuclear antibodies. Possible significance for the pathogenesis, clinical features and diagnosis of rheumatoid arthritis. Allergy 1980;35(4):263–89.
12. Wiik A. Neutrophil-specific autoantibodies in chronic inflammatory bowel diseases. Autoimmun Rev 2002;1(1–2):67–72.
13. Wiik A, Brimnes J, Heegaard N. Distinct differences in autoantigen specificity of antineutrophil cytoplasm antibodies in systemic vasculitides and other inflammatory diseases. Isr Med Assoc J 1999;1(1):4–7.

14. van der Woude FJ, Rasmussen N, Lobatto S, et al. Autoantibodies against neutrophils and monocytes: tool for diagnosis and marker of disease activity in Wegener's granulomatosis. Lancet 1985;1(8426):425–9.
15. Wiik A, van der Woude FJ. The new ACPA/ANCA nomenclature. Neth J Med 1990;36(3–4):107–9.
16. Wiik AS. Anti-neutrophil cytoplasmic antibodies in primary small vessel vasculitides. Scand J Rheumatol 1996;25(2):65–9.
17. Davies D, Moran ME, Niall JF, et al. Segmental glomerulonephritis with antineutrophil antibody: possible arbovirus aetiology. Br Med J 1982;285(6342):606.
18. Goldschmeding R, van der Schoot CE, Ten Bokkel Huininck D, et al. Wegener's granulomatosis autoantibodies identify a novel diiso-fluorophosphate-binding protein in the lysosomes of normal human neutrophils. J Clin Invest 1989;84(5): 1577–87.
19. Niles JL, McCluskey RT, Ahmad ME, et al. Wegener's granulomatosis autoantigen is a novel neutrophil serine proteinase. Blood 1989;74(6):1888–93.
20. Gupta SK, Niles JL, McCluskey RT, et al. Identity of Wegener's autoantigen (p29) with proteinase and myeloblastin. Blood 1990;76(10):2162.
21. Falk RJ, Jennette JC. Anti-neutrophil cytoplasmic autoantibodies with specificity for myeloperoxidase in patients with systemic vasculitis and idiopathic necrotizing and crescentic glomerulonephritis. N Engl J Med 1988;318(25):1651–7.
22. Bini P, Gabay JE, Teitel A. Antineutrophil cytoplasmic autoantibodies in Wegener's granulomatosis recognize conformational epitope(s) on proteinase 3. J Immunol 1992;149(4):1409–15.
23. Williams RC, Staud R, Malone CC, et al. Epitopes on proteinase-3 recognized by antibodies from patients with Wegener's granulomatosis. J Immunol 1994;152(9): 4722–37.
24. Griffith ME, Coulthart S, Pemberton A, et al. Anti-neutrophil cytoplasmic antibodies (ANCA) from patients with systemic vasculitis recognize restricted epitopes of proteinase 3 involving the catalytic site. Clin Exp Immunol 2001; 123(1):170–7.
25. Fujinaga M, Chernaia M, Halenbeck R, et al. The crystal structure of PR 3, a neutrophil serine proteinase antigen of Wegener's granulomatosis antibodies. J Mol Biol 1996;261(2):267–78.
26. Müller-Bérat N, Minowada J, Tsuji-Takayama K, et al. The phylogeny of proteinase 3/myeloblastin, the autoantigen in Wegener's granulomatosis, and myeloperoxidase as shown by immunohistochemical studies on human leukemic cell lines. Clin Immunol Immunopathol 1994;70(1):51–9.
27. Sturrock AB, Franklin KF, Rao G, et al. Structure, chromosomal assignment, and expression of the gene for proteinase 3, the Wegener's granulomatosis autoantigen. J Biol Chem 1992;267(29):21193–9.
28. Weiss SJ. Tissue destruction by neutrophils. N Engl J Med 1989;320(6):365–76.
29. Zeng J, Fenna RE. X-ray crystal structure of canine myeloperoxidase at 3 Å resolution. J Mol Biol 1992;226(1):185–207.
30. Chang KS, Schroeder W, Siciliano MJ. The localization of the human myeloperoxidase gene is in close proximity to the translocation breakpoint in acute promyelocytic leukemia. Leukemia 1987;1(5):458–62.
31. Falk RJ, Becker R, Terrell R, et al. Anti-myeloperoxidase autoantibodies react with native but not denatured myeloperoxidase. Clin Exp Immunol 1992;89(2):274–8.
32. Wiik A. Drug-induced vasculitis. Curr Opin Rheumatol 2008;20(1):35–9.
33. Kain R, Matsui K, Exner M, et al. A novel class of autoantigens of anti-neutrophil cytoplasmic antibodies in necrotizing and crescentic glomerulonephritis: the

lysosomal membrane glycoprotein h-lamp-2 in neutrophil granules and a related membrane protein in glomerular endothelial cells. J Exp Med 1995;181(2): 585–97.

34. Kain R, Exner M, Brandes R, et al. Molecular mimicry in pauci-immune focal necrotizing glomerulonephritis. Nat Med 2008;10(10):1088–96.

35. Bonaci-Nikolic B, Nikolic MM, Andrejevic S, et al. Antineutrophil cytoplasmic antibody (ANCA)-associated autoimmune diseases induced by antithyroid drugs: comparison with idiopathic ANCA vasculitides. Arthritis Res Ther 2005;7(5): R1072–81.

36. Wiik A. Clinical use of serological tests for ANCA: what do the studies say? Rheum Dis Clin North Am 2001;27(4):799–813.

37. Wiik A. Clinical and pathophysiological significance of anti-neutrophil cytoplasmic autoantibodies in vasculitis syndromes. Mod Rheumatol 2009;19(6): 590–9.

38. Hagen EC, Daha M, Hermans J, et al. The diagnostic value of standardized assays for anti-neutrophil cytoplasmic antibodies (ANCA) in idiopathic systemic vasculitis. Kidney Int 1998;53(3):743–53.

39. Fritzler MJ, Wiik A, Fritzler ML, et al. The use and abuse of commercial kits used to detect autoantibodies. Arthritis Res Ther 2003;5(4):192–201.

40. Jayne D. The diagnosis of vasculitis. Best Pract Res Clin Rheumatol 2009;23(3): 445–53.

41. Boomsma MM, Stegeman CA, van der Leij MJ, et al. Prediction of relapses in Wegener's granulomatosis by measurement of antineutrophil cytoplasmic antibody levels: a prospective study. Arthritis Rheum 2000;43(9):2025–33.

42. Segelmark M, Phillips BD, Hogan SL, et al. Monitoring proteinase 3 antineutrophil cytoplasmic antibodies for detection of relapses in small vessel vasculitis. Clin Diagn Lab Immunol 2003;10(5):769–74.

43. Terrier B, Saadoun D, Séne D, et al. Antimyeloperoxidase antibodies are a useful marker of disease activity in antineutrophil cytoplasmic antibody-associated vasculitides. Ann Rheum Dis 2009;68(19):1564–71.

44. Birck R, Schmidt WH, Kaelsch IA, et al. Serial ANCA determinations for monitoring disease activity in patients with ANCA-associated vasculitis: systematic review. Am J Kidney Dis 2006;47(1):15–23.

45. Franssen C, Gans R, Kallenberg C, et al. Disease spectrum of patients with antineutrophil cytoplasmic autoantibodies of defined specificity: distinct differences between patients with anti-proteinase 3 and anti-myeloperoxidase autoantibodies. J Intern Med 1998;244(3):209–16.

46. Wang F, Chen M, Zhao MH. Neutrophil degranulation in antineutrophil cytoplasmic antibody-negative pauci-immune crescentic glomerulonephritis. J Nephrol 2009;22(4):491–6.

47. Eisenberger U, Fakhouri F, Vanhille P, et al. ANCA-negative pauci-immune renal vasculitis: histology and outcome. Nephrol Dial Transplant 2005;29(7):1392–9.

48. Meroni PL, Del Papa N, Raschi E, et al. Antiendothelial cell antibodies (AECA): from laboratory curiosity to another useful autoantibody. In: Shoenfeld Y, editor. The decade of autoimmunity. Amsterdam: Elsevier Science; 1999. p. 285–94.

49. Holmen C, Christensson M, Liu J, et al. Wegener's granulomatosis is associated with organ-specific antiendothelial cell antibodies. Kidney Int 2004;66(3): 1049–60.

50. Yu F, Zhao MH, Zhang Y, et al. Anti-endothelial cell antibodies (AECA) in patients with propylthiouracil (PTU)-induced ANCA positive vasculitis are associated with disease activity. Clin Exp Immunol 2005;139(3):569–74.

51. Chanseaud Y, Pena-Lefebvre PG, Guilpain P, et al. IgM and IgG autoantibodies from microscopic polyangiitis patients but not those with other small- and medium-sized vessel vasculitides recognize multiple endothelial cell antigens. Clin Immunol 2003;109(2):165–78.
52. Del Papa N, Guidali L, Sironi M, et al. Anti-endothelial cell IgG antibodies from patients with Wegener's granulomatosis bind to human endothelial cells in vitro and induce adhesion molecule expression and cytokine secretion. Arthritis Rheum 1996;39(5):758–66.
53. Chan TM, Frampton G, Jayne DRW, et al. Clinical significance of anti-endothelial cell antibodies in systemic vasculitis: a longitudinal study comparing anti-endothelial cell antibodies and anti-neutrophil cytoplasm antibodies. Am J Kidney Dis 1993;22(3):387–92.
54. Gunnarsson A, Hellmark T, Wieslander J. Molecular properties of the Goodpasture epitope. Biol Chem 2000;275(40):30844–8.
55. Rutgers A, Heeringa P, Damoiseaux JG, et al. ANCA and anti-GBM antibodies in diagnosis and follow-up of vasculitic disease. Eur J Intern Med 2003;14(5): 287–95.
56. Lionaki S, Jennette JC, Falk RJ. Anti-neutrophil cytoplasmic (ANCA) and anti-glomerular basement membrane (GBM) autoantibodies in necrotizing and crescentic glomerulonephritis. Semin Immunopathol 2007;29(4):459–74.
57. Levy JB, Hammad T, Coulthart A, et al. Clinical features and outcome of patients with both ANCA and anti-GBM antibodies. Kidney Int 2004;66(4):1535–40.
58. Vecchi ML, Radice A, Renda F, et al. Anti-laminin autoantibodies in ANCA-associated vasculitis. Nephrol Dial Transplant 2000;15(10):1600–3.
59. Rees JD, Lanca S, Marques PV, et al. Prevalence of the antiphospholipid syndrome in primary systemic vasculitis. Ann Rheum Dis 2006;65(1):109–11.

Diagnostic Approach to ANCA-associated Vasculitides

Angelo L. Gaffo, MD, MSPH

KEYWORDS

- ANCA • Anti-neutrophil cytoplasmic antibody • Vasculitis
- Diagnosis • Differential diagnosis

Antineutrophil cytoplasmic antibody (ANCA)-associated vasculitides (AAVs) include Wegener's granulomatosis (WG), microscopic polyangiitis (MPA), and Churg-Strauss syndrome (CSS, also known as allergic granulomatous angiitis). Many investigators include a renal-limited form of vasculitis associated with ANCA manifested by an acute crescentic glomerulonephritis.[1] For the purpose of this article, renal-limited forms will be included with the other AAVs.

For the most part, these conditions share the characteristic of being aggressive and rapidly life threatening. Given their rarity, protean clinical manifestations, imperfect diagnostic tests, and wide differential diagnosis, they pose a diagnostic challenge even to experienced clinicians. On the other hand, because of the high toxicity of available therapies, all efforts should be exhausted toward a precise and definitive diagnosis before treatment is initiated. Classification criteria previously developed are of limited usefulness for clinical diagnosis of individual patients.[2–5]

This article presents diagnostic approaches for patients suspected of having an AAV. A general approach to AAV is initially presented, followed by specific considerations organized by organ system.

GENERAL APPROACH TO AAV
Suggestive Clinical Presentations

AAVs are usually multisystem diseases; however, there are cases in which these diseases could be limited to one organ system, as in renal-limited vasculitis with positive ANCA or the limited forms of WG. Despite these exceptions, most cases will involve more than one organ system during the course of the disease.[6–9] Systemic constitutional manifestations including fever, malaise, and asthenia are present in most patients. The identification of patterns in the clinical presentation is critical for

Disclosures: None.
Division of Clinical Immunology and Rheumatology, University of Alabama at Birmingham and Birmingham VA Medical Center, 700 South 19th Street, Birmingham, AL 35233, USA
E-mail address: agaffo@uab.edu

Rheum Dis Clin N Am 36 (2010) 491–506
doi:10.1016/j.rdc.2010.05.009
0889-857X/10/$ – see front matter. Published by Elsevier Inc.

rheumatic.theclinics.com

early diagnosis. For example, the concurrent development of pulmonary and renal manifestations of disease may suggest WG or MPA; onset of recurrent sinusitis or development of bilateral otitis media in a middle-age adult should trigger suspicion of WG, and new-onset refractory asthma with nasal polyposis should evoke consideration of CSS. As other diseases that could be more prevalent than AAV share these patterns, it is important to maintain a high index of suspicion for other conditions in the differential diagnosis of AAV. An overview of clinical syndromes associated with AAV and their differential diagnosis can be found in **Table 1**.

Pulmonary symptoms, including dyspnea, cough, hemoptysis, and symptoms of obstructive lung disease are among the most common forms of presentation for AAV.[10] The rapid onset of pulmonary hemorrhage induced by pulmonary capillaritis and diffuse alveolar hemorrhage (DAH) can be seen with WG and CSS, but is more characteristic of MPA. Cough productive of bloody sputum in the setting of progressive dyspnea is compatible with WG, but may be seen with a wide variety of other medical conditions such as bacterial pneumonia, pulmonary embolism, and many others. Recurrent obstructive pulmonary symptoms are suggestive of the predominantly eosinophilic involvement of CSS, but are not specific. Other presentations include pleuritis with or without pleural effusions and a more insidious onset of dyspnea caused by pulmonary hypertension or pulmonary fibrosis.[11,12] The differential diagnosis of these pulmonary manifestations of AAV includes infections or postinfectious complications, drug-induced lung injuries (mainly for DAH), other connective tissue diseases (rheumatoid arthritis with pulmonary nodules or systemic lupus erythematosus inducing DAH), and cardiac disease.

Renal involvement is one of the main features of MPA and WG, present at some point in 70% or more of the cases,[8,13] but it appears to be less common in CSS (about 25% of cases).[7] Most episodes of renal involvement are preceded by constitutional symptoms including malaise, myalgias, arthralgias, fever, anorexia, and weight loss.[14] Microscopic hematuria and proteinuria usually precede the deterioration in renal function, with a small proportion of patients presenting with gross hematuria or oliguria, as unilateral or bilateral ureteral stenoses can rarely occur with AAV.[15,16] The differential diagnosis includes other causes of glomerulonephritis such as systemic lupus erythematosus (SLE), other vasculitides (eg, Henoch-Schönlein purpura), and postinfectious or drug-induced syndromes. A common pattern for AAV is the pulmonary-renal syndrome that includes DAH and glomerulonephritis. Most of these cases have been described to be in association with AAV.[17,18] The differential diagnosis includes Goodpasture's disease, drug-induced vasculitis, SLE, antiphospholipid syndrome, infections, and neoplasms (the last 3 through a thrombotic microangiopathic mechanism).[17,18]

Head and neck involvement is the most common form of presentation in WG, but is virtually absent in MPA. In CSS, clinical series have reported that at least 50% of patients present with paranasal sinus disease, allergic rhinitis, or chronic rhinosinusitis with or without polyposis.[19] In WG, the forms of presentation are multiple and can involve the nose (with nasal obstruction, epistaxis, saddle-nose deformities, perforation of the nasal septum), eye (eg, red-eye syndromes with scleritis, keratitis, nasolacrimal disease, orbital disease, exophthalmos, diplopia),[20] ear (eg, tinnitus, hearing loss, otorrhea), and upper airway (eg, pain, hoarseness, stridor, cough).[21,22] In WG, the disease manifestations can be limited to the head and neck region, without including systemic constitutional symptoms. The presence of unexplained and recurrent nose or ear symptoms should raise suspicion for WG, although infectious and allergic conditions should be considered in the differential diagnosis. A condition to consider in cases of nasal septum damage is cocaine abuse, which can also present with

Table 1
Overview of clinical syndromes associated with ANCA-associated vasculitides and selected items in their differential diagnosis

Organ System	Clinical Syndrome	Differential Diagnosis
Pulmonary	Diffuse alveolar hemorrhage	SLE, infections (HIV, CMV, invasive aspergillosis), Goodpasture's disease, drug reactions, antiphospholipid syndrome, cryoglobulinemia
	Nodules and cavities	Infections (*Mycobacterium* spp, *Nocardia* spp, septic emboli), neoplasm, rheumatoid arthritis
	Pulmonary-renal syndrome	SLE, Goodpasture's disease, cryoglobulinemia
	Obstructive airway disease and eosinophilia	Asthma, allergic bronchopulmonary aspergillosis, drug or toxic reactions (leukotriene inhibitors)
	Pulmonary fibrosis	Idiopathic, connective tissue diseases (scleroderma, MCTD, myositis, SLE), rheumatoid arthritis
Head and neck	Recurrent sinusitis	Allergic, infections
	Nasal and septum damage	Relapsing polychondritis, cocaine abuse, psychiatric
	Ear disease	Infections, allergic
	Upper airway disease	Relapsing polychondritis, infections, neoplasms
	Eye and orbital disease	Malignancy (lymphoma), sarcoidosis, Graves disease, pseudolymphoma
Renal	Glomerulonephritis	SLE, postinfectious glomerulonephritis, IgA nephropathy, Goodpasture's disease, drug reactions
	Obstructive disease	Infections (tuberculosis), neoplasm
	Renal mass	Neoplasm
Nervous system	Peripheral neuropathy	Small and medium-size vasculitides (cryoglobulinemia, PAN), SLE, diabetes, toxic (heavy metals), metabolic,
	Meningitis	Multiple infections, drug reactions (NSAIDS)
	Focal CNS lesion	Multiple infections, neoplasms, demyelinating diseases
Cutaneous	Palpable purpura	Other vasculitides (LCV, cryoglobulinemia, HSP, PAN), embolic disease (RMSF, ecthyma, meningococcemia)
	Livedo racemosa	Antiphospholipid syndrome, SLE, vasculitis (PAN), embolic disease (cholesterol emboli)
	Urticaria, ulcers, or nodules	Infections (hepatitis B or C), medium vessel vasculitides (PAN), erythema nodosum, cutaneous SLE, sarcoidosis, lymphoma, amyloidosis, paniculitis

Abbreviations: ANCA, antineutrophil cytoplasmic antibodies; CMV, cytomegalovirus; HIV, human immunodeficiency virus; HSP, Henoch-Schönlein purpura; LCV, leukocytoclastic vasculitis; MCTD, mixed connective tissue disease; NSAIDS, nonsteroidal anti-inflammatory drugs; PAN, polyarteritis nodosa; RMSF, Rocky Mountain spotted fever; SLE, systemic lupus erythematosus.

false-positive serologic tests.[23] Atypical ANCA (with discordance between cytoplasmic ANCA and anti-proteinase 3 [anti-PR3] antibody or perinuclear ANCA with anti-myeloperoxidase [anti-MPO] antibody) in patients with nasal septal damage and history of cocaine abuse may be caused by ANCA with reactivity to human neutrophil elastase.[24–27]

Infections and other rheumatic conditions (eg, rheumatoid arthritis, sarcoidosis) should be considered in cases of scleritis. Endocrine (eg, hyperthyroidism) and neoplastic (eg, lymphoma) processes are in the differential in cases of exophthalmos and orbital pseudotumor.

Both the central and peripheral nervous systems can be affected by any of the AAVs. The clinical manifestations of central nervous system disease are a consequence of small-vessel vasculitis or granulomatous involvement and include strokelike symptoms with sensory or motor deficit, cognitive dysfunction,[28] epilepsy, cranial nerve involvement, and meningitis.[29] Peripheral nervous system involvement is common for all AAVs in the form of peripheral neuropathy, but seems to be more prevalent in CSS and MPA (50%–76%) than in WG (10%–50%).[6–8,30] Mononeuritis multiplex and symmetric polyneuropathies are described as the most common patterns of neurologic presentation in almost equal proportions.[29,31,32] These have a predilection for the lower extremities with the peroneal nerve being the most commonly involved although the cubital, median, and radial nerves in the upper extremities can also be affected.[7,29,33] Paresis, pain, and hypoesthesia are common features at presentation. The differential diagnosis in both the central and peripheral nervous system manifestations associated with AAV is extremely wide and includes infections causing focal lesions (eg, tuberculosis, nocardia) or seeding (eg, endocarditis), neoplasms (eg, lymphoma), demyelinating diseases (eg, acute demyelinating encephalomyelitis, multiple sclerosis), stroke or ischemic neuropathy, metabolic or toxic neuropathies, and other vasculitic or autoimmune conditions such as polyarteritis nodosa or SLE.

Cutaneous manifestations are common in all forms of AAV, affecting at least 40% to 50% of patients with WG, MPA, or CSS at some point of the disease.[7,8,34] Palpable purpura, digital ischemia or necrosis, and subcutaneous nodules with or without necrosis are frequent forms of presentation.[34–37] Livedo racemosa can be present in CSS and MPA, and oral or nasal ulcers are manifestations suggestive of WG especially in combination with gingival hyperplasia.[38] These cutaneous manifestations should be distinguished from those happening in other connective tissue diseases that frequently present with palpable purpura, such as cryoglobulinemia and Henoch-Schönlein purpura. Livedo racemosa, a syndrome closely related to livedo reticularis, can be a manifestation of SLE, antiphospholipid syndrome, or polyarteritis nodosa.[39] Hypersensitivity (cutaneous small vessel vasculitis) can be undistinguishable from AAVs that are otherwise asymptomatic. Finally, infections (eg, endocarditis), nutritional deficiencies (eg, scurvy), drug reactions, or paraneoplastic syndromes could present as cutaneous rashes simulating AAV.

Other clinical manifestations that may suggest the presence of an AAV include musculoskeletal symptoms such as myalgias, myositis, arthralgias, or frank arthritis. Cardiac involvement, as a result of vasculitic myocarditis, presents as dyspnea, chest pain, and palpitations in 23% to 45% of patients with CSS, although the prevalence of subclinical functional cardiac abnormalities is higher.[40,41] Episodes of recurrent deep venous thrombosis in a suggestive clinical setting could support a diagnosis of WG or CSS, as this complication has been reported to have an increased incidence in patients diagnosed with these conditions.[42,43]

Laboratory Testing and ANCA

The initial basic laboratory workup for suspected AAV must include a complete blood count with differential, a metabolic panel including serum creatinine and transaminases, a urinalysis, and inflammatory markers (sedimentation rate and/or C-reactive protein). The threshold should be very low for ordering tests to exclude hepatitis B and C, along with testing for cryoglobulins.

Normochromic, normocytic anemia is a feature common to all AAVs. Eosino-philia is suggestive of CSS, but can be also observed in WG and MPA. Throm-bocytosis or normal platelet counts are typical in AAV, whereas thrombocytopenia is uncommon in AAV and should raise suspicion for other conditions such as SLE or cryoglobulinemia related to hepatitis C infection. The urinalysis can reveal hematuria and/or proteinuria (usually in the non-nephrotic range) and may indicate renal involvement earlier in the course of the disease than the serum creatinine. Large amounts of proteinuria should increase suspicion for SLE or other diseases associated with glomerulonephritis. Elevation of serum transaminases should trigger prompt exclusion of hepatitis C (cryoglobulinemia) and hepatitis B (polyarteritis nodosa)–related diseases. Eleva-tions in inflammatory markers are common, but their absence does not rule out the presence of an AAV.

Depending on the clinical picture, tests for other autoimmune diseases should be ordered. For example, the absence of serum antinuclear antibody essentially rules out SLE as a possibility. Other examples include measurement of serum creatine-kinase tests as an initial screening in cases where there is a suspicion of autoimmune myositis; rheumatoid factor and anticyclic citrullinated peptide antibody testing in cases of suspected rheumatoid vasculitis; and serum comple-ment levels to assess for diseases characterized by complement deposition such as SLE or postinfectious glomerulonephritis. Antiglomerular basement membrane antibodies (anti-GBM) represent a special case, given that their utility is not limited to the differential diagnosis with Goodpasture's disease, but they confer valuable prognostic information (more severe disease) and have therapeutic impli-cations (possible indication for plasmapheresis) in cases of rapidly progressive glomerulonephritis and pulmonary-renal syndromes.[44,45]

Indirect immunofluorescence (IIF) testing for neutrophil cytoplasmic antibodies (ANCA) and enzyme-linked immunosorbent assays (ELISAs) for antibodies directed against PR3 and MPO are useful tests that, when applied in the right clinical setting, provide support for the diagnosis of an AAV.[46] The predictive values of these tests are greatly decreased when they are applied in inappropriate clinical scenarios,[47,48] as multiple conditions can have false positive tests in ANCA testing (**Table 2**). Commonly, IIF ANCA testing is ordered first; if positive, results are confirmed with ELISA tests for antibodies to PR3 and MPO.[49] However, the simultaneous ordering of these tests could also be advocated in view of the long turnaround times for these ELISA tests, the occasional occur-rence of negative IIF ANCA with positive ELISA PR3 or MPO,[50,51] and the reported added clinical value of the combination of tests.[46,52] Typically, the cyto-plasmic staining (c-ANCA) is associated with WG and the perinuclear staining (p-ANCA) is associated with MPA, although these patterns are not absolute, as cases of WG could present with positive p-ANCA and cases of MPA could present with positive c-ANCA tests.[50] Thus, positive IIF ANCA tests should always be confirmed with ELISA testing. IIF p-ANCA and ELISA MPO for MPA are regarded as less sensitive tests than their IIF and ELISA counterparts for WG.[46,53] "Atypical" ANCA patterns can present in association with AAV but these are more commonly seen with other autoimmune or inflammatory conditions.[50,51] ANCA testing is less sensitive in cases of CSS, with positive results in 26% to 48% of cases,[7,46,54] but patients with CSS and renal involvement have been reported to have positive ANCA test results in higher proportions (75%).[15] It is important to remember that at least 10% of patients with biopsy-confirmed AAV will not have a positive result for either IIF ANCA or ELISA tests.[46]

| Table 2 |
| Conditions associated with positive ANCA tests (IIF or ELISA) |

Category	Condition
Vasculitic	Cryoglobulinemia
	Leukocytoclastic cutaneous vasculitis
	Henoch-Schönlein purpura
	Polyarteritis nodosa
	Giant cell arteritis
	Takayasu's arteritis
	Behçet's syndrome
Other autoimmune	Systemic lupus erythematosus
	Goodpasture's disease
	Sjögren's syndrome
	Polymyositis and dermatomyositis
	Scleroderma
	Mixed-connective tissue disease
	Rheumatoid arthritis
	Spondyloarthropathies
	Inflammatory bowel disease (ulcerative colitis and Crohn's disease)
	Psoriatic arthritis
	Hashimoto's disease
	Multiple sclerosis
	Postinfectious glomerulonephritis
Infectious	Mycobacterium tuberculosis
	Human immunodeficiency virus
	Hepatitis C
	Pneumocystis carinii
	Poliomyelitis
	Endocarditis
Miscellaneous	Sarcoidosis
	Interstitial pulmonary fibrosis
	Myocardial infarction
	Cystic fibrosis
	Cocaine abuse
	Alport's syndrome

Abbreviations: ANCA, antineutrophil cytoplasmic antibodies; ELISA, enzyme-linked immunosorbent assay; IIF, indirect immunofluorescence.
Data from Refs. [48,49,53,90]

SPECIFIC DIAGNOSTIC CONSIDERATIONS PER ORGAN SYSTEM
Pulmonary

Radiologic evaluation is important in cases of suspected AAV involving the lungs. Findings on plain radiographs and computed tomography (CT) suggestive of WG include the presence of nodules or cavities with irregular and thin walls; these are usually multiple (in ~75% of cases) and bilateral, with a slight predilection for the subpleural and peribronchovascular regions.[55,56] These cavities could be easily mistaken for septic emboli, metastases, or lung abscesses.[57] In addition, WG can present with localized or diffuse patchy areas of air-space consolidation caused by pulmonary hemorrhage and thickening of the trachea or bronchi seen on radiographs or chest CT.[58] MPA usually presents with a pattern suggestive of DAH that includes the development of patchy or diffuse bilateral airspace opacities with a predilection for the lower lung zones.[55] Chest CT findings consistent with pulmonary fibrosis, including ground-glass and reticular opacities, septal thickening, and honeycombing, have been increasingly described in patients with MPA and are theorized to be secondary to recurrent subclinical pulmonary bleeding.[59] CSS usually presents with transient and symmetric areas of ground glass opacity or consolidation, with a predilection for the periphery of the lung fields, airway wall thickening, unilateral or bilateral pleural effusions, or nodules.[60,61]

The role of bronchoscopy is usually restricted to ruling out conditions in the differential diagnosis, evaluation of cases suspicious for DAH, and the assessment of endobronchial lesions. The samples provided by transbronchial biopsies are often insufficient to make a proper diagnostic assessment in cases of WG, although a good yield has been reported in cases of suspected CSS.[62] Unless a case is overwhelmingly characteristic and there is an absolute contraindication, surgical lung biopsy by video-assisted thoracoscopic surgery is the procedure of choice to establish diagnosis in cases suspected of pulmonary involvement by AAV. This procedure has low morbidity and mortality and the yield of the pulmonary tissue for precisely establishing the diagnosis and ruling out conditions in the differential of AAV is very good.[63–65]

Head and Neck

Ear, nose, and throat manifestations of WG, including sinusitis, septal perforations, and saddle-nose deformities, are commonly seen in the limited forms of the disease.[66] This has diagnostic and therapeutic implications, as patients with limited disease can have negative ANCA by IIF and negative anti-PR3 and anti-MPO by ELISA, even during active flares of their clinical disease[67]; therapeutic choices can be less aggressive in cases of limited AAV.[30]

CT of the head and neck is a sensitive test that can reveal changes in the sinus cavities of patients with WG, including mucosal thickening, sinus opacification, sclerosing otitis, and bony destruction or thickening.[68] CT or magnetic resonance imaging (MRI) evidence of involvement of the lacrimal region or retro-orbital masses can support ophthalmic compromise by WG. MRI could be helpful in demonstrating the inflammatory nature of retro-orbital masses in AAV.[20] Ophthalmologic examination in patients with suspected WG should include a slit-lamp examination and fundoscopy to assess for the presence of scleritis, keratitis, uveitis, and retinal lesions. Otolaryngologic examination in patients with suspected WG or CSS of the head and neck should include otoscopy, flexible fiberoptic laryngoscopy, nasal endoscopy, and audiometry. Tissue biopsy varies in its diagnostic yield according to the site involved by suspected AAV. In cases of retro-orbital masses it can help differentiating the granulomatous involvement of WG from other conditions such as lymphomas, sarcoidosis, Graves' disease, and orbital pseudotumor. The paranasal sinuses are additional areas where the biopsies for WG may be considered, but the diagnostic yield for findings specific for WG is relatively low. Similarly, biopsies of the oral cavity, larynx, external or middle ear, and subglottic region can be technically challenging and often nondiagnostic.[69] In cases of suspected CSS, biopsies of nasal polyps seem to have a low diagnostic yield when compared with other organ systems.[70]

Renal

Renal-limited forms of AAV without signs of systemic involvement are occasionally reported and are considered to be rare.[71,72] Besides the syndrome of glomerulonephritis, WG can rarely present with ureteral stenosis, papillary necrosis, perirenal hematomas, and renal masses.[73] An association between WG and a higher incidence of renal cell carcinoma has been described.[74] Thus, in cases of WG presenting in association with renal masses, the preferred procedure may be nephrectomy instead of fine-needle biopsy to avoid peritoneal seeding of the potential malignancy.[75]

Renal biopsy plays a crucial role in patients with glomerulonephritis and suspected AAV by allowing differentiation from conditions that induce deposition of immune complexes in the glomerulus. AAV induces glomerulonephritis by mechanisms that do not depend on immune-complex deposition and as a consequence are labeled as "pauci-immune" glomerulonephritis, as opposed to conditions such as SLE, post-infectious glomerulonephritis, and endocarditis that usually induce glomerulonephritis through immune-complex and complement deposition. Immunofluorescent staining of renal biopsy material usually allows for the differentiation of AAV from anti-GBM–induced disease, which is characterized by linear deposition of IgG in the basement membrane.

Features of AAV common in renal histopathology include fibrinoid necrosis, cellular and fibrous crescents, glomerulosclerosis, and periglomerular infiltrates. Features reflecting chronicity (eg, glomerulosclerosis, interstitial fibrosis, tubular atrophy, arteriosclerosis) are more commonly found in MPA and renal-limited AAV than in WG, possibly because of earlier diagnoses of the former two conditions than of the latter. Granulomatous reactions, although useful for establishing a diagnosis of AAV, are rarely found on kidney biopsy (2%–4% of cases).[76] CSS has histopathological features indistinguishable from the other AAVs, and even eosinophilic interstitial infiltrates, which are rarely present, are not specific for its diagnosis.[15] With the exception of granulomas, other histopathological characteristics of AAV do not allow for a differentiation of other conditions in the differential diagnosis, making immunoflorescence staining an essential feature of the renal biopsy.

Nervous System

Peripheral nervous system involvement could be the first manifestation of an AAV,[29,77] but in these cases the differential diagnosis is broad, including neuropathies of ischemic (eg, diabetic, amyloid), inflammatory (eg, sarcoidosis, idiopathic, medium-vessel vasculitis), infectious (eg, leprosy, HIV, Lyme disease), and malignant (eg, paraneoplastic) etiologies. Electromyographies with nerve conduction studies are helpful tools in better defining the neurologic syndromes (eg, mononeuropathy, mononeuritis multiplex, symmetric or asymmetric polyneuropathy) and identifying a nerve suitable for biopsy. Findings on nerve conduction studies reveal that the predominant pattern of involvement is indicative of axonal degeneration[32] and the needle electromyogram usually reveals denervation on the muscle groups supplied by the involved nerves. A controversy exists about the need to perform a muscle biopsy along with a nerve biopsy when vasculitis is in the differential. One point of view is that the muscle portion rarely provides the diagnosis when the nerve biopsy is negative,[78,79] but others conclude that the histopathology of the muscle may provide specific findings and increase the diagnostic yield.[80,81] The sural and peroneal nerves, along with the anterior tibialis and gastrocnemius muscles, are the preferred areas for biopsy. On nerve histopathology the findings are usually nonspecific, with perivascular infiltration of inflammatory cells, axonal degeneration, and necrotizing changes that can be active, inactive, or healed.[82]

All AAVs can involve the central nervous system and cause focal lesions through vasculitic involvement of central nervous system (CNS) vessels or granulomatous involvement of the brain parenchyma or meninges.[83–85] In WG, these granulomas can form primarily in the central nervous system, or they can be an extension from those in the ears or sinuses.[83] Even in cases of severe central nervous system involvement by AAV, ANCA testing can be consistently negative.[86,87] A rare but well-described presentation of WG is chronic pachymeningitis with negative or atypical testing for ANCA and positive ELISA tests MPO or PR3.[88,89] These cases of meningeal inflammation should be suspected in patients presenting with headache, encephalopathy, and cranial nerve involvement. Subclinical cognitive impairment is present in about 30% of patients with a small-vessel vasculitis and usually correlates with MRI findings.[28] MRI can demonstrate patterns of abnormalities consistent with vasculitic CNS involvement such as the forms of meningitis or parenchymal lesions with inflammation, hemorrhage, or ischemia; these findings are not specific for AAV or other forms of vasculitis. Lumbar puncture with cerebrospinal fluid analysis is important to aid in the differentiation between infectious and inflammatory conditions, including bacterial, viral, or tuberculous meningoencephalitis (the latter can present with positive IIF testing for ANCA and ELISA for PR3 and MPO[90]). Finally, a brain or meningeal biopsy is a procedure that, albeit invasive, is sometimes necessary when no other tissue can be feasibly biopsied.

Skin

Skin biopsy is a simple procedure that can be very informative in patients suspected of having AAV. An ideal biopsy extends to the subcutaneous tissue in the most tender, red, or purpuric lesion that is less than 48 hours old. The pathologic features of vasculitis are more likely to be present at this stage and the yield of the direct immunofluorescence (DIF) testing is optimal.[91] Deep biopsies will reveal involvement of larger vessels, which occasionally occurs in WG and should be expected in vasculitides that affect medium-size vessels, such as polyarteritis nodosa. Ulcerated lesions are not optimal for biopsy; the edge of superficial ulcers is preferred should biopsy be performed. DIF is an essential part of a cutaneous biopsy when vasculitis is in the differential diagnosis. The physician performing the procedure should be aware that the diagnosis of AAV is being entertained, as the processing of the sample for DIF is different than for routine histopathology. Ideally, 2 distinct biopsy samples for histopathology and DIF should be obtained, as splitting an individual sample could produce crush artifacts and significantly decrease the yield of the biopsy.[92]

Papular lesions in WG usually exhibit a pattern similar to a leukocytoclastic vasculitis, with neutrophilic infiltrates around dermal small vessels. Medium-sized vessel inflammation can be seen in ulcers and infarcts. Urticarial, granulomatous, and neutrophilic lesions (similar to pyoderma gangrenosum) are histopathological features that could also be found in WG.[93] The inflammatory neutrophilic infiltrates around small vessels will be similar in cases of CSS but could be enriched for eosinophils. The absence of granulomatous lesions will support a diagnosis of MPA, but given that this finding is rare even in proven cases of WG and other features are nonspecific, it is difficult to distinguish among the small and medium vessel vasculitides based solely on histopathological grounds.[94] Lack of deposition of immune complexes and complement on DIF examination can differentiate AAV from leukocytoclastic vasculitis, cryoglobulinemia, SLE, and Henoch-Schönlein purpura, in which different patterns of deposition are found.

OTHER DIAGNOSTIC CONSIDERATIONS
Multisystem Involvement

As previously mentioned, most cases of AAV involve more than one organ system, often simultaneously.[6–8] The diagnostic approach to patients with multisystem involvement will vary depending on the acuity of the presentation and the consistency of the clinical presentation with a diagnosis of AAV. In patients with low acuity or low pretest probability for AAV, diagnostic testing may be performed in a stepwise fashion. In acutely ill patients, the diagnostic evaluation (eg, serologies, nerve conduction testing, tissue biopsies) is oftentimes performed simultaneously while empiric treatment has been started. The diagnostic evaluation takes into consideration the turnaround time of the test, risk/benefit ratio, and diagnostic yield of the test. For example, a patient presenting with vague constitutional symptoms, sinus drainage, and mild peripheral neuropathy can await an initial laboratory evaluation and electrophysiologic testing as an outpatient with histopathological confirmation occurring later if clinically indicated. On the other hand, a patient with rapid onset of life-threatening pulmonary-renal syndrome may need to have serologies, histopathological diagnosis, and the initiation of empiric therapy performed simultaneously.

Histopathological Considerations

In cases of multisystem involvement, the choice of biopsy site should take into consideration the diagnostic yield of histopathology at the involved sites versus the potential risk imposed by the biopsy procedure. A sinus biopsy is associated with low risk; however, it also has a low yield for diagnostic purposes, oftentimes only revealing acute and chronic inflammation. A patient with an acute pulmonary-renal syndrome and high clinical suspicion for WG may benefit from information gained from lung biopsy; however, if the patient has a tenuous pulmonary status and would not tolerate the procedure, then another biopsy site may be considered, if confirmation is necessary. Histopathological confirmation may not be possible in some cases because of the lack of an accessible biopsy site, anticipated poor yield, or tenuous clinical status and therefore treatment will be based on clinical judgment.

Diagnostic Approach to Recurrent AAV

Recurrence of disease activity during or after the initial induction phase of treatment for AAV is common.[95–97] The diagnostic approach for suspected recurrences is complex but should start with confirmation of the primary disease activity versus medication toxicity, infection, or malignancy. For example, recurrence of hematuria in a patient with WG may be because of disease reactivation, a urinary tract infection, or bladder carcinoma from prior exposure to cyclophosphamide. Laboratory testing (ie, ANCA titers) as an aid in the prediction of recurrences is controversial and for the most part not well accepted.[98–101]

SUMMARY

ANCA-associated vasculitides represent a challenge to clinicians, given their rarity. Their diagnosis requires familiarity with the multiple clinical syndromes. Clinicians should also be aware of the conditions that are in the differential diagnoses of AAV and should keep in mind that mimics of AAV are often more common than AAV. The results of serologic tests must be interpreted in relation to the clinical presentation of the patient. Imaging studies are helpful in identifying suitable areas for biopsy but rarely establish the diagnoses by themselves. As a consequence, histopathological examination should be pursued in most cases unless a major contraindication exists. Empiric immunosuppression is often initiated in patients with severe disease manifestations while the diagnostic workup is performed, but this approach should not discourage clinicians from seeking histopathologic confirmation of the diagnosis.

REFERENCES

1. Jennette JC, Wilkman AS, Falk RJ. Anti-neutrophil cytoplasmic autoantibody-associated glomerulonephritis and vasculitis. Am J Pathol 1989;135:921.
2. Hunder GG, Arend WP, Bloch DA, et al. The American College of Rheumatology 1990 criteria for the classification of vasculitis. Introduction. Arthritis Rheum 1990;33:1065.
3. Jennette JC, Falk RJ, Andrassy K, et al. Nomenclature of systemic vasculitides. Proposal of an international consensus conference. Arthritis Rheum 1994;37:187.
4. Leavitt RY, Fauci AS, Bloch DA, et al. The American College of Rheumatology 1990 criteria for the classification of Wegener's granulomatosis. Arthritis Rheum 1990;33:1101.
5. Masi AT, Hunder GG, Lie JT, et al. The American College of Rheumatology 1990 criteria for the classification of Churg-Strauss syndrome (allergic granulomatosis and angiitis). Arthritis Rheum 1990;33:1094.
6. Gross WL, Csernok E. Wegener's granulomatosis: clinical and immunodiagnostic aspects. In: Ball GV, Bridges SL, editors. Vasculitis. 2nd edition. Oxford (UK); New York: Oxford University Press; 2008. p. xviii.
7. Guillevin L, Cohen P, Gayraud M, et al. Churg-Strauss syndrome. Clinical study and long-term follow-up of 96 patients. Medicine (Baltimore) 1999;78:26.
8. Guillevin L, Durand-Gasselin B, Cevallos R, et al. Microscopic polyangiitis: clinical and laboratory findings in eighty-five patients. Arthritis Rheum 1999;42:421.
9. Reinhold-Keller E, Herlyn K, Wagner-Bastmeyer R, et al. Stable incidence of primary systemic vasculitides over five years: results from the German vasculitis register. Arthritis Rheum 2005;53:93.
10. Pesci A, Pavone L, Buzio C, et al. Respiratory system involvement in ANCA-associated systemic vasculitides. Sarcoidosis Vasc Diffuse Lung Dis 2005; 22(Suppl 1):S40.
11. Hervier B, Pagnoux C, Agard C, et al. Pulmonary fibrosis associated with ANCA-positive vasculitides. Retrospective study of 12 cases and review of the literature. Ann Rheum Dis 2009;68:404.
12. Gomez-Puerta JA, Hernandez-Rodriguez J, Lopez-Soto A, et al. Antineutrophil cytoplasmic antibody-associated vasculitides and respiratory disease. Chest 2009;136:1101.
13. Kamali S, Erer B, Artim-Esen B, et al. Predictors of damage and survival in patients with Wegener's granulomatosis: analysis of 50 patients. J Rheumatol 2010;37:374.
14. Falk RJ, Hogan S, Carey TS, et al. Clinical course of anti-neutrophil cytoplasmic autoantibody-associated glomerulonephritis and systemic vasculitis. The Glomerular Disease Collaborative Network. Ann Intern Med 1990;113:656.
15. Sinico RA, Di Toma L, Maggiore U, et al. Renal involvement in Churg-Strauss syndrome. Am J Kidney Dis 2006;47:770.
16. Guillevin L, Pagnoux C, Texeira L. Microscopic polyangiitis. In: Ball GV, Bridges SL, editors. Vasculitis. 2nd edition. Oxford; New York: Oxford University Press; 2008. p. xviii.
17. Niles JL, Bottinger EP, Saurina GR, et al. The syndrome of lung hemorrhage and nephritis is usually an ANCA-associated condition. Arch Intern Med 1996;156:440.
18. Papiris SA, Manali ED, Kalomenidis I, et al. Bench-to-bedside review: pulmonary-renal syndromes—an update for the intensivist. Crit Care 2007;11:213.
19. Keogh KA, Specks U. Churg-Strauss syndrome: clinical presentation, antineutrophil cytoplasmic antibodies, and leukotriene receptor antagonists. Am J Med 2003;115:284.

20. Pakrou N, Selva D, Leibovitch I. Wegener's granulomatosis: ophthalmic manifestations and management. Semin Arthritis Rheum 2006;35:284.

21. Hoffman GS, Gross WL. Wegener's granulomatosis: clinical aspects. In: Hoffman GS, Weyand CM, editors. Inflammatory diseases of blood vessels. New York: Marcel Dekker; 2002. p. xvi.

22. Tsuzuki K, Fukazawa K, Takebayashi H, et al. Difficulty of diagnosing Wegener's granulomatosis in the head and neck region. Auris Nasus Larynx 2009; 36:64.

23. Rachapalli SM, Kiely PD. Cocaine-induced midline destructive lesions mimicking ENT-limited Wegener's granulomatosis. Scand J Rheumatol 2008; 37:477.

24. de Lange TE, Simsek S, Kramer MH, et al. A case of cocaine-induced panhypopituitarism with human neutrophil elastase-specific anti-neutrophil cytoplasmic antibodies. Eur J Endocrinol 2009;160:499.

25. Molloy ES, Langford CA. Vasculitis mimics. Curr Opin Rheumatol 2008;20:29.

26. Peikert T, Finkielman JD, Hummel AM, et al. Functional characterization of antineutrophil cytoplasmic antibodies in patients with cocaine-induced midline destructive lesions. Arthritis Rheum 2008;58:1546.

27. Wiesner O, Russell KA, Lee AS, et al. Antineutrophil cytoplasmic antibodies reacting with human neutrophil elastase as a diagnostic marker for cocaine-induced midline destructive lesions but not autoimmune vasculitis. Arthritis Rheum 2004;50:2954.

28. Mattioli F, Capra R, Rovaris M, et al. Frequency and patterns of subclinical cognitive impairment in patients with ANCA-associated small vessel vasculitides. J Neurol Sci 2002;195:161.

29. de Groot K, Schmidt DK, Arlt AC, et al. Standardized neurologic evaluations of 128 patients with Wegener granulomatosis. Arch Neurol 2001;58:1215.

30. Hoffman GS, Kerr GS, Leavitt RY, et al. Wegener granulomatosis: an analysis of 158 patients. Ann Intern Med 1992;116:488.

31. Kararizou E, Davaki P, Karandreas N, et al. Nonsystemic vasculitic neuropathy: a clinicopathological study of 22 cases. J Rheumatol 2005;32:853.

32. Oh SJ. Vasculitic neuropathy. In: Ball GV, Bridges SL, editors. Vasculitis. 2nd edition. Oxford (UK); New York: Oxford University Press; 2008. p. xviii.

33. Sugiura M, Koike H, Iijima M, et al. Clinicopathologic features of nonsystemic vasculitic neuropathy and microscopic polyangiitis-associated neuropathy: a comparative study. J Neurol Sci 2006;241:31.

34. Davis MD, Daoud MS, McEvoy MT, et al. Cutaneous manifestations of Churg-Strauss syndrome: a clinicopathologic correlation. J Am Acad Dermatol 1997; 37:199.

35. Nagai Y, Hasegawa M, Igarashi N, et al. Cutaneous manifestations and histological features of microscopic polyangiitis. Eur J Dermatol 2009;19:57.

36. Niiyama S, Amoh Y, Tomita M, et al. Dermatological manifestations associated with microscopic polyangiitis. Rheumatol Int 2008;28:593.

37. DeVore AE, Jorizzo JL. Cutaneous manifestations. In: Ball GV, Bridges SL, editors. Vasculitis. 2nd edition. Oxford (UK); New York: Oxford University Press; 2008. p. xviii.

38. Knight JM, Hayduk MJ, Summerlin DJ, et al. "Strawberry" gingival hyperplasia: a pathognomonic mucocutaneous finding in Wegener granulomatosis. Arch Dermatol 2000;136:171.

39. Kawakami T, Yamazaki M, Mizoguchi M, et al. Differences in anti-phosphatidylserine-prothrombin complex antibodies and cutaneous vasculitis

between regular livedo reticularis and livedo racemosa. Rheumatology (Oxford) 2009;48:508.

40. Dennert RM, van Paassen P, Schalla S, et al. Cardiac involvement in Churg-Strauss syndrome. Arthritis Rheum 2010;62:627.

41. Neumann T, Manger B, Schmid M, et al. Cardiac involvement in Churg-Strauss syndrome: impact of endomyocarditis. Medicine (Baltimore) 2009;88:236.

42. Merkel PA, Lo GH, Holbrook JT, et al. Brief communication: high incidence of venous thrombotic events among patients with Wegener granulomatosis: the Wegener's Clinical Occurrence of Thrombosis (WeCLOT) study. Ann Intern Med 2005;142:620.

43. Ames PR, Roes L, Lupoli S, et al. Thrombosis in Churg-Strauss syndrome. Beyond vasculitis? Br J Rheumatol 1996;35:1181.

44. Rutgers A, Slot M, van Paassen P, et al. Coexistence of anti-glomerular basement membrane antibodies and myeloperoxidase-ANCAs in crescentic glomerulonephritis. Am J Kidney Dis 2005;46:253.

45. Lindic J, Vizjak A, Ferluga D, et al. Clinical outcome of patients with coexistent antineutrophil cytoplasmic antibodies and antibodies against glomerular basement membrane. Ther Apher Dial 2009;13:278.

46. Hagen EC, Daha MR, Hermans J, et al. Diagnostic value of standardized assays for anti-neutrophil cytoplasmic antibodies in idiopathic systemic vasculitis. EC/BCR project for ANCA assay standardization. Kidney Int 1998;53:743.

47. Robinson PC, Steele RH. Appropriateness of antineutrophil cytoplasmic antibody testing in a tertiary hospital. J Clin Pathol 2009;62:743.

48. Mandl LA, Solomon DH, Smith EL, et al. Using antineutrophil cytoplasmic antibody testing to diagnose vasculitis: can test-ordering guidelines improve diagnostic accuracy? Arch Intern Med 2002;162:1509.

49. Stone JH, Talor M, Stebbing J, et al. Test characteristics of immunofluorescence and ELISA tests in 856 consecutive patients with possible ANCA-associated conditions. Arthritis Care Res 2000;13:424.

50. Savige J, Dimech W, Fritzler M, et al. Addendum to the International Consensus Statement on testing and reporting of antineutrophil cytoplasmic antibodies. Quality control guidelines, comments, and recommendations for testing in other autoimmune diseases. Am J Clin Pathol 2003;120:312.

51. Savige J, Gillis D, Benson E, et al. International consensus statement on testing and reporting of Antineutrophil Cytoplasmic Antibodies (ANCA). Am J Clin Pathol 1999;111:507.

52. Choi HK, Liu S, Merkel PA, et al. Diagnostic performance of antineutrophil cytoplasmic antibody tests for idiopathic vasculitides: metaanalysis with a focus on antimyeloperoxidase antibodies. J Rheumatol 2001;28:1584.

53. Schonermarck U, Lamprecht P, Csernok E, et al. Prevalence and spectrum of rheumatic diseases associated with proteinase 3-antineutrophil cytoplasmic antibodies (ANCA) and myeloperoxidase-ANCA. Rheumatology (Oxford) 2001;40:178.

54. Vinit J, Muller G, Bielefeld P, et al. Churg-Strauss syndrome: retrospective study in Burgundian population in France in past 10 years. Rheumatol Int 2009. [Epub ahead of print]. PMID: 20039171.

55. Castaner E, Alguersuari A, Gallardo X, et al. When to suspect pulmonary vasculitis: radiologic and clinical clues. Radiographics 2010;30:33.

56. Mayberry JP, Primack SL, Muller NL. Thoracic manifestations of systemic autoimmune diseases: radiographic and high-resolution CT findings. Radiographics 2000;20:1623.

57. Ananthakrishnan L, Sharma N, Kanne JP. Wegener's granulomatosis in the chest: high-resolution CT findings. AJR Am J Roentgenol 2009;192:676.
58. Cordier JF, Valeyre D, Guillevin L, et al. Pulmonary Wegener's granulomatosis. A clinical and imaging study of 77 cases. Chest 1990;97:906.
59. Tzelepis GE, Kokosi M, Tzioufas A, et al. Prevalence and outcome of pulmonary fibrosis in microscopic polyangiitis. Eur Respir J 2010;36(1):116.
60. Choi YH, Im JG, Han BK, et al. Thoracic manifestation of Churg-Strauss syndrome: radiologic and clinical findings. Chest 2000;117:117.
61. Kim YK, Lee KS, Chung MP, et al. Pulmonary involvement in Churg-Strauss syndrome: an analysis of CT, clinical, and pathologic findings. Eur Radiol 2007;17:3157.
62. Schnabel A, Holl-Ulrich K, Dalhoff K, et al. Efficacy of transbronchial biopsy in pulmonary vaculitides. Eur Respir J 1997;10:2738.
63. Frankel SK, Cosgrove GP, Fischer A, et al. Update in the diagnosis and management of pulmonary vasculitis. Chest 2006;129:452.
64. Travis WD, Hoffman GS, Leavitt RY, et al. Surgical pathology of the lung in Wegener's granulomatosis. Review of 87 open lung biopsies from 67 patients. Am J Surg Pathol 1991;15:315.
65. Mark EJ, Matsubara O, Tan-Liu NS, et al. The pulmonary biopsy in the early diagnosis of Wegener's (pathergic) granulomatosis: a study based on 35 open lung biopsies. Hum Pathol 1988;19:1065.
66. Stone JH. Limited versus severe Wegener's granulomatosis: baseline data on patients in the Wegener's granulomatosis etanercept trial. Arthritis Rheum 2003;48:2299.
67. Finkielman JD, Lee AS, Hummel AM, et al. ANCA are detectable in nearly all patients with active severe Wegener's granulomatosis. Am J Med 2007;120:643.e9.
68. Lohrmann C, Uhl M, Warnatz K, et al. Sinonasal computed tomography in patients with Wegener's granulomatosis. J Comput Assist Tomogr 2006;30:122.
69. Gubbels SP, Barkhuizen A, Hwang PH. Head and neck manifestations of Wegener's granulomatosis. Otolaryngol Clin North Am 2003;36:685.
70. Bacciu A, Bacciu S, Mercante G, et al. Ear, nose and throat manifestations of Churg-Strauss syndrome. Acta Otolaryngol 2006;126:503.
71. Oliet A, Praga M, Vidaur F, et al. Periglomerular granulomatosis. A limited form of Wegener's granulomatosis with exclusive renal involvement? Arch Intern Med 1988;148:1377.
72. Del Porto F, Proietta M, Stoppacciaro A, et al. Renal limited Wegener's granulomatosis. Lupus 2009;18:567.
73. Rich LM, Piering WF. Ureteral stenosis due to recurrent Wegener's granulomatosis after kidney transplantation. J Am Soc Nephrol 1994;4:1516.
74. Tatsis E, Reinhold-Keller E, Steindorf K, et al. Wegener's granulomatosis associated with renal cell carcinoma. Arthritis Rheum 1999;42:751.
75. Roussou M, Dimopoulos SK, Dimopoulos MA, et al. Wegener's granulomatosis presenting as a renal mass. Urology 2008;71:547,e1.
76. Hauer HA, Bajema IM, van Houwelingen HC, et al. Renal histology in ANCA-associated vasculitis: differences between diagnostic and serologic subgroups. Kidney Int 2002;61:80.
77. Cattaneo L, Chierici E, Pavone L, et al. Peripheral neuropathy in Wegener's granulomatosis, Churg-Strauss syndrome and microscopic polyangiitis. J Neurol Neurosurg Psychiatry 2007;78:1119.

78. Bennett DL, Groves M, Blake J, et al. The use of nerve and muscle biopsy in the diagnosis of vasculitis: a 5 year retrospective study. J Neurol Neurosurg Psychiatry 2008;79:1376.
79. Collins MP, Mendell JR, Periquet MI, et al. Superficial peroneal nerve/peroneus brevis muscle biopsy in vasculitic neuropathy. Neurology 2000;55:636.
80. Claussen GC, Thomas TD, Goyne C, et al. Diagnostic value of nerve and muscle biopsy in suspected vasculitis cases. J Clin Neuromuscul Dis 2000;1:117.
81. Vital C, Vital A, Canron MH, et al. Combined nerve and muscle biopsy in the diagnosis of vasculitic neuropathy. A 16-year retrospective study of 202 cases. J Peripher Nerv Syst 2006;11:20.
82. Wees SJ, Sunwoo IN, Oh SJ. Sural nerve biopsy in systemic necrotizing vasculitis. Am J Med 1981;71:525.
83. Seror R, Mahr A, Ramanoelina J, et al. Central nervous system involvement in Wegener granulomatosis. Medicine (Baltimore) 2006;85:54.
84. Kono H, Inokuma S, Nakayama H, et al. Pachymeningitis in microscopic polyangiitis (MPA): a case report and a review of central nervous system involvement in MPA. Clin Exp Rheumatol 2000;18:397.
85. Tokumaru AM, Obata T, Kohyama S, et al. Intracranial meningeal involvement in Churg-Strauss syndrome. AJNR Am J Neuroradiol 2002;23:221.
86. Reinhold-Keller E, de Groot K, Holl-Ulrich K, et al. Severe CNS manifestations as the clinical hallmark in generalized Wegener's granulomatosis consistently negative for antineutrophil cytoplasmic antibodies (ANCA). A report of 3 cases and a review of the literature. Clin Exp Rheumatol 2001;19:541.
87. Al Dhanhani A, Macaulay R, Maloney B, et al. Meningeal involvement in Wegener's granulomatosis. J Rheumatol 2006;33:364.
88. Nagashima T, Maguchi S, Terayama Y, et al. P-ANCA-positive Wegener's granulomatosis presenting with hypertrophic pachymeningitis and multiple cranial neuropathies: case report and review of literature. Neuropathology 2000;20:23.
89. Greco P, Palmisano A, Vaglio A, et al. Meningeal involvement in apparently ANCA-negative Wegener's granulomatosis: a role for PR3 capture-ELISA? Rheumatology (Oxford) 2007;46:1375.
90. Flores-Suarez LF, Cabiedes J, Villa AR, et al. Prevalence of antineutrophil cytoplasmic autoantibodies in patients with tuberculosis. Rheumatology (Oxford) 2003;42:223.
91. Carlson JA, Ng BT, Chen KR. Cutaneous vasculitis update: diagnostic criteria, classification, epidemiology, etiology, pathogenesis, evaluation and prognosis. Am J Dermatopathol 2005;27:504.
92. Chen KR, Carlson JA. Clinical approach to cutaneous vasculitis. Am J Clin Dermatol 2008;9:71.
93. Carlson JA. The histological assessment of cutaneous vasculitis. Histopathology 2010;56:3.
94. Kluger N, Pagnoux C, Guillevin L, et al. Comparison of cutaneous manifestations in systemic polyarteritis nodosa and microscopic polyangiitis. Br J Dermatol 2008;159:615.
95. Hogan SL, Falk RJ, Chin H, et al. Predictors of relapse and treatment resistance in antineutrophil cytoplasmic antibody-associated small-vessel vasculitis. Ann Intern Med 2005;143:621.
96. Jayne D, Rasmussen N, Andrassy K, et al. A randomized trial of maintenance therapy for vasculitis associated with antineutrophil cytoplasmic autoantibodies. N Engl J Med 2003;349:36.

97. Pagnoux C, Mahr A, Hamidou MA, et al. Azathioprine or methotrexate maintenance for ANCA-associated vasculitis. N Engl J Med 2008;359:2790.
98. Boomsma MM, Stegeman CA, van der Leij MJ, et al. Prediction of relapses in Wegener's granulomatosis by measurement of antineutrophil cytoplasmic antibody levels: a prospective study. Arthritis Rheum 2000;43:2025.
99. Finkielman JD, Merkel PA, Schroeder D, et al. Antiproteinase 3 antineutrophil cytoplasmic antibodies and disease activity in Wegener granulomatosis. Ann Intern Med 2007;147:611.
100. Sanders JS, Huitma MG, Kallenberg CG, et al. Prediction of relapses in PR3-ANCA-associated vasculitis by assessing responses of ANCA titres to treatment. Rheumatology (Oxford) 2006;45:724.
101. Savige J, Trevisin M, Hayman M, et al. Most proteinase3- and myeloperoxidase-antineutrophil cytoplasmic antibodies enzyme-linked immunosorbent assays perform less well in treated small-vessel vasculitis than in active disease. APMIS Suppl 2009;127:60–2.

Clinical Manifestations and Treatment of Wegener's Granulomatosis

Julia U. Holle, MD[a],*, Martin Laudien, MD[b],
Wolfgang L. Gross, MD, PhD[a]

KEYWORDS

- ANCA-associated vasculitis • Wegener's granulomatosis
- Clinical manifestations • Treatment

Wegener's granulomatosis (WG) is a rare autoimmune disorder of unknown etiology that is characterized by granulomatous inflammation and antineutrophil cytoplasmic antibodies (ANCA)-associated small-vessel vasculitis (AAV).[1,2] WG has a broad clinical spectrum that ranges from predominantly granulomatous manifestations restricted to the respiratory tract (localized disease) to severe, life-threatening necrotizing vasculitis affecting many organs, with a predilection for lung and kidney involvement (alveolar hemorrhage and crescentic glomerulonephritis). In WG, ANCA are mainly directed against Proteinase 3 (PR3); there is strong evidence from in vitro studies that ANCA play a crucial role in the mediation of small-vessel vasculitis.[3,4] It has been hypothesized that WG starts as localized disease of the respiratory tract with granulomatous inflammation that later generalizes into small-vessel vasculitis.[5,6] This concept has been endorsed by the EULAR (European League Against Rheumatism)/EUVAS (European Vasculitis Study Group) definition of disease stages[7] to facilitate consistent conduct of clinical trials and to provide evidence-based guidelines for stage-adapted therapy regimens.[8] As a result of EUVAS and other trials, recommendations for therapy for AAV have been published recently,[8] but new data are constantly available, providing evidence for the use of new therapies to reduce treatment toxicity and improve patients' outcome.

[a] Department of Rheumatology and Clinical Immunology, Vasculitis Center, University Hospital Schleswig-Holstein, Bad Bramstedt, Oskar-Alexander-Straße 26, 24576 Bad Bramstedt, Germany
[b] Department of Otorhinolaryngology, Head and Neck Surgery, University of Kiel, Arnold-Heller Straße 14, Kiel 24105, Germany
* Corresponding author.
E-mail address: Holle@klinikumbb.de

Rheum Dis Clin N Am 36 (2010) 507–526
doi:10.1016/j.rdc.2010.05.008
0889-857X/10/$ – see front matter © 2010 Elsevier Inc. All rights reserved.

CLINICAL MANIFESTATIONS
Classification Criteria, Epidemiology, Disease Stages, and Outcome

Incidence rates of 6 to 12 per million per year are reported for the United Kingdom, Germany, and Norway,[9–11] which have been confirmed at stable rates for the United Kingdom and Germany. Lower rates have been found in Southern Europe, such as in Spain (2.95/million/year).[12] In a recent United Kingdom study, the annual prevalence was reported to have increased from 28.8 per million in 1990 to 64.8 per million in 2005,[9] suggesting that survival is increasing due to improved therapy and care. WG is even more common in southern Sweden, with a point prevalence on January 1, 2003 of 160 per million.[13] Additional detailed data on the incidence and prevalence of WG are provided in the article by Holle and colleagues elsewhere in this issue.

Of interest is that a Japanese study reported an overall incidence of ANCA-associated renal vasculitis similar to that in Europe, but all patients were classified as microscopic polyangiitis (MPA); no cases of renal WG and Churg-Strauss syndrome were detected.[14] Nevertheless, there is evidence of WG occurring in Japan as described by Japanese ear/nose/throat (ENT) units.[15] Thus, Japanese patients may show a special phenotype of WG that does not progress to generalized renal vasculitis. Whether this phenotype corresponds to the definition of localized disease remains to be clarified.

According to a concept proposed by Fienberg,[5] WG starts as granulomatous disease and subsequently progresses to generalized vasculitis; this concept has been incorporated in the definition of disease stages introduced in 1995,[16] which has been updated several times. In the current definitions[7] (Table 1), the localized stage, defined as manifestations restricted to the upper and/or lower respiratory tract with no signs of systemic vasculitis, is differentiated from the systemic disease stages (early systemic, generalized, and severe disease). The early systemic stage is considered nonlife threatening, whereas in generalized disease organ function is at risk of compromise. In the severe disease stage, organ failure has already occurred (creatinine >500 μmol/L or approximately 5.7 mg/dL). Definitions of activity stages have also been updated lately and are intended to facilitate the conduct of clinical trials, and are very useful for treatment decisions in everyday practice.[7] Controlled trials initiated by the EUVAS have been performed for remission induction and maintenance for several disease stages in AAV and provide valuable evidence for stage-adapted therapy, and may also have an impact on the outcome of AAV.

Older age (>50 years), kidney involvement (with impaired renal function), pulmonary manifestations at diagnosis, and absence of ENT involvement are associated with an adverse outcome and increased mortality.[17–19] Whereas several studies published in the 1990s showed an increased mortality in WG patients compared with the general population with standardized mortality ratios (SMR) of 3.7 to 4.8,[20–23] a decrease in the SMR at 5 years' disease duration was reported from a recent Swedish population-based cohort of WG and MPA diagnosed before 1996 and after 1996 (from 2.5 to 1.6, respectively).[24] In addition, in a recent study assessing a population of patients with various vasculitides with disease onset in the 1990s, no increased SMR was reported for women younger than 60 years.[25]

The rate of end-stage renal disease (ESRD) varies among cohort studies, ranging from 23% of patients at 15 months to 23% at 10 years.[26] A decline in the rate of end-stage renal failures was reported[24] in a recent study, which may contribute to a reduction of mortality.

Shorter periods of remission induction and the increasing use of intravenous instead of oral cyclophosphamide (Cyc) or alternative treatments may account for a reduction

Table 1
Definition of disease stages in AAV according to EULAR

Clinical Subgroup	Systemic Vasculitis Outside ENT and Lung	Threatened Vital Organ Function	Other Definitions	Serum Creatinine (μmol/L)
Localized	No	No	no B-symptoms ANCA typically neg	<120
Early systemic	Yes	No	B-symptoms ANCA neg or pos	<120
Generalized	Yes	Yes	ANCA pos	<500
Severe	Yes	Organ failure	ANCA pos	>500
Refractory	Yes	Yes	Refractory to standard therapy	Any

Abbreviations: neg, negative; pos, positive.
Adapted from Mukhtyar C, Guillevin L, Cid MC, et al. EULAR recommendations for the management of primary small-vessel vasculitis. Ann Rheum Dis 2009;68:310–7; with permission.

in the cumulative Cyc dose as reported by Eriksson and colleagues[24] and to a reduction of Cyc-related side effects such as infections and malignancy. Using the current definition of remission,[7] this stage is achieved by 90% to 94% of patients, which highlights the efficacy of standard therapy for the induction of remission. Time to remission is usually less than 6 months,[26] but relapse is frequent (18%–40% at 24 months in WG) and remains a major issue: Eriksson and colleagues[24] found no decline in relapse rates in patients diagnosed before 1996 compared with after 1996.

Yet, an increased awareness of AAV may be a factor for improved survival, as a significant shortening of the interval from first symptoms to diagnosis was reported by recent studies.[24,27]

Localized Disease Manifestations/Upper and Lower Respiratory Tract Involvement

Upper respiratory tract involvement affecting the nasal and oral cavity, sinuses, trachea, and bronchi is reported to occur in 75% to 93% of patients at diagnosis[17,28] and in up to 99% of patients during the course of the disease.[17] Rhinosinusitis is the typical manifestation of WG leading to nasal bloody discharge, crusting, and epistaxis. Nasal crusting ("golden crusts") is a typical finding of endoscopic evaluation (**Fig. 1**), although it is not specific for WG. A standardized assessment to rate endonasal activity does not yet exist but is under investigation. Granulomatous inflammation/masses may also be found in the nasal cavity and sinuses, and may lead to bone erosion and cartilage destruction causing saddle nose deformity, which is reported in up to 28% of patients (**Fig. 2**).[17] Conductive hearing loss may be caused by direct involvement of the middle ear mucosa, or by dysfunction of the Eustachian tube due to mucosal involvement of the nasopharynx. The most dreaded granulomatous manifestation in localized disease is orbital granuloma/masses (seen in up to 15% of cases[29]). Orbital granuloma/masses may develop from inflammatory tissue invading from the sinuses, or may develop as a retroorbital mass in isolation. Orbital granuloma/masses are associated with severe complications such as infiltration or entrapment of ocular muscles and impairment of ocular motility, as well as optic nerve compression and atrophy with subsequent blindness. Orbital granuloma/masses are usually unilateral (>80%), but may affect both orbits in up to 14% of patients.[30] Some patients develop orbital

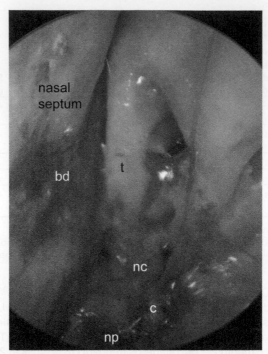

Fig. 1. Endoscopic view of the left nasal cavity (nc) of a WG patient demonstrating crusts (c) and bloody discharge (bd). np, nasopharynx; t, turbinate.

socket contracture, probably as a result of scar formation or fibrosis following immunosuppressive therapy.[31] Orbitonasal fistulas may also develop. Oral manifestations are rare and occur as ulcerative stomatitis (up to 10%[29]) or hyperplastic gingivitis; subglottic stenosis is the typical laryngeal involvement (12%–15%)[17,29]; and stenosis of smaller bronchi and mucosal ulcers of the tracheobronchial tree may also occur.

The overall incidence of pulmonary involvement is between 60% and 85%. The characteristic manifestations are granulomatous masses, alveolitis, and capillaritis, leading to diffuse alveolar hemorrhage (DAH). Pulmonary nodules and/or granuloma have been described on conventional radiography in around 60% of patients.[29] Alveolitis is related to diffuse or interstitial infiltrates. Active disease is associated with an increased neutrophil count in the bronchoalveolar lavage fluid (BAL fluid)[29,32] and diffuse infiltrates; an elevation of CD4+ T lymphocytes may also be found, mainly in conjunction with interstitial infiltrate.[32] DAH has been reported to occur in 7% to 45% of WG patients. Typically, hemoptysis and dyspnea are common symptoms, however, a significant proportion of patients have no history of hemoptysis. Chest radiographs usually reveal bilateral alveolar shadowing (**Fig. 3**); a ground-glass pattern is typically seen on computed tomography (CT). DAH can be confirmed by fiberoptic bronchoscopy, which shows diffuse bleeding arising from the pulmonary parenchyma with increasingly bloody lavage fluid and hemosiderin-laden macrophages. Bleeding may be severe, leading to hypovolemic shock and respiratory insufficiency. Mortality of DAH is estimated at 60%.[33,34]

In general, high-resolution CT (HRCT) may be a useful adjunctive diagnostic procedure to follow pulmonary manifestations. Cavitating nodules/masses with a diameter

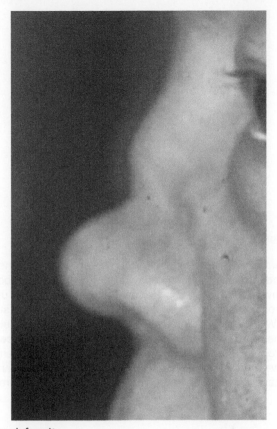

Fig. 2. Saddle nose deformity.

of greater than 3 cm on HRCT and parenchymal opacification are considered active lesions.[35,36]

Kidney Involvement

Glomerulonephritis is reported in 38% to 70% of patients[17,28,29,37] and is the hallmark of generalized disease (**Fig. 4**). Initial renal function may predict renal survival.[22] Approximately 10% to 20% of patients[17,22,29,37] develop end-stage renal failure requiring hemodialysis despite immunosuppressive therapy. Renal involvement/impairment is associated with poorer survival.[26] Diagnosis of renal involvement should be confirmed by biopsy, which usually reveals focal necrotizing glomerulonephritis with both intra- and extracapillary deposits.

Other Organ Manifestations

Most patients suffer from constitutional symptoms such as fever (23%–30% at presentation, 50% during disease course),[29,37] weight loss of more than 10% (50% during disease course),[29] and fatigue (61% at presentation)[37] when presenting with early systemic or generalized disease. Furthermore, musculoskeletal symptoms (arthralgia, arthritis, myalgia; 20%–60% at first presentation, up to 77% during disease course)[17,22,29,37] and ocular manifestations (52%–61%) are frequent complaints.[17,29]

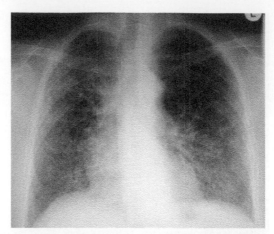

Fig. 3. Chest radiograph of a patient with diffuse alveolar hemorrhage.

Eye involvement manifests predominantly as (epi-)scleritis and conjunctivitis. Dacryocystitis and orbital granuloma may also develop (see above). Peripheral nervous system involvement occurs in 15% to 40% of patients,[17,29] usually as mononeuritis multiplex or sensorimotor polyneuropathy. In a prospective study on patients with generalized WG and standardized neurologic evaluations, most patients (83%) developed peripheral neuropathy within the first 2 years of the disease; symptoms of peripheral neuropathy may be the first signs of WG. Patients suffering from peripheral neuropathy were more often male (61%), older at onset (median age 53 years), had a larger disease extent, and had a higher ANCA titer compared with patients

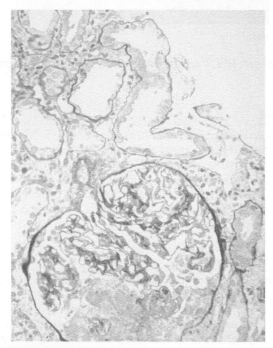

Fig. 4. Crescentic glomerulonephritis.

presenting without peripheral neuropathy. Symmetric polyneuropathy was slightly more frequent (55%) than mononeuritis multiplex (47%) in this study.[38] Skin manifestations such as palpable purpura, vesicles, papules, and subcutaneous nodules are also frequent (30%–46%)[17,29]; digital ischemic lesions or necrosis may develop.

Involvement of the central nervous system (CNS) is not common (7%–11%).[17,29,39] According to Drachman[40] and Seror and colleagues,[39] 3 distinct pathogenic mechanisms of CNS manifestations are described: First, there may be invasion of granulomatous tissue from the sinuses and/or orbit into surrounding tissues, thereby affecting CNS structures such as the optic nerve (by orbital granuloma), other cranial nerves (such as nervus facialis), meninges, and pituitary gland. Second, granulomatous inflammation can develop in CNS tissues itself, for example, in the meninges (hypertrophic pachymeningitis), the parietal bone, the pituitary gland, and the brain. Third, small-vessel vasculitis of cerebral and intraspinal vessels may occur. Pachymeningitis may be completely asymptomatic and develop without any signs of extracranial disease (in up to 40%), but is usually accompanied by chronic headache and sometimes cranial nerve palsies. Meningismus, seizures, limb palsies, and encephalopathy develop in less than 25% of patients. Meningitis of the spinal cord is also rare, but is typically associated with paraplegia. Meningitis may be demonstrated on magnetic resonance imaging (MRI); lumbar puncture usually reveals pleocytosis with lymphocytic predominance and/or increased protein. Granulomatous inflammation of the pituitary gland can induce central diabetes insipidus; manifestations such as intracerebral or subarachnoid hemorrhages, transient ischemic attacks, strokes, ischemic myelopathy, and arterial or venous thromboses may be caused by CNS vasculitis. Diagnosis of CNS involvement in WG may be challenging, as MRI changes and lumbar puncture may yield nonspecific results. Biopsy may be considered in unclear situations.

Clinically apparent heart involvement is rare in WG (6%–20%), but quite frequently reported on postmortem examination.[41] Thus, despite autopsy studies revealing pericarditis and coronary vasculitis in 50% of patients,[41,42] most patients have no clinical signs of cardiac disease. In a small series, subclinical pericardial effusions seen on transthoracic echocardiography were observed in 55%.[42] Tamponade of the pericardium requiring invasive procedures or myocardial infarction are only occasionally reported. Granulomatous myocarditis has been demonstrated in 25% of patients on autopsy; congestive heart failure and dilated cardiomyopathy are only rarely reported to occur. Valvulitis and arrhythmias have been published in case reports.[41,42]

Gastrointestinal manifestations are reported in only a few of the cohort studies[17,43] with rates between 1.7% and 5%; mesenteric vasculitis may lead to serious complications such as mesenteric ischemia and infarction. An overview of organ manifestations reported in cohort studies of more than 100 patients is shown in **Table 2**.

TREATMENT
Remission Induction

Cotrimoxazole (trimethoprim-sulfamethoxazole) is used by some for remission induction (and maintenance) in upper airway disease or localized disease; however, it is less effective in sustaining remission in generalized WG.[44,45]

For early systemic disease, methotrexate (MTX) has been shown to be effective in several open studies[46–50] and one controlled trial (NORAM, nonrenal alternative treatment with MTX[51]). Remission rates of 59% to 89.8% were reported with relapse rates of 37% to 89.8% after 10 to 29 months. Of importance is that the definition of early

Table 2
Organ manifestations developing during longitudinal follow-up of cohorts comprising more than 100 patients with Wegener's granulomatosis

Organ Involvement (%)	Hoffman et al, 1992[29] (n = 158)	Anderson et al, 1992[28] (n = 265)	Reinhold-Keller et al, 2000[17] (n = 155)	Abdou et al,[a] 2002[37] (n = 701)	Stone, 2003[43] (n = 180)
Upper respiratory tract	92	75	99	Sinus: 68 Nose: 51 Ear: 43	90
Lung	85	63	64	62	75
Kidney	72	60	70	38	68
Heart	6	<4	~20	N/A	3.7
Skin	46	25	>30	27	38.5
Central nervous system	8	N/A	<10	N/A	5
Peripheral nervous system	15	N/A	40	N/A	14
Gastrointestinal tract	N/A	N/A	<10	N/A	6.8
Joints	67	29	77	57	81
ANCA positive	N/A	N/A	84	77	73

Abbreviation: N/A, not available.
[a] Percentages are given for organ manifestations at diagnosis.

systemic disease varies among studies, and MTX dose and duration of therapy were variable in the studies, which therefore cannot be directly compared. Early systemic disease is currently defined as nonorgan threatening disease with a maximum creatinine level of less than 120 μmol/L (1.4 mg/dL). In the NORAM study, WG and MPA patients with even higher creatinine values (<150 μmol/L or 1.7 mg/dL) were enrolled. These patients were randomized to receive either oral cyclophosphamide (Cyc; at 2 mg/kg body weight/d) or oral MTX for 12 months plus glucocorticoids. After a follow-up of 18 months, relapse rates did not differ significantly (MTX group 89.8% vs Cyc group 93.5%); however, time to remission was longer in the MTX group in patients with extensive disease ($P = .04$) or pulmonary involvement ($P = .03$). Furthermore, the relapse at 18 months was more frequent in the MTX group (69.5% vs 46.5%) and occurred earlier (13 vs 15 months, $P = .023$), which should be taken into consideration when deciding on an individual patient's treatment in early systemic disease. In general, relapse rates were very high in the NORAM trial, probably as a result of the (early) cessation of therapy after 12 months.

In generalized disease, Cyc has been the mainstay for remission induction for many years, which is currently being challenged by recent preliminary data from controlled trials assessing the efficacy of rituximab compared with Cyc.[52,53] Cyc has been widely used for remission induction since the 1970s and its efficacy was suggested by open studies[54]; there are no controlled trials comparing Cyc with placebo to prove efficacy of this treatment, as this would be unethical. Four controlled trials addressed efficacy and toxicity between oral and intravenous Cyc,[55–58] with a meta-analysis of the first 3 trials also available.[59] In the first 3 trials, similar rates of remission were documented in both arms; however, intravenous Cyc had the advantage of a lower cumulative dose as well as fewer side effects such as infection and leukopenia. The meta-analysis confirmed these findings but also stated that intravenous Cyc may be associated with a higher relapse rate. In the latest trial,[58] CYCLOPS (Randomized Trial of Daily Oral versus Pulse cyclophosphamide as Therapy for ANCA-associated Vasculitis), 149 AAV patients with renal involvement (creatinine <500 μmol/L or 5.7 mg/dL) were randomized to intravenous pulse Cyc (15 mg/kg pulse every 2–3 weeks until remission plus 3 months) or to oral Cyc (initially 2 mg/kg/d until remission, then 1.5 mg/kg/d for 3 months) and then switched to azathioprine (Aza; 2 mg/kg/d plus low-dose glucocorticoid). There was no difference in the remission rate at 9 months (pulse Cyc 78.7% vs oral Cyc 88.1%) and in median time to remission (in both groups 3 months) as well as the development of end-stage renal disease, serious adverse events, and adverse events. There was a significant difference in the cumulative Cyc dose (8.2 vs 15.9 g, $P<.001$) and the episodes of leukopenia. Of note, there were 13 relapses in the pulse Cyc group compared with 6 in the oral Cyc group; however, the study was not powered to detect differences in relapse rates.

Very recent data, which have only been presented in abstract form to date,[52,53] showed equal efficacy of rituximab compared with Cyc, but need to be interpreted with caution as they are preliminary and long-term data are still lacking. The RAVE trial[52] compared oral Cyc (2 mg/kg/d for 3–6 months) for remission induction in AAV (creatinine <4 mg/dL) to 4 weekly infusions of 375 mg/m^2 of rituximab. In both arms, patients initially received 3 pulses of 1 g methylprednisolone, were tapered off glucocorticoids by 6 months, and received azathioprine for remission maintenance for 18 months. Of 197 patients included, 84 patients on rituximab and 81 patients on Cyc completed 6 months. After 6 months, there was no difference in the induction of remission (defined as BVAS/WG = 0 on no glucocorticoids): 64% of patients in the rituximab group and 55% of the Cyc group achieved this primary end point. Therefore, the RAVE trial demonstrates that rituximab is not inferior to oral Cyc in severe AAV for the induction of remission (see the article by Holle and colleagues elsewhere in this issue for further exploration of this topic). Similar results were demonstrated in the RIT-UXVAS trial,[53] assessing the efficacy of rituximab (375 mg/m^2 4 times weekly) plus 2 Cyc pulses compared with Cyc pulses for 3 to 6 months alone (44 patients, 3:1 randomization). Patients in both arms received concomitant glucocorticoids, which were stopped after 12 months; furthermore, patients on Cyc pulse therapy were switched to remission maintenance with azathioprine after 3 to 6 months. In this trial there were no differences in the primary end point (remission at 12 months) (76% vs 82%). From this trial it was concluded that the combined Cyc-Rituximab regimen is not inferior to Cyc pulse alone and that rituximab was efficient in sparing Cyc pulses. Data from these 2 studies provide the first evidence for an alternative, noninferior treatment to Cyc for remission induction of severe AAV. This new treatment option should be especially considered in young patients to preserve fertility. Nevertheless, further studies and long-term data will be needed to confirm these preliminary data.

The efficacy of mycophenolate mofetil (MMF) for remission induction in generalized AAV with creatinine levels less than 500 μmol/L (5.7 mg/dL) has been assessed in a small randomized controlled trial of 35 patients,[60] in which patients received either MMF or Cyc. Surprisingly, complete remission was achieved in 77.8% in the MMF group versus 47% in the Cyc group, and renal recovery was 44% versus 15%, respectively. At present, MMF is being investigated for remission induction in active, newly diagnosed MPA and WG and is being compared with pulse Cyc therapy in a larger randomized controlled trial (randomized clinical trial of mycophenolate mofetil versus cyclophosphamide for remission induction in ANCA-associated vasculitis, MYCYC) initiated by the EUVAS.

Severe (generalized) disease is defined as organ failure, in particular occurring as respiratory or renal failure (creatinine >500 μmol/L or 5.7 mg/dL). Plasma exchange (PE), in addition to standard remission induction, has been shown to improve renal survival compared with methylprednisolone (MP) pulses (MEPEX trial).[61] In 137 newly diagnosed WG and MPA patients with a creatinine level greater than 500 μmol/L, dialysis independence at 3 months was significantly higher in the PE group compared with the MP group (69% vs 49%) and the difference was sustained after 1 year; however, there was no difference in patient survival between the 2 groups. This is in line with former studies,[62,63] which showed benefit in renal but not overall survival in patients with initial dialysis dependence or high creatinine levels. No controlled trials are available with respect to alveolar hemorrhage and PE; however, a retrospective analysis of 20 patients with alveolar hemorrhage who received PE reported resolution of alveolar hemorrhage in all patients.[64] PE is currently recommended by the EUVAS in the treatment of severe renal disease (creatinine >500 mmol/L) in addition to standard remission induction. The British Society of Rheumatology suggests PE be used in the treatment of alveolar hemorrhage.[65] A randomized controlled trial initiated by the EUVAS and the American VCRC (Vasculitis Clinical Research Consortium) to investigate the efficacy of PE in less severe generalized disease (creatinine <500 μmol/L) is currently underway (PEXIVAS trial).

Maintenance

Maintenance therapy is essential because of high relapse rates, which have been documented even under maintenance therapy (18%–40% at 24 months). MTX, Aza, leflunomide (Lef), and MMF have been suggested as options for maintenance therapy in the EUVAS recommendations, mainly based on randomized controlled trials such as CYCAZAREM (for Aza) and LEM (for Lef).[66–68] Shortly after the EUVAS recommendations, the results of WEGENT, a randomized controlled trial comparing MTX and

Aza, were published.[68] In CYCAZAREM (Randomized Trial of Cyclophosphamide vs Azathioprine during Remission in ANCA-positive Systemic Vasculitis), 144 AAV patients with WG, MPA, or renal limited disease in the generalized disease stage (creatinine <500 μmol/L) initially received remission induction with oral Cyc at 1.5 mg/kg/d plus glucocorticoids, and were then randomized (after successful remission induction) to either continue Cyc or to be switched to Aza (2 mg/kg/d). After 18 months, there was no difference in relapse (13.3% vs 15%), renal function, and rate of end-stage renal failure, demonstrating that Aza is a safe option for (short-term) maintenance therapy in AAV. Long-term data from retrospective studies suggest that maintenance with Aza may be associated with a higher relapse rate compared with Cyc, particularly if the ANCA status remains positive, but long-term Cyc is definitely not an option for remission maintenance due to its toxicity. In the future, intermittent use of rituximab may be an alternative for maintenance therapy; this is currently being investigated in the MAINRITSAN trial (Maintenance of Remission using Rituximab in Systemic AAV): After remission induction with oral or pulse Cyc, patients receive either rituximab 500 mg every 6 months or azathioprine 2 mg/kg/d. Recruitment is ongoing.

In the WEGENT study, 126 patients with WG or MPA received either oral MTX or Aza for maintenance after remission induction with intravenous Cyc. There was no significant difference in relapse-free survival and toxicity between the 2 treatment regimens. The data from this study were not included in the EUVAS recommendations, as this study was published later. Based on this study, the authors believe that the level of recommendation and grade of evidence for MTX should be upgraded from level 2b, grade B to level grade 1b, grade A. In a smaller controlled trial (LEM) including only WG patients (64 patients) comparing MTX with Lef for maintenance, the relapse rate was significantly higher in the MTX group (20 mg/wk orally) compared with the Lef group (30 mg/d orally) (46% vs 23%), which led to an early termination of the study.

MMF is not considered in the EUVAS recommendations but may be used for maintenance of remission. However, it should not be considered as first- or second-choice option, as preliminary data from a controlled EUVAS trial (IMPROVE) demonstrated significantly higher relapse rates for MMF (55%) compared with Aza (38%).[69] In uncontrolled prospective and retrospective trials, the use of MMF for maintenance was associated with high relapse rates (48% and 49%, respectively).[70–72]

Cotrimoxazole (trimethoprim-sulfamethoxazole) may be an option for maintenance of upper airway manifestations in WG, but is less efficient in preventing relapse than MTX.[73]

Maintenance therapy should be continued for at least 18 months. The British Society of Rheumatology recommends to continue maintenance therapy for 24 months and, if the ANCA status remains positive, for even as long as 5 years.

Wegener's Granulomatosis Etanercept Trial

The Wegener's Granulomatosis Etanercept Trial (WGET) trial investigated the effect of etanercept as additional treatment to standard therapy during remission induction and maintenance.[74] One hundred and eighty patients were randomized to etanercept; there were no significant improvements in remission rates and time to remission at the end of follow-up. In addition, there were more treatment-related complications in the etanercept-treated patients; 6 patients who received etanercept and standard therapy with Cyc developed solid malignancies. Etanercept should therefore not be used in addition to standard therapy for remission induction and maintenance. No conclusion can be drawn, however, as to whether etanercept may or may not be useful as an alternative treatment by itself for remission induction and maintenance or in refractory disease.

Treatment of Refractory Disease

Treatment options in refractory disease include rituximab and infliximab as well as intravenous immunoglobulins (IVIG), deoxyspergualin, and antithymocyte globulin (ATG); however, most of the treatments lack evidence from controlled trials.

At present, rituximab is probably the most frequently used drug in refractory disease. Sixteen open-label studies on rituximab in refractory disease have been published so far.[75–89] In the largest study[88] comprising 65 patients, 75% achieved complete remission, 23% partial remission, and there was no efficacy in only 2%. Furthermore, rituximab enabled glucocorticoid reduction from a median of 12.5 mg/d to 9 mg/d (at 6 months) and the withdrawal of immunosuppression in 62% of subjects. Nevertheless, relapse occurred in half of the patients who achieved full remission. First reports on the use of rituximab in granulomatous manifestations pointed to a lack of effectiveness,[80] but recent studies report remission rates of up to 80% in granulomatous manifestations such as retroorbital granuloma.[89] Further studies are needed to clarify this issue.

Remission rates of 70% to 88% have been reported from 4 open-label studies of infliximab in refractory AAV,[90–93] but patient numbers were small and treatment duration as well as follow-up was short. Moreover, in the largest study (32 patients),[93] a high rate of infections (21%) was noted. Remission in 13 of 15 patients was observed in an open study of ATG in refractory AAV patients.[94] However, relapse rates and side effects were high (relapse in 7 patients after 21.8 months, infections in 5 patients, serum sickness in 2 patients).

Deoxyspergualin was investigated in 3 open trials,[95–97] with remission rates of 70% to 100% (after 6 cycles of therapy) reported. In the largest study[97] a high rate of side effects and relapses were documented (43% relapse after median 170 days of remission despite maintenance with Aza).

IVIG represents another treatment option. Apart from 3 open studies demonstrating a beneficial effect on AAV, a small randomized placebo-controlled trial (34 AAV patients)[98] showed a significantly higher rate of remission in the IVIG-treated group compared with placebo (15 vs 6 remissions, $P = .015$); however, this effect was not maintained beyond 3 months. IVIG may in particular be used in refractory situations and concomitant infection to treat both conditions.

MMF was efficient in the induction of remission in recurrent, cyclophosphamide-resistant AAV or in patients with contraindications for Cyc, as shown by small open studies.[72,99,100] It should not be considered as a first-line option, because preliminary results of the IMPROVE trial (see Maintenance section) may cast doubts on the efficacy of MMF not only for maintenance but also for remission induction, especially in refractory disease.

Concomitant Glucocorticoid Therapy

Glucocorticoid (GC) therapy is a mainstay of therapy for remission induction and maintenance. For remission induction, prednisolone/prednisone at 1 mg/kg/d is recommended[7] for 1 month, followed by a stepwise tapering to less than 15 mg/d after 3 months of therapy. There are no clear guidelines on the cessation of glucocorticoids; during remission, GC doses should not exceed 10 mg/d. The practice of an early cessation of GC in recent United States studies may be responsible for higher relapse rates (eg, in WGET) compared with EULAR/EUVAS studies. However, no evidence is available from controlled trials to answer which amount of GC is required for safe remission induction and maintenance and when GC can safely be stopped. Patients on GC are recommended to receive prophylaxis against osteoporosis.[7] (See **Table 3** for the EULAR recommendations for treatment of AAV.)

Supportive Care

Exposure to Cyc is associated with an increased risk of hemorrhagic cystitis and bladder cancer,[101–103] which may occur several years after the cessation of Cyc. Fluids and mesna should be administered on the day of the Cyc pulse, as recommended by EULAR/EUVAS,[7] and may also be considered in patients receiving oral Cyc.[7] Monitoring for nonglomerular hematuria and regular cystoscopy in case of hemorrhagic cystitis is useful.[7]

Table 3
Summary of the current recommendation for treatment of AAV according to EULAR

Disease Stage	Treatment
Induction of remission	
Early systemic	MTX 15 mg/wk oral/parenteral, increase to 20–25 mg/wk + GC (level 1B, grade B) Folic acid supplementation
Generalized	Cyclophosphamide IV/oral + GC (level 1A/ 1B, grade A) Duration: 3–6 mo (oral) or 6–9 pulses (IV) (Rituximab may be an alternative)[a]
Severe (Creatinine >500 μmol/L)	Standard therapy for generalized disease + plasma exchange
Concomitant GC	Prednisolone/prednisone 1 mg/kg/d oral Taper to 15 mg/d or less within 3 mo
Maintenance of remission	
After successful induction of remission	Azathioprine 2 mg/kg/d oral (level 1B, grade A) + low-dose GC Leflunomide 20 mg/d oral (level 1B, grade B) + low-dose GC MTX 20–25 mg/wk (level 1B, grade A)[b] + low-dose GC Duration: at least 18 mo
Concomitant GC	Prednisolone/prednisone less than 10 mg/d
Refractory, relapsing and persistent disease	
After failed standard remission induction	IVIG 2 g/kg IV for 5 d Rituximab IV Infliximab 3–5 mg/kg IV 1–2 monthly MMF 2 g/d oral 15-Deoxyspergualin 0.5 mg/kg/d SC until nadir; then stop until leukocyte recovery (6 cycles) ATG 2.5 mg/kg/d IV for 10 d (adjusted to lymphocyte count)

Abbreviations: ATG, antithymocyte globulin; GC, glucocorticoids; IVIG, intravenous immunoglobulins; MMF, mycophenolate mofetil; MTX, methotrexate.

[a] Rituximab is not included in the EULAR recommendations, as results from controlled trials became available later and have so far been published in abstract form.[51,52]

[b] Level 2B, grade B in EULAR recommendations, should be upgraded to level 1B, grade A due to evidence from WEGENT study.[67]

Adapted from Mukhtyar C, Guillevin L, Cid MC, et al. EULAR recommendations for the management of primary small-vessel vasculitis. Ann Rheum Dis 2009;68:310–7; with permission.

As Cyc and GC are independently associated with an increased risk of major infections, close surveillance of patients is necessary. Although rates of infections declined in the 1990s, major infections still pose a common problem. Major infections were documented in 24% of patients in a retrospectively analyzed cohort[104]; bacterial infections, especially pneumonias, herpes zoster recurrences, opportunistic infections such as cytomegalovirus reactivation, and pneumocystis pneumonia were most common. In Europe, the use of pneumocystis prophylaxis with Cotrimoxazole (trimethoprim-sulfamethoxazole) is encouraged[7] in all patients receiving Cyc. It may also be useful for patients on high-dose GC.[104] Mupirocin may be used as topical antibiotic treatment for chronic relapsing nasal activity[7] for *Staphylococcus aureus* eradication, but must be considered carefully, as widespread use may lead to resistance against methicillin-resistant *Staphylococcus aureus*. Apart from medication, patient education is an important issue in supportive care. Preliminary data suggest an increase in the patients' knowledge regarding the disease and its therapy after standardized training increases health-related quality of life, self-efficacy, and patient-assessed health status,[105] even if formal proof of an improved outcome of educated vasculitis patients is still lacking.

SUMMARY

WG is characterized by granulomatous lesions and vasculitic disease manifestations. Granulomatous lesions are found in the upper and lower respiratory tract (eg, granulomatous sinusitis, orbital masses, and pulmonary granuloma), whereas vasculitic manifestations occur frequently in lung (alveolar hemorrhage) and kidney (glomerulonephritis). Vasculitis is typically associated with ANCA directed against proteinase 3. WG has been traditionally associated with a poor outcome and increased mortality, as documented by numerous studies; however, recent cohort studies report an improved outcome. Some studies even suggest that the SMR that is no longer increased as compared with the normal population. The improved outcome is probably a consequence of increased awareness leading to an earlier diagnosis and to improved treatment strategies derived from evidence from controlled trials. The treatment regimen is adapted to disease stage and activity. In generalized disease, Cyc is recommended for induction of remission; preliminary evidence from controlled trials suggests that rituximab may be an effective alternative to Cyc, but long-term data are not yet available. PE should be adjunctive treatment in severe disease. In early systemic disease, MTX may be a safe alternative to Cyc for remission induction. Options for maintenance including MTX, Aza, and Lef or MMF may be considered when other maintenance medications are associated with contraindications or have side effects. It is not clear for how long maintenance therapy is required, but periods from 18 months to 5 years have been suggested. Despite maintenance therapy, relapse remains a major problem in the course of WG.

REFERENCES

1. Fries JF, Hunder GG, Bloch DA, et al. The American College of Rheumatology 1990 criteria for the classification of vasculitis. Summary. Arthritis Rheum 1990;33:1135–6.
2. Jennette JC, Falk RJ, Andrassy K, et al. Nomenclature of systemic vasculitides. Proposal of an international consensus conference. Arthritis Rheum 1994;37(2): 187–92.

3. Falk RJ, Terrell RS, Charles LA, et al. Antineutrophil cytoplasmic autoantibodies induce neutrophils to degranulate and produce oxygen radicals in vitro. Proc Natl Acad Sci U S A 1990;87:4115–9.
4. Calderwood JM, Williams JM, Morgan MD, et al. ANCA induces beta2 integrin and CXC chemokine-dependent neutrophil-endothelial cell interactions that mimic those of highly cytokine-activated endothelium. J Leukoc Biol 2005;77: 33–43.
5. Fienberg R. Pathergic granulomatosis. Am J Med 1955;19:829–31.
6. Mueller A, Holl-Ulrich K, Lamprecht P, et al. Germinal centre-like structures in Wegener's granuloma: the morphological basis for autoimmunity? Rheumatology 2008;47:1111–3.
7. Hellmich B, Flossman O, Gross WL, et al. EULAR recommendations for conducting clinical studies and/or clinical trials in systemic vasculitis: focus on anti-neutrophil cytoplasm antibody-associated vasculitis. Ann Rheum Dis 2007;66:605–17.
8. Mukhtyar C, Guillevin L, Cid MC, et al. EULAR recommendations for the management of primary small vessel vasculitis. Ann Rheum Dis 2009;68:310–7.
9. Watts RA, Al-Taiar A, Scott DG, et al. Prevalence and incidence of Wegener's granulomatosis in the UK general practice research database. Arthritis Rheum 2009;61(10):1412–26.
10. Reinhold-Keller E, Herlyn K, Wagner-Bastmeyer R, et al. Stable incidence of systemic vasculitides over five years: results from the Germany vasculitis register. Arthritis Rheum 2005;53:93–9.
11. Koldingsnes W, Nossent H. Epidemiology of Wegener's granulomatosis in northern Norway. Arthritis Rheum 2000;43:2481–7.
12. Gonzalez-Gay MA, Garcia-Porrua C, Guerrero J, et al. The epidemiology of the primary systemic vasculitides in northwest Spain: implications of the Chapel Hill Conference definitions. Arthritis Rheum 2003;49:388–93.
13. Mohammad AJ, Jacobsson LT, Mahr AD, et al. Prevalence of Wegener's granulomatosis, microscopic polyangiitis, polyarteritis nodosa and Churg-Strauss syndrome within a defined population in southern Sweden. Rheumatology 2007;46:1329–37.
14. Fujimoto S, Uezono S, Hisanga S, et al. Incidence of ANCA-associated primary renal vasculitis in the Miyazaki Prefecture: the first population-based, retrospective epidemiologic survey in Japan. Clin J Am Soc Nephrol 2006;1:1016–22.
15. Aozasa K, Ohsawa M, Tajima K, et al. Nation-wide study of lethal mid-line granuloma in Japan: frequencies of Wegener's granulomatosis, polymorphic reticulosis, malignant lymphoma and other related conditions. Int J Cancer 1989;44:63–6.
16. Rasmussen N, Jayne RWD, Abramowicz D, et al. European therapeutic trials in ANCA-associated systemic vasculitis: disease scoring, consensus regimens and proposed clinical trials. Clin Exp Immunol 1995;101(Suppl 1):29–34.
17. Reinhold-Keller E, Beuge N, Latza U, et al. An interdisciplinary approach to the care of patients with Wegener's granulomatosis: long-term outcome in 155 patients. Arthritis Rheum 2000;43:1021–32.
18. Mahr AD, Girard T, Agher R, et al. Analysis of factors predictive of survival based on 49 patients with systemic Wegener's granulomatosis and prospective follow-up. Rheumatology 2001;40:492–8.
19. Bligny D, Mahr AD, Toumelin PL, et al. Predicting mortality in systemic Wegener's granulomatosis: a survival analysis based on 93 patients. Arthritis Rheum 2004;51:83–91.

20. Matteson EL, Gold KN, Bloch DA. Long-term survival of patients with Wegener's granulomatosis from the American College of Rheumatology Wegener's granulomatosis classification cohort. Am J Med 1996;101:129–34.
21. Lane SE, Watts RA, Shepstone L, et al. Primary systemic vasculitis: clinical features and mortality. QJM 2005;98:97–111.
22. Aasarod K, Iversen BM, Hammerstrom J, et al. Wegener's granulomatosis: clinical course in 108 patients with renal involvement. Nephrol Dial Transplant 2000; 15:611–8.
23. Knight A, Askling J, Ekbom A. Cancer incidence in a population-based cohort of patients with Wegener's granulomatosis. Int J Cancer 2002;100:82–5.
24. Eriksson P, Jacobsson L, Lindell A, et al. Improved outcome in Wegener's granulomatosis and microscopic polyangiitis? A retrospective analysis of 95 cases in two cohorts. J Intern Med 2009;265:496–506.
25. Stratta P, Marcuccio C, Campo A, et al. Improvement in relative survival of patients with vasculitis: study of 101 cases compared to the general population. Int J Immunopathol Pharmacol 2008;21:631–42.
26. Mukhtyar C, Flossmann O, Hellmich B, et al. Outcomes from studies of antineutrophil cytoplasm antibody associated vasculitis: a systematic review by the European League Against Rheumatism systemic vasculitis task force. Ann Rheum Dis 2008;67:1004–10.
27. Takala KH, Kautiainen H, Malmberg H, et al. Wegener's granulomatosis in Finland in 1981-2000: clinical presentation and diagnostic delay. Scand J Rheumatol 2008;37:435–8.
28. Anderson G, Coles ET, Crane M, et al. Wegener's granuloma. A series of 265 British cases seen between 1975 and 1985. A report by a sub-committee of the British Thoracic Society Research Committee. Q J Med 1992;83:427–38.
29. Hoffman GS, Kerr GS, Leavitt RY, et al. Wegener granulomatosis: an analysis of 158 patients. Ann Intern Med 1992;116:488–98.
30. Provenzale JM, Allen NB. Wegener granulomatosis: CT and MR findings. AJNR Am J Neuroradiol 1996;17:785–92.
31. Talar-Williams C, Sneller MC, Langford CA, et al. Orbital socket contracture: a complication of inflammatory orbital disease in patients with Wegener's granulomatosis. Br J Ophthalmol 2005;89:493–7.
32. Schnabel A, Reuter M, Gloeckner K, et al. Bronchoalveolar lavage cell profiles in Wegener's granulomatosis. Respir Med 1999;93:498–506.
33. Haworth SJ, Savage CO, Carr D, et al. Pulmonary haemorrhage complicating Wegener's granulomatosis and microscopic polyarteritis. Br Med J 1985;290:1775–8.
34. Thickett DR, Richter AG, Nathani N, et al. Pulmonary manifestations of antineutrophil cytoplasmic antibody (ANCA-) positive vasculitis. Rheumatology 2006;45:261–8.
35. Reuter M, Schnabel A, Wesner T, et al. Pulmonary Wegener's granulomatosis: correlation between high-resolution CT findings and clinical scoring of disease activity. Chest 1998;114:500–6.
36. Komocsi A, Reuter M, Heller M, et al. Active disease and residual damage in treated Wegener's granulomatosis: an observational study using pulmonary high-resolution computed tomography. Eur Radiol 2003;13:36–42.
37. Abdou NI, Kullmann GJ, Hoffman GS, et al. Wegener's granulomatosis: survey of 701 patients in North America. Changes in outcome in the 1990s. J Rheumatol 2002;29:309–16.
38. de Groot K, Schmidt DK, Arlt AC, et al. Standardized neurologic evaluations of 128 patients with Wegener's granulomatosis. Arch Neurol 2001;58:1215–21.

39. Seror R, Mahr A, Ramanoelina J, et al. Central nervous system involvement in Wegener's granulomatosis. Medicine 2006;85:54–65.
40. Drachman DA. Neurological complication of Wegener's granulomatosis. Arch Neurol 1963;8:145–55.
41. Korantzopulos P, Papaioannides D, Siogas K. The heart in Wegener's granulomatosis. Cardiology 2004;102:7–10.
42. Morelli S, Gurgo Di Castelmenardo AM, Conti F, et al. Cardiac involvement in patients with Wegener's granulomatosis. Rheumatol Int 2000;19:209–12.
43. Stone JH, Wegener's Granulomatosis Etanercept Trial Research Group. Limited versus severe Wegener's granulomatosis: baseline data on patients in the Wegener's granulomatosis etanercept trial. Arthritis Rheum 2003;48:2299–309.
44. Stegeman CA, Tervaert JW, de Jong PE, et al. Trimethoprimsulfamethoxazole (co-trimoxazole) for the prevention of relapses of Wegener's granulomatosis. Dutch Co-Trimoxazole Wegener Study Group. N Engl J Med 1996;335(1): 16–20.
45. Reinhold-Keller E, De Groot K, Rudert H, et al. Response to trimethoprim/sulfamethoxazole in Wegener's granulomatosis depends on the phase of disease. QJM 1996;89(1):15–23.
46. Hoffman GS, Leavitt RY, Kerr GS, et al. The treatment of Wegener's granulomatosis with glucocorticoids and methotrexate. Arthritis Rheum 1992;35:1322–9.
47. Sneller MC, Hoffman GS, Talar-Williams C, et al. An analysis of forty-two Wegener's granulomatosis patients treated with methotrexate and prednisone. Arthritis Rheum 1995;38:608–13.
48. de Groot K, Müller M, Reinhold-Keller E, et al. Induction of remission in Wegener's granulomatosis with low dose methotrexate. J Rheumatol 1998;25:492–5.
49. Stone JH, Tun W, Hellman DB. Treatment of non-life-threatening Wegener's granulomatosis with methotrexate and daily prednisone as the initial therapy of choice. J Rheumatol 1999;26:1134–9.
50. Langford CA, Talar-Williams C, Sneller MC. Use of methotrexate and glucocorticoids in the treatment of Wegener's granulomatosis. Long-term renal outcome in patients with glomerulonephritis. Arthritis Rheum 2000;43:1836–40.
51. De Groot K, Rasmussen N, Bacon PA, et al. Randomized trial of cyclophosphamide versus methotrexate for induction of remission in early systemic antineutrophil cytoplasmic antibody-associated vasculitis. Arthritis Rheum 2005;52(8): 2461–9.
52. Stone JH, Merkel PA, Seo P, et al. Rituximab versus cyclophosphamide for the induction of remission in ANCA-associated vasculitis: a randomized controlled trial (RAVE) [abstract 550]. Arthritis Rheum 2009;60(Suppl 10):S204.
53. Jones R, Cohen-Tervaert JW, Hauser T, et al. Randomized trial of rituximab vs. cyclophosphamide for ANCA-associated renal vasculitis: RITUXVAS [abstract A24]. APMIS 2009;117(Suppl 127):78.
54. Fauci AS, Haynes BF, Katz P, et al. Wegener's granulomatosis: prospective clinical and therapeutic experience with 85 patients for 21 years. Ann Intern Med 1983;98:76–85.
55. Adu D, Pall A, Luqmani RA, et al. Controlled trial of pulse versus continuous prednisolone and cyclophosphamide in the treatment of systemic vasculitis. QJM 1997;90(6):401–9.
56. Guillevin L, Cordier JF, Lhote F, et al. A prospective, multicenter, randomized trial comparing steroids and pulse cyclophosphamide versus steroids and oral cyclophosphamide in the treatment of generalized Wegener's granulomatosis. Arthritis Rheum 1997;40(12):2187–98.

57. Rihova Z, Jancova E, Merta M, et al. Daily oral versus pulse intravenous cyclophosphamide in the therapy of ANCA-associated vasculitis—preliminary single center experience. Prague Med Rep 2004;105(1):64–8.

58. de Groot K, Harper L, Jayne DR, et al. Pulse versus daily oral cyclophosphamide for induction of remission in antineutrophil cytoplasmic antibody-associated vasculitis: a randomized trial. Ann Intern Med 2009;150:670–80.

59. de Groot K, Adu D, Savage CO. The value of pulse cyclophosphamide in ANCA-associated vasculitis: meta-analysis and critical review. Nephrol Dial Transplant 2001;16(10):2018–27.

60. Hub W, Liu C, Xian H, et al. Mycophenolate mofetil versus cyclophosphamide for inducing remission of ANCA vasculitis with moderate renal involvement. Nephrol Dial Transplant 2008;23(4):1307–12.

61. Jayne DR, Gaskin G, Rasmussen N, et al. Randomized trial of plasma exchange or high-dosage methylprednisolone as adjunctive therapy for severe renal vasculitis. J Am Soc Nephrol 2007;18(7):2180–8.

62. Pusey CD, Rees AJ, Evans DJ, et al. Plasma exchange in focal necrotizing glomerulonephritis without anti-GBM antibodies. Kidney Int 1991;40(4):757–63.

63. Frasca GM, Soverini ML, Falaschini A, et al. Plasma exchange treatment improves prognosis of antineutrophil cytoplasmic antibody-associated crescentic glomerulonephritis: a case-control study in 26 patients from a single center. Ther Apher Dial 2003;7(6):540–6.

64. Klemmer PJ, Chalermskulrat W, Reif MS, et al. Plasmapheresis therapy for diffuse alveolar hemorrhage in patients with small-vessel vasculitis. Am J Kidney Dis 2003;42(6):1149–53.

65. Lapraik C, Watts R, Bacon P, et al. BSR and BHPR guidelines for the management of adults with ANCA associated vasculitis. Rheumatology 2007;46:1615–6.

66. Jayne D, Rasmussen N, Andrassy K, et al. A randomized trial of maintenance therapy for vasculitis associated with antineutrophil cytoplasmic autoantibodies. N Engl J Med 2003;349(1):36–44.

67. Metzler C, Miehle N, Manger K, et al. Elevated relapse rate under oral methotrexate versus leflunomide for maintenance of remission in Wegener's granulomatosis. Rheumatology 2007;46:1087–91.

68. Pagnoux C, Mahr A, Hamidou MA, et al. Azathioprine of methotrexate maintenance for ANCA-associated vasculitis. N Engl J Med 2008;359:2790–803.

69. Hiemstra T, Walsh M, de Groot K, et al. Randomized trial of mycophenolate mofetil vs. azathioprine for maintenance therapy in ANCA-associated vasculitides (AAV) [abstract A23]. APMIS 2009;117(Suppl 127):77.

70. Nowack R, Gobel U, Klooker P, et al. Mycophenolate mofetil for maintenance therapy of Wegener's granulomatosis and microscopic polyangiitis: a pilot study in 11 patients with renal involvement. J Am Soc Nephrol 1999;10(9): 1965–71.

71. Langford CA, Talar-Williams C, Sneller MC. Mycophenolate mofetil for remission maintenance in the treatment of Wegener's granulomatosis. Arthritis Rheum 2004;51(2):278–83.

72. Koukoulaki M, Jayne DR. Mycophenolate mofetil in anti-neutrophil cytoplasm antibodies-associated systemic vasculitis. Nephron Clin Pract 2006;102(3–4): c100–7.

73. de Groot K, Reinhold-Keller E, Tatsis E, et al. Therapy for the maintenance of remission in sixty-five patients with generalized Wegener's granulomatosis. Methotrexate versus trimethoprim/sulfamethoxazole. Arthritis Rheum 1996;39: 2052–61.

74. Wegener's Granulomatosis Etanercept Trial (WGET) Research Group. Etanercept plus standard therapy for Wegener's granulomatosis. N Engl J Med 2005;352(4):351–61.
75. Keogh KA, Wylam ME, Stone JH, et al. Induction of remission by B lymphocyte depletion in eleven patients with refractory antineutrophil cytoplasmic antibody-associated vasculitis. Arthritis Rheum 2005;52(1):262–8.
76. Keogh KA, Ytterberg SR, Fervenza FC, et al. Rituximab for refractory Wegener's granulomatosis: report of a prospective, open-label trial. Am J Respir Crit Care Med 2006;173:180–7.
77. Eriksson P. Nine patients with anti-neutrophil cytoplasmic antibody positive vasculitis successfully treated with rituximab. J Intern Med 2005;257(6):540–8.
78. Stasi R, Stipa E, Del Poeta G, et al. Longterm observation of patients with anti-neutrophil cytoplasmic antibody-associated vasculitis treated with rituximab. Rheumatology (Oxford) 2006;45(11):1432–6.
79. Omdal R, Wildhagen K, Hansen T, et al. Anti-CD20 therapy of treatment-resistant Wegener's granulomatosis: favourable but temporary response. Scand J Rheumatol 2005;34:229–32.
80. Aries PM, Hellmich B, Voswinkel J, et al. Lack of efficacy of rituximab in Wegener's granulomatosis with refractory granulomatous manifestations. Ann Rheum Dis 2006;65(7):853–8.
81. Smith KG, Jones RB, Burns SM, et al. Long-term comparison of rituximab treatment for refractory systemic lupus erythematosus and vasculitis: remission, relapse and re-treatment. Arthritis Rheum 2006;54(9):2970–82.
82. Brihaye B, Aouba A, Pagnoux C, et al. Adjunction of rituximab to steroids and immunosuppressants for refractory/relapsing Wegener's granulomatosis: a study on 8 patients. Clin Exp Rheumatol 2007;25(1 Suppl 44):S23–7.
83. Sanchez-Cano D, Callejas-Rubio JL, Ortego-Centeno N. Effect of rituximab on refractory Wegener granulomatosis with predominant granulomatous disease. J Clin Rheumatol 2008;14(2):92–3.
84. Lovric S, Erdbruegger U, Kümpers P, et al. Rituximab as rescue therapy in anti-neutrophil cytoplasmic antibody-associated vasculitis: single centre experience with 15 patients. Nephrol Dial Transplant 2009;24:179–85.
85. Roccatello D, Baldovino S, Alpa M, et al. Effects of anti-CD20 monoclonal antibody as a rescue treatment for ANCA-associated idiopathic systemic vasculitis with or without overt renal involvement. Clin Exp Rheumatol 2008;26(3 Suppl 49):S67–71.
86. Seo P, Specks U, Keogh KA. Efficacy of rituximab in limited Wegener's granulomatosis with refractory granulomatous manifestations. J Rheumatol 2008;35(10):2017–23.
87. Taylor SR, Salama AD, Joshi L, et al. Rituximab is effective in the treatment of refractory ophthalmic Wegener's granulomatosis. Arthritis Rheum 2009;60:1540–7.
88. Jones RB, Ferraro AJ, Chaudhry AN, et al. A multicenter survey of rituximab therapy for refractory antineutrophil cytoplasmic antibody-associated vasculitis. Arthritis Rheum 2009;60:2156–68.
89. Martinez del Pero M, Chaudhry A, Jones RB, et al. B-cell depletion with rituximab for refractory head and neck Wegener's granulomatosis: a cohort study. Clin Otolaryngol 2009;34:328–35.
90. Booth AD, Jefferson HK, Ayliffe W, et al. Safety and efficacy of TNFalpha blockade in relapsing vasculitis. Ann Rheum Dis 2002;61:559.

91. Bartolucci P, Ramanoelina J, Cohen P, et al. Efficacy of the anti-TNF-alpha antibody infliximab against refractory systemic vasculitides: an open pilot study on 10 patients. Rheumatology 2002;41(10):1126–32.

92. Lamprecht P, Voswinkel J, Lilienthal T, et al. Effectiveness of TNF-alpha blockade with infliximab in refractory Wegener's granulomatosis. Rheumatology 2002;41(11):1303–7.

93. Booth A, Harper L, Hammad T, et al. Prospective study of TNF alpha blockade with infliximab in anti-neutrophil cytoplasmatic antibody-associated systemic vasculitis. J Am Soc Nephrol 2004;15(39):717–21.

94. Schmitt WH, Hagen EC, Neumann I, et al. Treatment of refractory Wegener's granulomatosis with antithymocyte globulin (ATG): an open study in 15 patients. Kidney Int 2004;65(4):1440–8.

95. Birck R, Warnatz K, Lorenz HM, et al. 15- Deoxyspergualin in patients with refractory ANCA-associated systemic vasculitis: a six-month open-label trial to evaluate safety and efficacy. J Am Soc Nephrol 2003;14(2):440–7.

96. Schmitt WH, Birck R, Heinzel PA, et al. Prolonged treatment of refractory Wegener's granulomatosis with 15-deoxyspergualin: an open study in seven patients. Nephrol Dial Transplant 2005;20(6):1083–92.

97. Flossmann O, Baslund B, Bruchfeld A, et al. Deoxyspergualin in relapsing and refractory Wegener's granulomatosis. Ann Rheum Dis 2009;68:1125–30.

98. Jayne DR, Chapel H, Adu D, et al. Intravenous immunoglobulin for ANCA-associated systemic vasculitis with persistent disease activity. QJM 2000; 93(7):433–9.

99. Stassen PM, Cohen Tervaert JW, Stegeman CA. Induction of remission in active anti-neutrophil cytoplasmic antibody-associated vasculitis with mycophenolate mofetil in patients who cannot be treated with cyclophosphamide. Ann Rheum Dis 2007;66(6):798–802.

100. Joy MS, Hogan SL, Jennette JC, et al. A pilot study using mycophenolate mofetil in relapsing or resistant ANCA small vessel vasculitis. Nephrol Dial Transplant 2005;20(12):2725–32.

101. Hellmich B, Kausch I, Doehn C, et al. Urinary bladder cancer in Wegener's granulomatosis undergoing immunosuppressive therapy. Arthritis Rheum 2000; 43(8):1841–8.

102. Talar-Williams C, Hijazi YM, Walther MM, et al. Cyclophosphamide-induced cystitis and bladder cancer in patients with Wegener's granulomatosis. Ann Intern Med 1996;124:477–84.

103. Knight A, Askling J, Granath F, et al. Urinary bladder cancer in Wegener's granulomatosis: risks and relation to cyclophosphamide. Ann Rheum Dis 2004;63: 1307–11.

104. Charlier C, Henegar C, Launay O, et al. Risk factors for major infections in Wegener's granulomatosis: analysis of 113 patients. Ann Rheum Dis 2009; 68:658–63.

105. Herlyn K, Gross WL, Reinhold-Keller E. Longitudinal effects of structured patient education programs for vasculitis patients. Z Rheumatol 2008;67:206–10.

Clinical Manifestations and Treatment of Churg-Strauss Syndrome

Chiara Baldini, MD, PhD, Rosaria Talarico, MD, PhD,
Alessandra Della Rossa, MD, PhD, Stefano Bombardieri, MD*

KEYWORDS

- Churg-Strauss syndrome - Clinical manifestations
- Therapy - Vasculitis - ANCA

Churg-Strauss syndrome (CSS) is a systemic necrotizing vasculitis named after the two pathologists, Churg and Strauss, who first described the disease in 1951.[1] In their original work, Churg and Strauss described 13 patients presenting with a clinical syndrome characterized by asthma, hypereosinophilia, and evidence of vasculitis affecting several extrapulmonary organs and identified the disorder as a separate disease distinguishable from panarteritis nodosa and from the other systemic vasculitides.[1] Over time, the clinical picture of CSS has been progressively delineated and classification/diagnostic criteria have been elaborated to better define the particular aspects of the disease. In 1990, the American College of Rheumatology developed a set of diagnostic criteria for the disease, including asthma, eosinophilia greater than 10% on differential white blood cell count, mononeuropathy (including multiplex mononeuritis multiplex) or polyneuropathy, nonfixed pulmonary infiltrates on roentgenography, paranasal sinus abnormality, and biopsy containing a blood vessel with extravascular eosinophils. The presence of 4 or more of these 6 criteria yielded a sensitivity of 85% and a specificity of 99.7%.[2] More recently, the Chapel Hill Consensus Conference defined CSS as an eosinophil-rich and granulomatous inflammation involving the respiratory tract and a necrotizing vasculitis affecting small to medium-sized vessels, associated with asthma and eosinophilia.[3] Finally, CSS has been classified along with Wegener's granulomatosis (WG) and microscopic polyangiitis (MPA) as one of the antineutrophil cytoplasmic antibodies (ANCAs)–associated vasculitides because of the presence of ANCAs, which have been documented in

Rheumatology Unit, Department of Internal Medicine, University of Pisa, via Roma 67, 56126 Pisa, Italy
* Corresponding author.
E-mail address: s.bombardieri@int.med.unipi.it

Rheum Dis Clin N Am 36 (2010) 527–543
doi:10.1016/j.rdc.2010.05.003
0889-857X/10/$ – see front matter © 2010 Elsevier Inc. All rights reserved.

approximately 40% of patients.[4,5] So far, a few large clinical series have been published assessing the clinical features of the disease and the long-term outcome of CSS patients. In all these series CSS has been described as a complex systemic disorder sharing the features of a systemic small-vessel vasculitis and those of an allergic hypereosinophilic disorder, with vasculitis and hypereosinophilia variously involved in the pathogenesis of the different manifestations of the disease.[6,7] From a therapeutic point of view, there is a wide consensus that the use of systemic corticosteroids, in combination with immunosuppressants for the most severe cases, seems to be the effective cornerstone of the treatment of the disease, which has a good prognosis compared with other small vessel systemic vasculitides.[8] This review provides a clinical overview of CSS and a summary of the current treatment as well as novel therapies for the disease.

WHAT HAVE WE LEARNED FROM LARGE CLINICAL SERIES?

CSS is a rare disorder characterized by an incidence of 0.11 to 2.66 new cases per million population per year and an overall prevalence of 10.7 to 14 per 1,000,000 adults.[9–11] The male-to-female ratio ranges from 0.3 to 2.3 and the mean age at the onset reported in the literature varies from 38 to 52 years (range 7–74 years).[12,13] Due to its rarity, the number of published large clinical series of CSS is limited.[14–27] Nonetheless, there is a general agreement in the clinical description of the disease among the different series. The reported frequencies of organ manifestations and clinical features of CSS are summarized in **Fig. 1**.

CSS is usually described as a 3-stage disorder characterized by a prodromal phase dominated by asthma, rhinosinusitis, and nasal polyposis followed by a second phase characterized by peripheral blood and tissue eosinophilia, and, finally, a third, properly defined, vasculitic phase. Although these 3 phases do not necessarily have to follow one another, all the largest clinical series justified their patients' clinical and serologic features on the pathogenetic background of these stages of the disease.[6,12,13] Among the possible clinical manifestations of the disease, a few features have been recognized as distinctive for CSS and

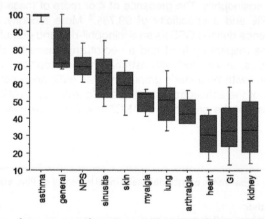

Fig. 1. Frequencies of organ manifestations and clinical features of CSS. The box-and-whisker plot displays the frequencies of CSS clinical manifestations as reported in the literature largest series. Frequencies are expressed in terms of quartiles (Q1 and Q3), statistical median, and minimum and maximum values.

are considered able to differentiate CSS from the other systemic vasculitides and from the other hypereosinophilic syndromes (HESs).

Late-Onset Asthma and Other CSS Distinguishing Features

Asthma seems to be the unifying feature of all CSS patients (96%–100%) and it is the main feature of the prodromal phase. Anecdotally, the development of asthmatic symptoms after the onset of the vasculitic phase has also been reported, but it represents the exception and not the rule.[20,23] The typical latency between asthma and the vasculitic phase of the disease is estimated to last for an average of 3 to 9 years but has been reported as long as 30 years.[14–27] This latency could be explained in part by treatments used for asthma control. For example, oral corticosteroids might partially suppress full-blown vasculitis for long periods of time, leading to forme frustes of CSS, which are unrecognized until corticosteroid tapering.[28] The relationship between leukotriene receptor antagonists and other antiasthmatic drugs with the development of CSS is under debate.[24,29,30] Although some investigators believe these drugs play a causative role in CSS, some believe that antileukotrienes and other drugs, such as the anti-IgE monoclonal antibody, omalizumab, simply make it possible for the patients to taper corticosteroids, thereby unmasking the underlying vasculitic process.[24,29–31]

In comparison with patients with common atopic asthma, CSS patients typically have an adult-onset asthma, which usually becomes more severe with time and is often refractory to the traditional inhalation treatment.[32] Up to three-quarters of patients require oral corticosteroids for adequate asthma control before the diagnosis of CSS.[14] Asthma is often associated with moderate or severe blood eosinophilia. Airway inflammation in CSS may be severe, because eosinophil levels in induced sputum are higher than in asthma.[32]

Asthmatic symptoms might exacerbate, but more commonly decrease, when the vasculitic phase arises.[12,14] Nonetheless, asthma tends to be a persistent manifestation of the disease and is one of the most important factors that negatively influence the quality of life of the patients, even when the other disease manifestations are under therapeutic control.[19–21]

Asthma is frequently associated with allergic rhinitis (47%–93%), nasal polyps, obstruction, and chronic or recurrent paranasal sinusitis (62%–77%) as seen on radiographs or CT scan.[14–27] Nasal polyps, in particular, are widely considered a distinct feature of the disease and may cause the chronic airway obstruction, which is a classic manifestation of damage in CSS.[6,12,14] Unlike WG, however, the presence of nasal pain, crusting, or hemorrhage is uncommon, and, overall, granulomas with eosinophilic infiltrates are less common than symptoms attributable to allergic rhinitis.[33]

The role of common allergens in the prodromal phase of CSS as a common background for asthma and allergic rhinitis is debated. Recently, evidence of respiratory allergy, as demonstrated by specific IgE consistent with the clinical history, was found in less than one-third of 51 consecutive unselected CSS patients. This supports the hypothesis that allergy might be only one of the several mechanisms triggering exacerbation of asthma or upper airways symptoms in CSS.[34]

In addition to upper airway involvement, the lung is a typical target organ in CSS.[35,36] Pulmonary symptoms occur in 37% to 77% of patients and represent the result of a vasculitic process combined with varying degrees of eosinophilic infiltration.[14–27] Transient pulmonary infiltrates with asthma and eosinophilia precede systemic vasculitis in 40% of cases but can occur in the prodromal phase or the vasculitic phase.[14] During the first 2 phases, the histologic picture is generally that of extensive eosinophilic infiltration, whereas during the latter phase, necrotizing vasculitis and granulomas are more common.[12] Bronchial alveolar lavage usually reveals a normal total cell count but with a dramatic increase in the percentage of eosinophils. Radiologically, infiltrates are generally patchy, asymmetric, or diffuse, without lobar or segmental distribution. Bilateral nodular infiltrates can also occur, but in contrast to WG, they rarely cavitate. The most common abnormalities on high-resolution CT scanning consist of bilateral ground-glass opacities and bronchial wall thickening. Infiltrates can be associated with pleural effusion in approximately 20% to 30% of cases.[37]

Another distinctive feature of CSS is the involvement of the neurologic system.[38] Peripheral neuropathy is the most important feature of the vasculitic process in CSS, occurring in up to 75% to 81% of patients.[14–27] Neurologic symptoms may also be the presenting symptoms in approximately 20% of CSS patients.[20] The vasculitic process typically involves the peripheral nerves, resulting in mononeuritis multiplex. Patients may present with sudden weakness or foot or wrist drop along with sensory deficits in the distribution of one or more distal nerves. In some patients, distal symmetric sensorimotor peripheral neuropathies have also been described. The common peroneal nerve and the internal popliteal nerve are the most frequently involved nerves; nonetheless, nerves of the upper limbs (ie, ulnar and radial nerves) might be involved as well. Sural nerve biopsy is the gold standard test in documenting the involvement of peripheral nervous system (PNS) in systemic vasculitis, but pathologic confirmation of necrotizing vasculitis and perineural infiltration of eosinophils and inflammatory cells have been reported only in half of the cases, with axonal degeneration the most common finding. The severity of neurologic manifestations varies, but even when severe, neurologic symptoms usually tend to respond promptly to the standard therapy.[6–38] Some years ago, the authors described the case of a patient with an extremely severe peripheral involvement, tetraparesis, complete loss of strength (the patient was unable to move even in the absence of gravity), and a complete denervation pattern on electroneurography. The patient recovered almost completely after immunosuppressive therapy with only a mild residual motor deficit.[23] Similar data are reported by others, emphasizing that PNS involvement may be dramatic but usually tends to resolve. Among residual minor symptoms, hyperesthesia or neuropathic pain, sometimes associated with mild motor deficit, seems common.[20] Central nervous system involvement is less frequent but has been associated with a significant morbidity and mortality. Central vasculitis may predispose to hemorrhagic cerebrovascular events, especially in association with uncontrolled hypertension. Cranial nerve palsies are infrequent, but involvement of cranial nerves II, III, VII, and VIII has been described. The most common cranial nerve lesion is an ischemic optic neuritis.[38,39]

Other Clinical Manifestations of the Eosinophilic and Vasculitic Phases of CSS

Constitutional symptoms

The early stages of CSS are often marked by general nonspecific constitutional symptoms consisting of malaise, significant and rapid weight loss (>5% body weight), and fever. Diffuse myalgia and polyarthralgia have been also reported in 37% to 57% of CSS patients, especially at the onset of the disease.[12,40] Polyarthralgias have been described as mostly migratory and involving all the joints. Arthritis and synovitis have been reported in a smaller percentage of patients (<20%).[6,13]

Skin involvement

More than half of patients (53%–68%) experience cutaneous manifestations, which reflects the predominant vasculitic involvement of small vessels.[41,42] Palpable purpura on the lower extremities is the most frequent skin lesion along with subcutaneous skin nodules of the scalp and of the limbs, urticarial rashes, cutaneous infarction, and livedo reticularis.[42] The skin is the most commonly biopsied tissue due to the ease of biopsy. Although there are no findings specific for CSS, skin biopsy frequently allows clinicians to confirm the diagnosis in the appropriate clinical setting.[43]

Heart involvement

In their original cohort of patients, Churg and Strauss found myocardial abnormalities in more than 50% of the autopsies, ranging from the extensive replacement of myocardium by granulomas and scar tissue to coronary vessel vasculitis.[1] Myocardial damage might be caused by toxic mediators released by activated infiltrating eosinophils or by vasculitic lesions in myocardium and in the coronary vessels. Myocarditis may lead to postinflammatory fibrosis and restrictive cardiomyopathy or congestive cardiac failure whereas coronary vasculitis may result in ischemic heart disease.[40] The spectrum of cardiac manifestations includes acute pericarditis, constrictive pericarditis, restrictive or dilated cardiomyopathy, myocarditis, arrhythmias, and sudden death. When these manifestations are present, they are associated with a worse prognosis, accounting for approximately 50% of deaths.[8] Considering the potential adverse outcomes associated with heart involvement in CSS, early detection is of clinical importance. Recently, cardiac MRI (CMRI) has been proposed as a useful tool to characterize myocardial involvement in CSS patients with or without clinical symptoms,and is purported to identify histologically proved fibrosis and active myocarditis. The frequency of abnormalities on CMRI is concordant with the reported percentage of myocardial involvement found during autopsy examinations of CSS patients and suggests a high incidence of cardiac manifestations in CSS patients even during remission. It is, however, debated whether or not CMRI should be performed in asymptomatic patients given the high frequency of false-positive CMRI results.[44,45]

Gastrointestinal involvement

Digestive tract symptoms, including abdominal pain, intestinal obstruction, nausea, vomiting, diarrhea, and bleeding are common in CSS patients, reported in up to one–third of cases.[6,12,13,40] From a pathogenetic point of view, these gastrointestinal manifestations may be related to 2 different mechanisms: eosinophilic infiltration of the bowel wall and mesenteric vasculitis. Eosinophilic intestinal infiltration may mimic most of the other forms of eosinophilic gastroenteritis and may precede or coincide with the vasculitic phase of CSS. Submucosal infiltrates can produce obstructive nodular masses, whereas mucosal involvement may result in diarrhea and bleeding.[13] Serosal disease can produce an eosinophilic peritonitis with ascites with the ascitic fluid typically containing large numbers of eosinophils.[46] Small and medium-sized mesenteric vessel vasculitis can cause bowel ischemia and may lead to mucosal ulcerations and possibly perforation, eventually requiring emergency laparotomy.[47] Pancreatitis, necrotizing acalculous cholecystitis, and liver eosinophilic infiltrates have also been reported.[48]

Renal involvement

The kidney is not frequently involved in CSS. Overall, renal involvement occurs in less than one-quarter of CSS patients, far less common than in WG or MPA.[6] The characteristic glomerular lesion of CSS is focal segmental glomerulonephritis with necrotizing features indistinguishable from the other ANCA-associated vasculitis; however, renal disease is considered milder and rarely causes renal failure.[49] Investigators from the United Kingdom have reported higher frequencies of renal involvement in CSS (50%–80%) than other series, and in their experience renal outcome seemed similar to that of MPA. A possible explanation for this discrepancy is that their patients were all drawn from a kidney disease unit.[16] Finally, other renal lesions have been described in CSS, including eosinophilic interstitial infiltrates and IgA nephropathy.[23]

Miscellaneous

Other organ systems may also be affected in CSS. Central retinal artery and vein occlusion, salivary gland enlargement, myositis, and vasculitic involvement of the breast have been described.[50] Patients with CSS also seem to have a propensity for thromboembolic events, similar to that seen in patients with WG.[51]

Clinical Significance of ANCAs in CSS: Just One Disease Entity?

CSS has been traditionally included in ANCA-associated vasculitis together with WG and MPA. The prevalence of ANCAs in CSS is less consistent than in WG or MPA, reported in approximately 40% of cases.[6,12,13,20] The ANCA immunofluorescence pattern is usually perinuclear with specificity for myeloperoxidase (MPO) by enzyme-linked immunosorbent assay. Only a minority of patients have cytoplasmic ANCAs with antibodies to proteinase 3.[12] Recently, it has been shown that different clinical phenotypes could be observed according to the presence or absence of ANCA, thereby suggesting different disease pathogenetic mechanisms in CSS. In 2005, for the first time, 2 different studies, one from the French Vasculitis Study Group[25] and the other from Italy,[26] compared CSS patients' demographic, clinical, and laboratory features according to their ANCA status at diagnosis and described different disease phenotypes according to the presence or absence of ANCAs. Previously, only Keogh and Specks,[24] retrospectively studying 74 CSS patients, had found an increased prevalence of central nervous system involvement in ANCA-positive patients. In all other series, no correlation was detected between ANCAs and CSS clinical manifestations, perhaps due to the small number of patients enrolled.

Sablé-Fourtassou and colleagues with the French Vasculitis Study Group described the clinical and serologic features of 112 CSS patients. Forty-three of 112 patients (38%) were ANCA positive and their positive ANCA status was associated with renal involvement, peripheral neuropathy, and biopsy-proved vasculitis. In the same series, a negative ANCA status was associated with heart disease and fever.[25] Similar results were also found by Sinico and colleagues[26] and published in the same year. ANCAs were present in 35 of the 93 Italian patients (37.6%) included in the study. ANCA positivity was significantly associated with higher prevalence of renal disease and pulmonary hemorrhage and, to a lesser extent, with other organ system manifestations (purpura and mononeuritis multiplex) but with lower frequencies of lung disease and heart disease. ANCA-positive patients also tended to relapse more frequently. Furthermore, in both studies, vasculitis was documented less frequently in histologic specimens from ANCA-negative patients in comparison with ANCA-positive patients.[26]

On the basis of these findings, it has been hypothesized that, as in WG and MPA, ANCAs might contribute directly to the endothelial vasculitic damage in the ANCA-positive subset, whereas in the ANCA-negative subgroup, eosinophils might be directly responsible for tissue damage by the release of harmful cationic proteins, such as the eosinophilic cationic protein (implicated in cardiotoxicity), and the eosinophil-derived neurotoxin.[52] Overall, these data suggest that CSS, when presenting as a form of necrotizing small-vessel vasculitis, is a true ANCA-associated disease characterized by the positivity for MPO ANCAs. Alternatively, the ANCA-negative subset seems clinically characterized by eosinophil tissue infiltration resulting in fibrotic organ damage and seems to belong more to the spectrum of HESs rather than to the spectrum of ANCA-vasculitis. The hypothesis of the existence of 2 subsets in CSS is now indirectly supported by the findings of an increased frequency of HLA-DRB4 in CSS patients and its association with the ANCA-positive disease subset.[53] Although the existence of 2 clinical phenotypes may reveal the existence of different pathogenetic pathways in CSS, it should be stressed, that in these studies, the ANCA-positive and ANCA-negative dichotomy is not absolute and overlap between the 2 phenotypes is common. Moreover, the therapeutic implications in distinguishing these 2 subsets are far from clarified, because ANCA had no obvious effect on remission or survival. Thus, it is premature to propose different therapeutic strategies, according to pathogenic subsets.

CSS Laboratory Features and the Lack of Disease Biomarkers

Apart from ANCAs, many other laboratory abnormalities have been described in CSS.[14–27] Nonetheless, the vast majority of these laboratory features are largely nonspecific and include normochromic normocytic anemia and elevated erythrocyte sedimentation rate (ESR) or C-reactive protein, especially during the phase of active vasculitis. In addition, elevated serum IgE has been observed in up to 75% of patients and serum rheumatoid factor has been detected in as many as 60% of patients.[14]

Alternatively, peripheral blood eosinophilia (>10% on differential white blood cell count or >1.5 × 10^9/L) is probably the hallmark of CSS and may characterize any stage of the disease.[6] At the onset of the disease, the absence of eosinophilia may be explained by prior corticosteroid treatment for asthma. There is sometimes a close association between the degree of eosinophilia and the activity of the vasculitic disease. A rise in the eosinophilic count may precede a relapse of the vasculitis; however, these 2 features may be dissociated and peripheral blood eosinophilia might not recur during relapse.[12] There is also evidence that peripheral blood eosinophils count may correlate with serum eosinophil cationic protein.[54] Overall, despite the fact that hypereosinophilia and eosinophil cationic protein may be hallmarks of CSS, their diagnostic value is limited because they do not distinguish CSS from the other HESs. Moreover, no laboratory tests serve as reliable, feasible, and standardized disease biomarkers that reflect disease activity over time and can guide therapeutic intervention.

CSS, HES, and Other Systemic ANCA-Associated Vasculitis: Elements of Differential Diagnosis

The differential diagnosis of CSS includes several different diseases, mainly HES and the other forms of ANCA-associated vasculitis, such as MPA and WG.

HES is chronic condition characterized by a persistent and sustained peripheral blood eosinophilia, exceeding 1500 cells/μL for more than 6 consecutive months, which is responsible for the development of organ dysfunction or damage.[55] HES shares several clinical and histologic features with CSS. The target organs in the 2 syndromes are similar. The clinical picture of HES might be characterized by lung, cardiac, PNS, gastrointestinal, and skin involvement. The organ involvement and damage is directly related to eosinophilic infiltration; signs of vasculitis and ANCA are completely absent in HES. No clinical manifestations are considered pathognomonic of HES or CSS (**Table 1**).[6,32] Late-onset asthma, however, is rare in HES (even though bronchial hyperactivity may be present) whereas endomyocardial fibrosis is widely considered a more typical finding of HES rather than of CSS.[32] Recently, the diagnosis of HES has been facilitated by molecular biology techniques because specific mutations have been identified in some subsets of this syndrome. The identification of FIP1-like 1 platelet-derived growth factor receptor-alpha in cases

Table 1
Churg-Strauss syndrome and hypereosinophilic syndrome: elements of differential diagnosis

Clinical Manifestations	Hypereosinophilic Syndrome	Churg-Strauss Syndrome
Heart involvement	Endocardial fibrosis, restrictive cardiomyopathy	Pericardial involvement, myocardial involvement Small vessel vasculitis
Asthma	Rare	Almost always present
Sinusitis	Rare	Common
PNS involvement	Rare	Common
Skin involvement	Urticaria	Purpura, urticaria
Elevated ESR	Rare	Common
Elevated IgE	Rare	Common
Biopsy proved vasculitis	Absent	Present (especially in late phase)
ANCAs	Absent	Present in approximately 40% patients

of HES or T-cell antigen receptor rearrangements can be used routinely to differentiate the 2 conditions.[56,57] There is an area of uncertainty that includes patients with CSS without the histologic evidence of vasculitis or ANCA and HES with negative molecular genetic testing. In these cases, it may be difficult to distinguish CSS from HES. Additional research may make it easier to differentiate the two conditions.

As far as other systemic vasculitides are concerned, it is widely known that WG and MPA may involve the same organs as CSS and may also be ANCA positive (MPA is characterized by the same positivity of anti-MPO ANCA antibodies), but the presence of asthma and eosinophilia is uncommon.[6,12] Moreover, in contrast to WG, extrapulmonary lesions are more commonly found in the gastrointestinal tract, spleen, and heart rather than in the kidney in CSS.[1,12,13,40] The typical upper respiratory necrotizing lesions of WG are rare in CSS[33] as well as the cavitations, which have been reported in WG.[58] CSS may cause a pauci-immune glomerulonephritis, which could be similar to WG or MPA, but renal involvement is uncommon in CSS and generally more benign, with few reports of renal failure.[49]

LONG-TERM OUTCOMES AND PROGNOSIS: A BENIGN DISORDER WITH A GRUMBLING COURSE

Before the use of corticosteroids, the mortality rate of CSS was approximately 50% within 3 months of the diagnosis.[8,20,21,59] CSS is now generally considered a mild benign disorder with an overall lower mortality compared with other systemic vasculitides.[8,59] In 2007, the European League Against Rheumatism systemic vasculitis task force undertook a systematic literature review to define specific outcomes in primary systemic vasculitis. According to the reported data, the remission rate in CSS has been reported as approximately 81% to 91%, in line with WG and higher than in MPA (75%–89%), respectively.[60] The relapse rate has been estimated at approximately 20% to 30% (lower than MPA 34% and WG 30%–40%) and seemed to increase with time. Gastrointestinal involvement, ANCA persistent positivity, and a rise of the ANCA titers are reported as risk factors for relapse in CSS. Relapses have been widely described as minor and defined as the occurrence or reappearance of CSS features (for example, fever, arthralgias, and constitutional symptoms) without evidence of major organ involvement. Major relapses, defined as the development of major organ involvement, such as alveolar hemorrhage, abdominal pain, or neuropathy, have been reported less frequently. Exacerbations of asthma or sinusitis, with or without a rise in the peripheral eosinophil count, were explicitly not considered relapses but fluctuating levels of disease activity (grumbling disease). These symptoms were often difficult to verify, persisted for an extended period of time, and were difficult to distinguish from damage. In clinical practice, this low activity disease state usually did not warrant an escalation of therapy beyond a modest increase in the dose of the usual medication or addition of low-dose corticosteroids.[60]

Despite the good prognosis of CSS, in comparison with other systemic vasculitis, many patients with CSS require long-term therapy with corticosteroids for asthma control.[21] This prolonged use of corticosteroids has been reported as responsible for the higher rate of therapy side effects.[21–23] In the series by Solans and colleagues,[22] hypercortisolism, corticosteroid-induced diabetes mellitus, corticosteroid-induced myopathy, osteoporosis with vertebral fractures, and osteonecrosis of the femoral head were observed in 50% of the patients during follow-up. Other damage manifestations were directly related to the disease and included neurologic and cardiac manifestations, such as hypoesthesia of the lower limbs, atrophy and muscular weakness with an abnormal gait, neuropathic pain, and cardiac insufficiency.[22]

Patient survival in CSS has been reported as 93% to 94% at 1 year and 60% to 97% at 5 years (higher than MPA: 82%–92% and 45%–76%, respectively, at 1 and 5 years, and comparable with WG: 85%–97% and 69%–91%).[8,60] Among all the clinical, biologic, immunologic, and therapeutic factors associated with the prognosis of CSS, Guillevin and colleagues[20,21] identified 5 factors responsible for higher mortality: proteinuria (>1 g per day), renal insufficiency (serum creatinine >1.58 mg/dL), cardiomyopathy, gastrointestinal tract, and central nervous system involvement. These factors have become the basis of the so-called five-factor score (FFS), which is a score that defines poor prognosis and higher mortality in patients with CSS. The absence of any of the 5 factors carries a good prognosis (RR 0.52; 95% CI, 0.42 to 0.62; $P<.03$) and the presence of 2 or more increases the risk of mortality (RR 1.36; 95% CI, 1.10 to 1.62; $P<.001$). Of the 5 factors, cardiomyopathy is an independent risk factor in CSS (hazard ratio 3.39; 95% CI, 1.6 to 7.3). Proteinuria (>1g per day) was not associated with poorer survival in a prospective cohort.[60] In addition to disease-related mortality, iatrogenic mortality must also be taken into account and may range from 28% to 47%, usually linked to the adverse effects of long-term immunosuppression.[8,14,15,20,22,60]

In the authors' experience, the mortality rate seems lower than in other series because no deaths were originally reported in their first case series description, and they have registered only 1 death out of 47 patients regularly followed in a 10-year period. This death was disease related and attributable to CSS cardiac involvement.[23]

TREATMENT OF CSS
The Earlier the Better

CSS may be characterized by an abrupt onset and a multisystemic involvement with potentially life-threatening manifestations, followed by a relapsing-remitting course punctuated by minor or major disease flares. Corticosteroids and immunosuppressants, especially cyclophosphamide (CYC), have considerably improved the prognosis and overall survival rates in patients with CSS by controlling the disease manifestations if promptly administered.[6,12,13,40] Corticosteroids, in particular, have dramatically changed the natural history of CSS, being able to inhibit the prolongation of eosinophil survival in extravascular tissues and to effect a prompt reduction of the peripheral eosinophil count to within the normal range in most patients. The induction of remission by early use of corticosteroids and CYC may be one of the most important factors in positively influencing patients' prognosis.[61] Traditionally, the initial management of CSS patients consists of the use of corticosteroids (at a dosage of 1 mg/kg per day of prednisone or its equivalent). For the induction of remission, the administration of methylprednisolone pulses has been limited to the more severe patients, usually in association with CYC, administered by oral or intravenous route, or in combination with other immunosuppressive drugs.[12] In the authors' experience, methylprednisolone pulses in combination with CYC were largely used for the induction of remission in most of the patients and were generally preferred to the daily oral administration of moderate corticosteroid doses.[23] The authors are more inclined to believe that in acute-onset CSS, the early administration of pulse corticosteroid therapy and CYC could be safer and more effective in controlling the disease than the long-term administration of medium or high doses of the same drugs. Methotrexate (MTX) plus low-dose prednisolone has been proposed as a valuable alternative for induction of remission in non–life- or organ-threatening courses and for remission maintenance in CSS. In an open-label study, 11 patients were treated with MTX for induction of remission at initial diagnosis and relapse. Twenty-five patients received MTX for maintenance of remission. Although safe and effective for the induction of remission, the ability of MTX to prevent relapses in this study seemed limited and the investigators concluded that the identification of an optimal maintenance regimen and prognostic factors for treatment response required trials with larger numbers of patients.[62]

The French Vasculitis Study Group conducted 2 randomized controlled trials, one in patients with poor-prognosis factors (FFS ≥1), the other in patients without poor-prognosis factors (FFS = 0) (**Table 2**).[63,64] The results of these trials have shown that in patients without poor-prognosis factors,[63] clinical remission could be obtained with corticosteroids alone, adding oral azathioprine or CYC pulses only in cases of relapse or treatment failure. Corticosteroids alone as first-line treatment induced remission in 93% of the 72 patients included in the study. The proportion of patients in this trial, however, who required second-line drugs for initial therapeutic failure or relapse (35%) was higher than has been previously reported (22.9%–28.1%). Relapses occurred mostly during tapering of corticosteroids and were less frequent after the first year of treatment. Moreover, after a mean follow-up of 5 years, approximately 80% of the patients whose disease was in remission were still taking systemic corticosteroids to control asthma and sinusitis. The investigators concluded that even if remission of CSS in the absence of poor-prognosis factors can be achieved by therapy with corticosteroids alone, other therapeutic strategies aimed at limiting the high rate of relapses and the widespread need for CS over the long term remain to be assessed.

The second prospective multicenter therapeutic trial[64] was conducted in 48 patients with poor-prognosis factors (FFS ≥1) to compare the efficacy of corticosteroids with 6 or with 12 adjunctive CYC pulses for the treatment of severe CSS. This study demonstrated that in patients with poor-prognosis factors, 12 CYC pulses added to corticosteroids were more able to control severe CSS than a 6-pulse regimen, with mild relapses more frequent in the latter group. There was no statistically significant difference, however, between the 2 treatment groups with respect to the percentage of clinical remission, failure treatment, survival, and major relapse. A short-term course (3–6 months) of CYC

Table 2	
Induction of remission, maintenance, and novel treatments in Churg-Strauss syndrome	
	Treatment of Churg-Strauss Syndrome
Induction of remission	*Without poor prognosis*[63] Oral prednisone 1 mg/kg daily for 3 wk, tapering 5 mg every 10 d to 0.5 mg/kg. Then, taper 2.5 mg every 10 d to the minimal effective dosage or, until definitive withdrawal *or* 1 intravenous methylprednisolone pulse (15 mg/kg) *followed by* oral prednisone (as above) *In case of relapse in the first year or treatment failure add:* Oral azathioprine 2/mg/kg daily for at least 6 mo *or* 6 CYC pulses (600 mg/m^2) every 2 wk for 1 mo, then every 4 wk thereafter *With poor prognosis*[64] 3 consecutive methylprednisolone pulses (15 mg/kg) on d 1–3 *plus* oral prednisone (see above) *plus* *either* 12 CYC pulses (600 mg/m^2) every 2 wk for 1 mo, then every 4 wk thereafter *or* short-course of CYC (oral 2 mg/kg for 3 mo *or* 6 CYC pulses [600 mg/m^2] every 2 wk for 1 mo, then every 4 wk thereafter), followed by azathioprine 2 mg/kg for 1 y or more
Maintenance of remission	MTX (10–25 mg/wk) Cyclosporin A (1.5–2.5 mg/kg/d) Azathioprine (2 mg/kg/d)
Refractory disease[a]	Plasma exchange IVIG (0.4 g/kg/d for 5 d) Interferon-alfa (3 million IU 3 times/wk subcutaneously) TNF inhibitors: infliximab, etanercept, adalimumab Rituximab (325 mg/m^2 for 4 consecutive wk)

[a] The following drugs may be considered but have not been proved efficacious in CSS: mepolizumab (anti–IL-5) (5 monthly infusions of 750 mg each); omalizumab (anti-IgE) (0.016 mg/kg per IU of IgE every 4 wk, administered subcutaneously at 4-wk or 2-wk intervals).

followed by maintenance with azathioprine might be equivalent to long-term treatment with CYC in other ANCA-associated vasculitides but has not been formally addressed in CSS. As in other ANCA-associated vasculitides, oral administration of CYC is restricted to the most severe forms, because it has been shown that oral CYC can be efficacious where pulses have failed. The use of CYC (oral or pulses) has also been proposed in patients with mononeuritis multiplex (even though PNS involvement is not part of the FFS) to prevent disability and damage.

The Challenge of Maintaining Remission and Prevent Disease Damage

CSS is widely recognized as a systemic vasculitis with a remission rate higher than WG and MPA. Nonetheless, the maintenance of remission is a challenge and the relapse rate of CSS during the disease course is considerable.[21,40,61] The maintenance of remission is usually accomplished with corticosteroids alone or in conjunction with other immunosuppressants, such as methotrexate, cyclosporine A, or azathioprine, analogous to what is used in WG or MPA (see **Table 2**).[65] It has to be clarified, however, how long to continue corticosteroids or immunosuppressants, which drug to stop first, and how to deal with the minor relapses/grumbling disease manifestations that characterize the clinical course of CSS. Novel therapies could help to spare corticosteroids, thereby preventing the well-known adverse effects (ie, osteoporosis, fractures, hypertension, obesity, diabetes, and cataracts).[66]

Refractory Disease and Novel Therapies

In refractory or frequently relapsing patients, several alternative therapies have been recently proposed (see **Table 2**). Plasma exchange may be efficacious in refractory disease and should be used in cases of rapidly progressive glomerulonephritis or alveolar hemorrhage, which are the most severe expressions of the disease.[61] Intravenous immunoglobulin (IVIG) therapy may also be considered as a second-line treatment for CSS patients, particularly in the case of neuropathy or cardiomyopathy, which are resistant to conventional therapy.[67] There is not much evidence supporting the effectiveness of IVIG in CSS, however, and the mechanisms underlying the action of IVIG remain unclear. Recently, after anecdotal case reports, a prospective open-label trial was performed with interferon-alfa (3 million IU 3 times weekly subcutaneously) for induction of remission in seven CSS patients refractory to CYC. Although data on the mode of action of interferon-alfa in CSS in vivo are lacking, several lines of evidence suggest that it modulates the overproduction of eosinophil-activating cytokines in CSS. Interferon-alfa reduces expression of both interleukin (IL)-5 and IL-13 by differentiated Th2 cells in vitro. Thus, given the overproduction of IL-5 in CSS, downregulation of IL-5-released by activated T cells is a potential explanation for the therapeutic effect of interferon-alfa in CSS.[68]

In addition to IVIG and interferon-alfa, tumor necrosis factor (TNF) inhibitors[69] and rituximab[70] have been used as alternative or adjunctive therapies in small case series. The experience with anti-TNF agents in CSS is limited and consists of isolated reports. Arbach and colleagues[71] treated 3 cases with heart and central nervous system involvement and that were refractory to CYC and corticosteroid therapy. One patient was treated with etanercept and the other 2 with infliximab. This experimental treatment proved effective and safe and induced complete remission in one patient and partial remission in the second and stopped disease progression in the third. Despite encouraging results, there are few published data on the treatment of CSS with anti-TNF drugs Recently, rituximab has been successfully used to treat another ANCA-associated vasculitis, WG. A phase II/III trial was started in the United States in December 2007 for CSS. Two recent reports of bronchospasm during anti-CD20 therapy in patients with CSS suggest that rituximab should be used cautiously in this population, because it might trigger hypersensitivity reactions or could release proinflammatory cytokines that might trigger bronchospasm. In the specific setting of CSS, more experience is needed along with mandatory close respiratory monitoring, especially during the first minutes of rituximab infusion.[72]

Among the novel therapies, a final mention should be made of 2 monoclonal drugs: mepolizumab and omalizumab. The first is an anti–IL-5 monoclonal antibody, which is currently being evaluated for the treatment of severe asthma, nasal polyposis and HES, and eosinophilic esophagitis.[73] Omalizumab is a recombinant humanized monoclonal anti-IVIG E antibody, which is indicated as an add-on therapy in patients with inadequately controlled moderate to severe persistent allergic asthma, despite treatment with high-dose inhaled corticosteroids and long-acting inhaled β_2-agonists.[74,75] In some asthma patients, the steroid-sparing effects of these agents resulted in unmasking of symptoms of CSS, raising concerns about the use of these drugs in CSS. Encouraging reports in refractory CSS have been recently published for both drugs.[76,77]

In conclusion, CSS seems to be a pleiotropic systemic vasculitis that shares many clinical characteristics with other ANCA-associated vasculitis, potentially causing a necrotizing process that can dramatically involve any organs or systems. At the same time, the clinical picture of CSS reflects the pathogenic role of peripheral blood and tissue hypereosinophilia, which can directly contribute to the damage of the main target organs. This dual face of the disease complicates its diagnostic algorithm, making it difficult to start early pharmacologic treatment. Alternatively, if promptly and aggressively treated, CSS has proved a relatively mild disorder characterized by high remission rate and low mortality. Two recent clinical trials have extensively investigated induction of remission in CSS. Nonetheless, maintenance treatment, prevention of relapses, and better control of the grumbling manifestations of the disease are a challenge. It is hoped that the novel therapies that may become available for CSS together with a better understanding of the pathogenesis of the clinical manifestations of the disease might improve the therapeutic armamentarium for CSS, permitting better long-term control of the disease.

ACKNOWLEDGMENTS

We wish to thank Wendy Doherty and Miss Luisa Marconcini for their valuable contribution in reviewing the text.

REFERENCES

1. Churg J, Strauss L. Allergic granulomatosis, allergic angiitis, and periarteritis nodosa. Am J Pathol 1951;27(2):277–301.
2. Masi AT, Hunder GG, Lie JT, et al. The American College of Rheumatology 1990 criteria for the classification of Churg-Strauss syndrome (allergic granulomatosis and angiitis). Arthritis Rheum 1990;33(8):1094–100.
3. Jennette JC, Falk RJ, Andrassy K, et al. Nomenclature of systemic vasculitides. Proposal of an international consensus conference. Arthritis Rheum 1994;37: 187–92.
4. Watts RA, Scott DG. Recent developments in the classification and assessment of vasculitis. Best Pract Res Clin Rheumatol 2009;23(3):429–43.
5. Luqmani RA. Towards diagnostic criteria for the ANCA-associated vasculitides. Clin Exp Rheumatol 2007;25(1 Suppl 44):S57.
6. Pagnoux C, Guillevin L. Churg-Strauss syndrome: evidence for disease subtypes? Curr Opin Rheumatol 2010;22(1):21–8.
7. Chen M, Kallenberg CG. New advances in the pathogenesis of ANCA-associated vasculitides. Clin Exp Rheumatol 2009;27(1 Suppl 52):S108–14.
8. Phillip R, Luqmani R. Mortality in systemic vasculitis: a systematic review. Clin Exp Rheumatol 2008;26(5 Suppl 51):S94–104.
9. Gatenby PA, Lucas RM, Engelsen O, et al. Antineutrophil cytoplasmic antibody-associated vasculitides: could geographic patterns be explained by ambient ultraviolet radiation? Arthritis Rheum 2009;61(10):1417–24.
10. Mohammad AJ, Jacobsson LT, Mahr AD, et al. Prevalence of Wegener's granulomatosis, microscopic polyangiitis, polyarteritis nodosa and Churg-Strauss syndrome within a defined population in southern Sweden. Rheumatology (Oxford) 2007;46(8):1329–37.
11. Mahr A, Guillevin L, Poissonnet M, et al. Prevalence of polyarteritis nodosa, microscopic polyangiitis, Wegener's granulomatosis, and Churg-Strauss syndrome in a French urban multiethnic population in 2000: a capture-recapture estimate. Arthritis Rheum 2004;51:92–9.

12. Sinico RA, Bottero P. Churg-Strauss angiitis. Best Pract Res Clin Rheumatol 2009; 23(3):355–66.
13. Kahn JE, Blétry O, Guillevin L. Hypereosinophilic syndromes. Best Pract Res Clin Rheumatol 2008;22(5):863–82.
14. Chumbley LC, Harrison EG Jr, DeRemee RA. Allergic granulomatosis and angiitis (Churg-Strauss syndrome). Report and analysis of 30 cases. Mayo Clin Proc 1977;52(8):477–84.
15. Lanham JG, Elkon KB, Pusey CD, et al. Systemic vasculitis with asthma and eosinophilia: a clinical approach to the Churg-Strauss syndrome. Medicine (Baltimore) 1984;63(2):65–81.
16. Gaskin G, Clutterbuck EJ, Pusey CD. Renal disease in the Churg-Strauss syndrome. Diagnosis, management and outcome. Contrib Nephrol 1991;94: 58–65.
17. Abu-Shakra M, Smythe H, Lewtas J, et al. Outcome of polyarteritis nodosa and Churg–Strauss syndrome. An analysis of twenty-five patients. Arthritis Rheum 1994;37:1798–803.
18. Reid AJ, Harrison BD, Watts RA, et al. Churg-Strauss syndrome in a district hospital. QJM 1998;91(3):219–29.
19. Lhote F, Cohen P, Guillevin L. Polyarteritis nodosa, microscopic polyangiitis and Churg-Strauss syndrome. Lupus 1998;7(4):238–58.
20. Guillevin L, Cohen P, Gayraud M, et al. Churg-Strauss syndrome. Clinical study and long-term follow-up of 96 patients. Medicine (Baltimore) 1999;78(1):26–37.
21. Gayraud M, Guillevin L, le Toumelin P, et al, French Vasculitis Study Group. Long-term follow-up of polyarteritis nodosa, microscopic polyangiitis, and Churg-Strauss syndrome: analysis of four prospective trials including 278 patients. Arthritis Rheum 2001;44(3):666–75.
22. Solans R, Bosch JA, Pérez-Bocanegra C, et al. Churg-Strauss syndrome: outcome and long-term follow-up of 32 patients. Rheumatology (Oxford) 2001; 40(7):763–71.
23. Della Rossa A, Baldini C, Tavoni A, et al. Churg-Strauss syndrome: clinical and serological features of 19 patients from a single Italian centre. Rheumatology (Oxford) 2002;41(11):1286–94.
24. Keogh KA, Specks U. Churg-Strauss syndrome: clinical presentation, antineutrophil cytoplasmic antibodies, and leukotriene receptor antagonists. Am J Med 2003;115(4):284–90.
25. Sablé-Fourtassou R, Cohen P, Mahr A, et al, French Vasculitis Study Group. Antineutrophil cytoplasmic antibodies and the Churg-Strauss syndrome. Ann Intern Med 2005;143(9):632–8.
26. Sinico RA, Di Toma L, Maggiore U, et al. Prevalence and clinical significance of antineutrophil cytoplasmic antibodies in Churg-Strauss syndrome. Arthritis Rheum 2005;52(9):2926–35.
27. Oh MJ, Lee JY, Kwon NH, et al. Churg-Strauss syndrome: the clinical features and long-term follow-up of 17 patients. J Korean Med Sci 2006;21(2):265–71.
28. Churg A, Brallas M, Cronin SR, et al. Formes frustes of Churg-Strauss syndrome. Chest 1995;108(2):320–3.
29. Nathani N, Little MA, Kunst H, et al. Churg-Strauss syndrome and leukotriene antagonist use: a respiratory perspective. Thorax 2008;63(10):883–8.
30. Bibby S, Healy B, Steele R, et al. Association between leukotriene receptor antagonist therapy and Churg-Strauss syndrome: an analysis of the FDA AERS database. Thorax 2010;65(2):132–8.

31. Puéchal X, Rivereau P, Vinchon F. Churg-Strauss syndrome associated with oma-lizumab. Eur J Intern Med 2008;19(5):364–6.

32. Thomson CC, Tager AM, Weller PF. Clinical problem-solving. More than your average wheeze. N Engl J Med 2002;346(6):438–42.

33. Papadimitraki ED, Kyrmizakis DE, Kritikos I, et al. Ear-nose-throat manifestations of autoimmune rheumatic diseases. Clin Exp Rheumatol 2004;22(4):485–94.

34. Bottero P, Bonini M, Vecchio F, et al. The common allergens in the Churg-Strauss syndrome. Allergy 2007;62(11):1288–94.

35. Eustace JA, Nadasdy T, Choi M. Disease of the month. The Churg Strauss syndrome. J Am Soc Nephrol 1999;10(9):2048–55.

36. Del Pero MM, Sivasothy P. Vasculitis of the upper and lower airway. Best Pract Res Clin Rheumatol 2009;23(3):403–17.

37. Kim YK, Lee KS, Chung MP, et al. Pulmonary involvement in Churg-Strauss syndrome: an analysis of CT, clinical, and pathologic findings. Eur Radiol 2007; 17(12):3157–65.

38. Zhang W, Zhou G, Shi Q, et al. Clinical analysis of nervous system involvement in ANCA-associated systemic vasculitides. Clin Exp Rheumatol 2009;27(1 Suppl 52): S65–9.

39. Ferro JM. Vasculitis of the central nervous system. J Neurol 1998;245(12):766–76.

40. Lamprecht P, Holle J, Gross WL. Update on clinical, pathophysiological and ther-apeutic aspects in ANCA-associated vasculitides. Curr Drug Discov Technol 2009;6(4):241–51.

41. Crowson AN, Mihm MC Jr, Magro CM. Cutaneous vasculitis: a review. J Cutan Pathol 2003;30(3):161–73.

42. Rashtak S, Pittelkow MR. Skin involvement in systemic autoimmune diseases. Curr Dir Autoimmun 2008;10:344–58.

43. Jennette JC, Falk RJ. The role of pathology in the diagnosis of systemic vasculitis. Clin Exp Rheumatol 2007;25(1 Suppl 44):S52–6.

44. Marmursztejn J, Vignaux O, Cohen P, et al. Impact of cardiac magnetic reso-nance imaging for assessment of Churg-Strauss syndrome: a cross-sectional study in 20 patients. Clin Exp Rheumatol 2009;27(1 Suppl 52):S70–6.

45. Dennert RM, van Paassen P, Schalla S, et al. Cardiac involvement in Churg-Strauss syndrome. Arthritis Rheum 2010;62(2):627–34.

46. Pagnoux C, Mahr A, Cohen P, et al. Presentation and outcome of gastrointestinal involvement in systemic necrotizing vasculitides: analysis of 62 patients with polyar-teritis nodosa, microscopic polyangiitis, Wegener granulomatosis, Churg-Strauss syndrome, or rheumatoid arthritis-associated vasculitis. Medicine (Baltimore) 2005;84(2):115–28.

47. Sharma MC, Safaya R, Sidhu BS. Perforation of small intestine caused by Churg-Strauss syndrome. J Clin Gastroenterol 1996;23(3):232–5.

48. Boggi U, Mosca M, Giulianotti PC, et al. Surviving catastrophic gastrointestinal involvement due to Churg-Strauss syndrome: report of a case. Hepatogastroen-terology 1997;44(16):1169–71.

49. Sinico RA, Di Toma L, Maggiore U, et al. Renal involvement in Churg-Strauss syndrome. Am J Kidney Dis 2006;47(5):770–9.

50. De Salvo G, Li Calzi C, Anastasi M, et al. Branch retinal vein occlusion followed by central retinal artery occlusion in Churg-Strauss syndrome: unusual ocular mani-festations in allergic granulomatous angiitis. Eur J Ophthalmol 2009;19(2):314–7.

51. Allenbach Y, Seror R, Pagnoux C, et al, French Vasculitis Study Group. High frequency of venous thromboembolic events in Churg-Strauss syndrome, Wegener's granulomatosis and microscopic polyangiitis but not polyarteritis

nodosa: a systematic retrospective study on 1130 patients. Ann Rheum Dis 2009; 68(4):564–7.

52. Kallenberg CG. Churg-Strauss syndrome: just one disease entity? Arthritis Rheum 2005;52(9):2589–93.

53. Vaglio A, Martorana D, Maggiore U, et al, Secondary and Primary Vasculitis Study Group. HLA-DRB4 as a genetic risk factor for Churg-Strauss syndrome. Arthritis Rheum 2007;56(9):3159–66.

54. Guilpain P, Auclair JF, Tamby MC, et al. Serum eosinophil cationic protein: a marker of disease activity in Churg-Strauss syndrome. Ann N Y Acad Sci 2007;1107:392–9.

55. Roufosse F. Hypereosinophilic syndrome variants: diagnostic and therapeutic considerations. Haematologica 2009;94(9):1188–93.

56. Pugliese N, Bruzzone M, Della Rossa A, et al. Churg-Strauss vasculitis and idiopathic hypereosinophyl syndrome: role of molecular biology in the differential diagnosis of hypereosinophyl syndrome. Reumatismo 2008;60(2):120–4.

57. Tefferi A, Gotlib J, Pardanani A. Hypereosinophilic syndrome and clonal eosinophilia: point-of-care diagnostic algorithm and treatment update. Mayo Clin Proc 2010;85(2):158–64.

58. Manganelli P, Fietta P, Carotti M, et al. Respiratory system involvement in systemic vasculitides. Clin Exp Rheumatol 2006;24(2 Suppl 41):S48–59.

59. Bourgarit A, Le Toumelin P, Pagnoux C, et al, French Vasculitis Study Group. Deaths occurring during the first year after treatment onset for polyarteritis nodosa, microscopic polyangiitis, and Churg-Strauss syndrome: a retrospective analysis of causes and factors predictive of mortality based on 595 patients. Medicine (Baltimore) 2005;84(5):323–30.

60. Mukhtyar C, Flossmann O, Hellmich B, et al, European Vasculitis Study Group (EUVAS). Outcomes from studies of antineutrophil cytoplasm antibody associated vasculitis: a systematic review by the European League Against Rheumatism systemic vasculitis task force. Ann Rheum Dis 2008;67(7):1004–10.

61. Guillevin L. Advances in the treatments of systemic vasculitides. Clin Rev Allergy Immunol 2008;35(1–2):72–8.

62. Metzler C, Hellmich B, Gause A, et al. Churg Strauss syndrome—successful induction of remission with methotrexate and unexpected high cardiac and pulmonary relapse ratio during maintenance treatment. Clin Exp Rheumatol 2004;22(6 Suppl 36):S52–61.

63. Ribi C, Cohen P, Pagnoux C, et al, French Vasculitis Study Group. Treatment of Churg-Strauss syndrome without poor-prognosis factors: a multicenter, prospective, randomized, open-label study of seventy-two patients. Arthritis Rheum 2008; 58(2):586–94.

64. Guillevin L, Cohen P, Mahr A, et al. Treatment of polyarteritis nodosa and microscopic polyangiitis with poor prognosis factors: a prospective trial comparing glucocorticoids and six or twelve cyclophosphamide pulses in sixty-five patients. Arthritis Rheum 2003;49(1):93–100.

65. Jayne D, Rasmussen N, Andrassy K, et al, European Vasculitis Study Group. A randomized trial of maintenance therapy for vasculitis associated with antineutrophil cytoplasmic autoantibodies. N Engl J Med 2003;349(1):36–44.

66. Pagnoux C, Guillevin L. How can patient care be improved beyond medical treatment? Best Pract Res Clin Rheumatol 2005;19(2):337–44.

67. Taniguchi M, Tsurikisawa N, Higashi N, et al. Treatment for Churg-Strauss syndrome: induction of remission and efficacy of intravenous immunoglobulin therapy. Allergol Int 2007;56(2):97–103.

68. Metzler C, Schnabel A, Gross WL, et al. A phase II study of interferon-alpha for the treatment of refractory Churg-Strauss syndrome. Clin Exp Rheumatol 2008; 26(3 Suppl 49):S35–40.
69. Hellmich B, Gross WL. Recent progress in the pharmacotherapy of Churg-Strauss syndrome. Expert Opin Pharmacother 2004;5(1):25–35.
70. Roccatello D, Baldovino S, Alpa M, et al. Effects of anti-CD20 monoclonal antibody as a rescue treatment for ANCA-associated idiopathic systemic vasculitis with or without overt renal involvement. Clin Exp Rheumatol 2008;26(3 Suppl 49): S67–71.
71. Arbach O, Gross WL, Gause A. Treatment of refractory Churg-Strauss-Syndrome (CSS) by TNF-alpha blockade. Immunobiology 2002;206(5):496–501.
72. Bouldouyre MA, Cohen P, Guillevin L. Severe bronchospasm associated with rituximab for refractory Churg-Strauss syndrome. Ann Rheum Dis 2009;68(4):606.
73. Walsh GM. Mepolizumab and eosinophil-mediated disease. Curr Med Chem 2009;16(36):4774–8.
74. Giavina-Bianchi P, Kalil J. Omalizumab administration in Churg-Strauss syndrome. Eur J Intern Med 2009;20(6):e139.
75. Spina MF, Miadonna A. Role of omalizumab and steroids in Churg-Strauss syndrome. J Allergy Clin Immunol 2009;124(3):600–1.
76. Pabst S, Tiyerili V, Grohé C. Apparent response to anti-IgE therapy in two patients with refractory "forme fruste" of Churg-Strauss syndrome. Thorax 2008;63(8): 747–8.
77. Kahn JE, Grandpeix-Guyodo C, Marroun I, et al. Sustained response to mepolizumab in refractory Churg-Strauss syndrome. J Allergy Clin Immunol 2010; 125(1):267–70.

Microscopic Polyangiitis

Sharon A. Chung, MD, MAS[a], Philip Seo, MD, MHS[b],*

KEYWORDS

- Microscopic polyangiitis • Vasculitis
- Antineutrophil cytoplasmic autoantibodies
- Pulmonary-renal syndrome

Microscopic polyangiitis (MPA) is an idiopathic autoimmune disease characterized by a systemic vasculitis that predominantly affects small-caliber blood vessels and is associated with the presence of antineutrophil cytoplasmic autoantibodies (ANCA). Because of its relationship to ANCA, it is often claxssified as a form of ANCA-associated vasculitis, an important subset of the primary systemic vasculitides that includes Wegener's granulomatosis (WG), the Churg-Strauss syndrome (CSS), and renal-limited vasculitis. Because it can lead to both pulmonary capillaritis and glomerulonephritis, MPA is also a prime cause of the pulmonary–renal syndrome, a group of disorders that includes Goodpasture's syndrome (which is associated with antiglomerular basement membrane [GBM] antibodies), systemic lupus erythematosus, and WG. This article discusses the history, pathogenesis, clinical manifestations, and treatment of MPA.

HISTORICAL OVERVIEW AND EPIDEMIOLOGY

Although syphilitic aneurysms had been recognized since the 1500s, the first complete description of a primary systemic vasculitis came in 1866, when Kussmaul and Maier described the plight of Carl Seufarth, a 27-year-old journeyman tailor who had rapidly become incapacitated by fevers, myalgias, renal insufficiency, neuropathy, and abdominal pain. At autopsy, they described "[p]eculiar mostly nodular thickening . . .

Funding: The National Institutes of Health/National Institute of Arthritis and Musculoskeletal and Skin Diseases (1K23AR052820-01). American College of Rheumatology Physician Scientist Development Award. National Institutes of Health/National Center for Research Resources (5 KL2 RR024130-04). Dr Seo is a Lowe Family Scholar in the Johns Hopkins University Center for Innovative Medicine.
[a] Division of Rheumatology, Department of Medicine, Rosalind Russell Medical Research Center for Arthritis, University of California, San Francisco, CA, USA
[b] Division of Rheumatology, Johns Hopkins University School of Medicine, the Johns Hopkins Vasculitis Center, 5501 Hopkins Bayview Circle, JHAAC Room 1B.1A, Baltimore, MD 21224, USA
* Corresponding author.
E-mail address: seo@jhmi.edu

Rheum Dis Clin N Am 36 (2010) 545–558
doi:10.1016/j.rdc.2010.04.003
0889-857X/10/$ – see front matter © 2010 Elsevier Inc. All rights reserved.
rheumatic.theclinics.com

of countless arteries of and below the caliber of the liver artery and the major branches of the coronary arteries of the heart, principally in the bowel, stomach, kidneys, spleen, heart, and voluntary muscles, and to a lesser extent also in the liver, subcutaneous cell tissue and the bronchial and phrenic arteries."[1] Although the significance of these findings, which they dubbed *periarteritis nodosa*, was not immediately clear, this is now widely recognized as the archetypal description of polyarteritis nodosa.[2]

For years after this description, all patients with a noninfectious arteritis were classified as having polyarteritis nodosa. In 1923, Friedrich Wohlwill[3] described two patients who seemed to have a novel form of this disease, characterized by the presence of glomerulonephritis and nongranulomatous inflammation of the small-caliber blood vessels. This "microscopic form of periarteritis nodosa" was gradually recognized as a new entity, distinct from classic polyarteritis nodosa. In 1953, Pearl Zeek[4] noted that this disease was pathologically similar to hypersensitivity vasculitis, preferentially involving the arterioles and venules of the visceral organs (including the lung) but often sparing the medium-caliber blood vessels. In 1950, Wainwright and Davson[5] used the phrase *microscopic polyarteritis* to describe this phenotype.

In 1985, Caroline Savage and colleagues[6] defined microscopic polyarteritis as a small-vessel vasculitis associated with focal segmental glomerulonephritis and hemoptysis. In 1994, the Chapel Hill Consensus Conference proposed the term *microscopic polyangiitis* to describe patients with a small-vessel vasculitis characterized by the absence of immune complex deposition on immunofluorescence, and the presence of pulmonary capillaritis and glomerulonephritis.[7] The new name emphasized the differences between this phenomenon and classic polyarteritis nodosa, which was defined as a medium-vessel vasculitis that spared the arterioles and venules.

Despite this clear distinction, distinguishing these two phenomena clinically is not always straightforward; the classic description of polyarteritis nodosa by Kussmaul and Maier,[8] for example, includes evidence of a small-vessel vasculitis. Moreover, the Chapel Hill Consensus Conference criteria do not always clearly distinguish MPA from other forms of vasculitis, such as WG.[9] Regardless, the introduction of this nomenclature resulted in a rapid reduction in the prevalence of polyarteritis nodosa, because many of these patients were reclassified as having MPA.[10]

In 1954, Godman and Churg[11] noted that the "microscopic form of periarteritis" was closely related to WG and CSS. In the ensuing years, it gradually became clear that these three forms of systemic vasculitis were also linked by the presence of anticytoplasmic antibodies directed against neutrophils. ANCA were first reported in association with focal segmental glomerulonephritis in the 1980s.[12] Subsequent work showed that these antibodies were associated with distinct staining patterns when alcohol-fixed neutrophils were used as a substrate. In 1988, Jennette and Falk[13] reported that serum from patients with WG, renal-limited vasculitis, and MPA was associated with antibodies that created a perinuclear staining pattern (p-ANCA). This p-ANCA pattern is caused by antibodies against myeloperoxidase (MPO). Some authors have suggested that MPO-ANCA be used to distinguish MPA from polyarteritis nodosa,[14] although these antibodies are also found in other forms of vasculitis, including drug-induced ANCA-associated vasculitis, CSS, and WG.

Regardless, ANCA has become a useful tool for the diagnosis of vasculitis, and may be partially responsible for the perceived increase in prevalence of the primary systemic vasculitides.[15] Southern Sweden has the highest reported prevalence of MPA, with 94 cases per million.[16] Overall, however, the incidence of MPA is higher in southern Europe than in northern Europe; for example, the incidence of MPA in Norway is 2.7 per million,[17] but 11.6 per million in Spain (**Table 1**).[18] The incidence

Table 1 Incidence of microscopic polyangiitis in Europe	
	Cases Per Million Population
Norway	2.7
United Kingdom	5.8
Germany	2.6
Spain	11.6

Data from Lane SE, Watts R, Scott DG. Epidemiology of systemic vasculitis. Curr Rheumatol Rep 2005;7(4):270–5.

and prevalence of MPA in other parts of the world is less clear, but the prevalence seems to be higher in European populations.[19]

PATHOGENESIS

Growing evidence indicates that ANCA play a role in the pathogenesis of MPA. In theory, this might occur in two steps. In the first step, neutrophils are primed by exposure to low levels of proinflammatory cytokines, such as interleukin-1 or tumor necrosis factor-α.[20] This process leads to surface expression of MPO, followed by adherence of neutrophils to the endothelial surface of blood vessels or glomeruli. In the second step, neutrophils are activated by interaction with MPO-ANCA, either through binding of its substrate[21] or interaction with neutrophil Fc receptors.[22]

Two animal models support a potential role for MPO-ANCA in the pathogenesis of MPA,[23,24] showing that MPO-ANCA are sufficient to induce pulmonary capillaritis and glomerulonephritis given the correct biologic milieu. Also in support of this role is a case report describing pulmonary hemorrhage and renal insufficiency in a newborn infant, presumably mediated by passage of MPO-ANCA from mother to fetus.[25] A subsequent case report, however, documents that placental transmission of MPO-ANCA is not sufficient to induce disease.[26] The development of vasculitis likely requires the presence of several cofactors, including genetic predisposition, in order for ANCA to be pathogenic.

This model fails to address the substantial number of patients who are ANCA-negative at diagnosis.[27] Not all patients with active vasculitis are ANCA-positive, and MPO-ANCA titers themselves correlate poorly with disease activity in MPA. These observations imply that ANCA are not essential to pathogenesis in all patients with MPA, or that more than one mechanism can lead to the same clinical diagnosis. For example, recent work indicates that ANCA directed against lysosomal membrane protein-2 (LAMP-2), possibly induced by exposure to FimH-expressing gram-negative bacteria, may play a key role in the development of vasculitis in some patients[28] (although this work has not yet been widely replicated).

CLINICAL FEATURES

MPA has a slight male predominance (male:female ratio of 1.8:1),[14,29,30] with an average age of onset between 50 and 60 years.[14,19,29] As expected for an illness that affects multiple organ systems, patients with MPA can present with a myriad of different symptoms. However, more than 70% of patients have constitutional symptoms, such as fever or weight loss at diagnosis.[6,29] Patients can present acutely (ie, experiencing symptoms from days to weeks) or have an indolent course before diagnosis. For example, nonspecific symptoms such as a flu-like illness[6] or arthralgias can be present for months to years before diagnosis.[30] This section discusses the major clinical manifestations of MPA, presented by organ system.

Renal Manifestations

Renal involvement, characterized by rapidly progressive glomerulonephritis (RPGN), is the major clinical feature of MPA. Previous studies report that 80% to 100% of patients with MPA experience renal manifestations,[6,14] which can range from an asymptomatic urinary sediment to end-stage renal disease requiring dialysis.[30] Consistent with glomerulonephritis, the most common clinical manifestations of renal involvement are proteinuria (in the nephrotic range in up to 50% of patients), microscopic hematuria, and urinary granular or red blood cell casts.[6]

The hallmark finding on renal biopsy is focal segmental necrotizing glomerulonephritis, which is seen in up to 100% of patients with renal involvement (**Fig. 1**).[6] Glomerular crescents are also common, and can be present in approximately 90% of patients.[6] Frank vasculitis and fibrinoid necrosis are seen less frequently, and are observed in fewer than 20% of patients.[6] Areas away from the glomeruli also can be affected; for example, interstitial nephritis and tubular atrophy are seen in approximately half of the patients with MPA.[6] Immunofluorescence shows minimal deposition of immunoglobulins or complement in the glomeruli and renal vessels (hence the descriptive term *pauci-immune*), unlike other forms of small-vessel vasculitis, such as Henoch-Schönlein purpura, cryoglobulinemic vasculitis, or anti-GBM disease.[31] The changes seen on renal biopsy are similar for the three ANCA-associated vasculitides (MPA, WG, and CSS), and thus cannot be used to distinguish among these entities.

The mainstay of treatment for renal involvement in MPA is glucocorticoids and cyclophosphamide. With this therapy, approximately 90% of patients experience a complete or partial remission.[32] However, despite immunosuppression, approximately 20% of patients in one series progressed to end-stage renal disease and required renal replacement therapy, either in the form of kidney transplant or dialysis. Not surprisingly, a low serum creatinine at diagnosis in this group predicted a better renal survival rate.[32]

ANCA and anti-GBM antibodies can coexist. Approximately 30% of patients with anti-GBM antibodies have circulating ANCA.[33,34] Conversely, a lower percentage (5%–14%) of patients with a positive ANCA test have evidence of anti-GBM

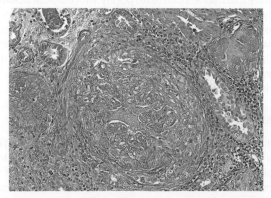

Fig. 1. Crescentic glomerulonephritis in a patient with microscopic polyangiitis (hematoxylin and eosin stain).

antibodies.[33,35] In patients with concurrent ANCA and anti-GBM antibodies, most of the ANCA are directed against MPO (66%–100%).[33-35]

In a series of 22 patients with both antibodies who underwent renal biopsy, all showed linear deposition of IgG and C3 on immunofluorescence. Of the 22 biopsies, 4 (18.2%) also showed granular deposition of IgG, IgM, and C3. Patients with both ANCA and anti-GBM antibodies are sometimes treated with plasma exchange in addition to conventional immunouppression.[33] Studies of whether these double-positive patients have worse renal outcomes than those with only ANCA or anti-GBM antibodies have conflicting results.[33] Some suggest that these patients are more likely to experience relapse than those with anti-GBM antibodies alone.[34,36] Regardless, lower serum creatinine at diagnosis is associated with an increased renal survival rate.[33]

Pulmonary Manifestations

Pulmonary involvement can be seen in 25% to 55% of patients. Manifestations include hemoptysis and alveolar hemorrhage, infiltrates, pleural effusion, pulmonary edema, pleuritis, and interstitial fibrosis.[6,14,30] The classic pulmonary manifestation of MPA is diffuse alveolar hemorrhage caused by pulmonary capillaritis, which has been reported in 12% to 55% of patients.[37-39] Common presenting symptoms of alveolar hemorrhage include dyspnea, cough, hemoptysis, and pleuritic chest pain.[40]

In patients with alveolar hemorrhage, chest radiographs show patchy, bilateral airspace opacities, usually involving the upper and lower lung fields.[37,39] The most common finding on CT is ground-glass attenuation (seen in >90% of patients), which corresponds to alveolar hemorrhage, interstitial chronic inflammation of the alveolar septa, and capillaritis (**Fig. 2**). Consolidation is seen in approximately 80% of patients with pulmonary involvement. Thickening of the bronchovascular bundles and honeycombing are also observed.[37,39]

Patients often undergo bronchoscopy to evaluate the cause of bleeding. For patients with alveolar hemorrhage, bronchoalveolar lavage (BAL) fluid is usually grossly hemorrhagic, and on sequential lavage the fluid remains bloody.[37,39,41] Perls Prussian blue staining of the BAL fluid shows elevated numbers of hemosiderin-laden macrophages, which are present in more than 30% of patients with MPA.[37,39]

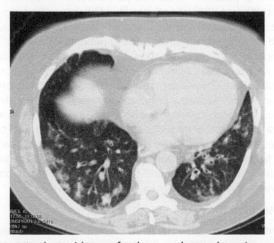

Fig. 2. CT scan demonstrating evidence of pulmonary hemorrhage in a patient with microscopic polyangiitis.

Biopsy of areas of the lung demonstrating alveolar hemorrhage can show intra-alveolar and interstitial red blood cells; pauci-immune, hemorrhagic, necrotizing alveolar capillaritis;[38] neutrophilic infiltration resulting in fibrinoid necrosis and dissolution of the arterial and venular walls;[41] and intra-alveolar hemosideroisis.[37] Granulomatous inflammation is usually not observed in MPA and its presence suggests an alternative diagnosis, such as WG.

Pulmonary function testing can show either restrictive or obstructive patterns. The most frequent abnormality is reduced carbon monoxide diffusing capacity, which can increase dramatically during active alveolar hemorrhage.[38]

Treatment options for patients with alveolar hemorrhage from MPA include aggressive immunosuppression and plasma exchange.[39] In severe cases, mechanical ventilation can be required to maintain oxygenation. A few case reports show successful use of extracorporeal membrane oxygenation.[39] However, alveolar hemorrhage is associated with a worse prognosis in patients with MPA. Patients with pulmonary hemorrhage are nine times more likely to die and have higher rates of relapse.[39]

Given the predominance of pulmonary and renal manifestations in MPA, MPA is a well-recognized cause of pulmonary–renal syndromes, along with other autoimmune diseases such as WG, anti-GBM disease, and systemic lupus erythematosus. One study suggests that MPA is the most common cause of pulmonary–renal syndromes.[42]

Pulmonary fibrosis is a less well-recognized pulmonary manifestation of MPA.[43–45] Fibrosis can present months to years before, at, or years after the diagnosis of MPA.[45,46] Although the cause of the fibrosis is unclear, chronic subclinical alveolar hemorrhage has been presented as a possible cause.[44] The prognosis for patients with pulmonary fibrosis is poor[45] but may be improved by the institution of immunosuppressive agents.[38,44]

More unusual pulmonary manifestations attributed to MPA include pulmonary artery aneurysms[47] and panbronchiolitis.[48]

Skin Manifestations

Skin lesions are found in 30% to 60% of patients,[6,14,30,49] and are the initial presenting sign in 15% to 30% of patients.[49] Palpable purpura is the most common manifestation, and occurs in 30% to 40% of patients.[49,50] Other manifestations include livedo reticularis, nodules, urticaria, and skin ulcers with necrosis.[49] Dermatologic manifestations have been associated with arthralgias in patients with MPA.[49]

Biopsies of palpable purpura often show leukocytoclastic vasculitis, with neutrophilic infiltration of the small-caliber vessels in the superficial dermis, fibrinoid necrosis, and nuclear dust.[50] However, a nonspecific perivascular lymphocytic infiltration can also be seen.[49,51] Biopsies of cutaneous nodules generally show vasculitis involving vessels of the deep dermis or subcutis.[49] Immunofluorescence studies are generally negative or show few deposits of immunoglobulins and complement.[49,51] Although nodules are seen more frequently in polyarteritis nodosa, and palpable purpura is more frequent in MPA, both dermatologic manifestations occur in both diseases. Thus, these manifestations and their histologic findings cannot be used to differentiate between polyarteritis nodosa and MPA.

Gastrointestinal Manifestations

The most frequently reported gastrointestinal symptom in MPA is abdominal pain,[52] which can occur in 30% to 58% of patients.[14,30] Although gastrointestinal bleeding occurs in up to 21% to 29% of patients,[52,53] massive hemorrhage is rare.[54]

Angiographic studies, although not routinely performed, have shown arterial aneur-syms[54,55] as a potential source of bleeding. Other gastrointestinal manifestations have been reported, such as colonic ulcerations,[56] intestinal ischemia,[52,57] and bowel perforation.[52] However, they are likely less frequent in MPA than in polyarteritis nodosa, because the published literature reflects fewer reports of these manifestations in patients with MPA.

Involvement of the liver occurs rarely in MPA. Liver dysfunction in MPA may present as elevated liver enzymes, with alkaline phosphatase and γ-glutamyl transferase more affected than aspartate or alanine transaminase. These abnormal findings can precede the development of glomerulonephritis or pulmonary hemorrhage.[58–61] Histologic findings from liver biopsies performed from these cases have shown fibrinoid degeneration of an interlobular arteriole[60] and necrotizing arteritis and lymphocytic infiltration of portal tracts.[61] In addition, primary biliary cirrhosis has been reported in patients with MPA,[62,63] but whether the association is causal is unknown.

Neurologic Manifestations

Neurologic involvement in MPA is common, and affects between 37% and 72% of patients.[14,29,64] Peripheral neuropathy occurs more frequently than central nervous system involvement, with mononeuritis multiplex and distal symmetric polyneuropathy as the predominant peripheral nervous system manifestations. Necrotizing vasculitis can be seen on sural nerve biopsy in up to 80% of affected patients, and nerve conduction studies typically show acute axonopathy.[65] Some studies suggest that relapse rates of peripheral neuropathy are low,[65,66] but this area warrants further investigation.

Central nervous system manifestations account for 17% to 30% of the neurologic involvement seen in MPA.[14,64] Manifestations are quite varied, and can include cerebral hemorrhage,[29] pachymeningitis,[67] and non-hemorrhagic cerebral infarctions.[68]

Laboratory Testing

Currently, no laboratory test has diagnostic specificity for MPA. Because ANCA are detected in only 50% to 75% of patients with MPA,[14,30] the absence of circulating ANCA does not exclude this diagnosis. ANCA associated with MPA generally has a perinuclear staining pattern (p-ANCA) caused by antibodies against MPO (MPO-ANCA), which can be detected using enzyme-linked immunoassays (ELISA). Immuno-fluorescence has greater sensitivity, but the ELISA has greater specificity for diagnosing MPA. Unfortunately, neither test is specific for MPA, because these antibodies can be found in patients with the other ANCA-associated vasculitides in addition to other inflammatory diseases,[69] such as drug-induced ANCA-associated vasculitis,[70] cystic fibrosis,[71] and various infections.[72,73]

Nonspecific markers of inflammation are also observed in patients with MPA. The most common findings are an elevated erythrocyte sedimentation rate and C-reactive protein. Other findings include elevated white blood cell and platelet counts, and a normochromic normocytic anemia.[53]

TREATMENT

Given that most patients will present with glomerulonephritis, initial therapy of MPA generally entails the use of glucocorticoids and a cytotoxic agent such as cyclophosphamide. This regimen produces remission in 90% of patients. The regimen, first described by Fauci and Wolff[74] for the treatment of WG, used daily oral cyclophosphamide (2 mg/kg per day) for years, both to induce and maintain remission. Although effective, this regimen is associated with substantial toxicity, including infertility, malignancy, and hemorrhagic cystitis.[75] For this reason, substantial effort has been expended to find ways to minimize cyclophosphamide exposure, either through developing alternate dosing regimens or identifying subsets of patients who can be treated without resorting to cytotoxic agents.

Remission Maintenance Strategies

The Cyclophosphamide Versus Azathioprine for Early Remission Phase of Vasculitis trial (CYCAZAREM) treated 60 subjects with MPA and 95 with WG who had involvement of the kidneys or another vital organ.[76] All subjects were treated with a remission induction regimen of daily oral cyclophosphamide (2 mg/kg per day) and prednisolone for 3 to 6 months, after which they were randomized to undergo continued therapy with either cyclophosphamide (1.5 mg/kg per day) or azathioprine (2 mg/kg per day). Patients who had been randomized to receive cyclophosphamide were transitioned to azathioprine after 1 year of therapy. The primary end point of the trial was relapse rate, which was shown to be equivalent among both groups (15% vs 10%; $P = .94$).

CYCAZAREM effectively showed that induction of remission with cyclophosphamide, followed by remission maintenance with azathioprine, was as effective at preventing disease flare as a prolonged course of cyclophosphamide. However, whether other remission maintenance agents, such as methotrexate, might be equally effective was less clear. This question was addressed by the French Vasculitis Study Group, which treated 30 patients with MPA and 96 with WG with intravenous cyclophosphamide (0.6 mg/m^2 every 2 weeks for three doses, then 0.6 mg/m^2 every 3 weeks until remission was achieved, then an additional 0.7 mg/m^2 every 3 weeks for three additional doses).[77] These subjects were subsequently randomized to undergo remission maintenance therapy with either oral methotrexate (titrated to 25 mg/wk) or azathioprine (2 mg/kg per day). The relapse rate was again determined to be equivalent in both groups (33% vs 36%; $P = .71$).

Taken together, these trials indicate that for the treatment of MPA, remission induction with a limited course of cyclophosphamide, followed by remission maintenance with an antimetabolite such as methotrexate or azathioprine, is an appropriate treatment strategy for patients with severe disease. This reasoning leaves open the question, however, of whether adjunctive therapies, such as plasma exchange, might further augment the response to immunosuppression.

This possibility was examined by the Methylprednisolone versus Plasma Exchange as Additional Therapy for Severe, ANCA-Associated Glomerulonephritis trial (MEPEX), which enrolled 95 patients with MPA and 24 with WG, all of whom had biopsy-proven glomerulonephritis and a serum creatinine of 5.8 mg/dL or greater.[78] All patients underwent treatment with oral glucocorticoids and cyclophosphamide (2.5 mg/kg per day for 3 months, then 1.5 mg/kg per day for an additional 3 months) followed by azathioprine (2 mg/kg per day). In addition, patients were randomized to undergo adjunctive therapy with either intravenous methylprednisolone (1 g/d for 3 days) or a series of seven plasma exchange procedures over 14 days. The primary end point of renal recovery at 3 months occurred more frequently among patients who had received plasma exchange (49% vs 69%; $P = .02$). Randomization to plasma exchange resulted in a 24% risk reduction of end-stage renal disease at 12 months (43% vs 19%). However, mortality was equivalent in both groups, and long-term follow-up studies show no difference in mortality or renal survival.

Remission Induction Strategies

Because of the toxicities inherent to the use of cyclophosphamide, investigators have focused on developing strategies to treat MPA that avoid using cytotoxic agents altogether. One strategy involves identifying patients with milder disease, who may not require aggressive treatment to experience remission. Silva and colleagues[79] recruited 17 patients with MPA with mild to moderate renal involvement (defined as a serum creatinine ≤ 3 mg/dL) for treatment with glucocorticoids and mycophenolate mofetil (2–3 g total dose daily). Thirteen of these patients (76%) met the primary end point and 12 remained in remission until month 18. Regimens that avoid the use of cyclophosphamide for disease that does not affect life or the function of a vital organ may be valuable to help some patients avoid cytotoxic agents; research in analogous patients with WG indicates that methotrexate[80] and leflunomide[81] may also be effective.

Rituximab may represent an important alternative to cyclophosphamide for patients with higher levels of disease activity that may not respond adequately to antimetabolite therapies. The multicenter, double-blinded Rituximab Versus Cyclophosphamide for Induction of Remission in ANCA-Associated Vasculitis trial (RAVE) randomized 48 patients with MPA and 147 with WG to undergo either standard therapy or treatment with rituximab.[82] Standard therapy included a remission induction regimen of daily oral cyclophosphamide (2 mg/kg per day) for 3 to 6 months, followed by a remission maintenance regimen of azathioprine (2 mg/kg per day). Rituximab was administered using a standard lymphoma protocol (375 mg/m^2 intravenously weekly for 4 weeks).

This trial showed that rituximab is noninferior to cyclophosphamide for the induction of remission at 6 months (63.6% vs 53.1%; $P = .089$). Remission rates at 6 months increase when subjects who were allowed to remain on low-dose glucocorticoids are included in the calculations (70.7% vs 62.2%; $P = .103$). Post hoc analysis indicates that rituximab may be especially effective for patients with relapsing disease (66.7% vs 42.0%; $P = .013$). Although the long-term consequences associated with rituximab treatment are not entirely clear for this patient population,[83] this trial strongly supports rituximab as an alternative to cyclophosphamide for the treatment of MPA.

SUMMARY

MPA is a systemic necrotizing vasculitis with significant renal and pulmonary manifestations. The pathogenesis of MPA has not been clearly defined, although current evidence supports a role for ANCA. Diagnosis can be challenging, and relies on the physician drawing together elements of the patient's clinical history and symptoms with diagnostic tests such as tissue biopsy and autoantibody testing. Prognosis for MPA has greatly improved with the use of cyclophosphamide and glucocorticoids. The future of MPA treatment seems bright, as newer medications such as rituximab show great promise as effective alternative therapeutic agents with potentially less toxicity.

REFERENCES

1. Matteson E. Commemorative translation of the 130-year anniversary of the original article by Adolf Kussmaul and Rudolf Maier. Rochester (NY): Mayo Foundation; 1996. Anonymous.
2. Matteson EL. Historical perspective on the classification of vasculitis. Arthritis Care Res 2000;13(2):122–7.

3. Wohlwill F. Über die nur mikroskopisch erkennbare Form der Periarteritis nodosa. Virchows Arch Pathol Anat Physiol 1923;246:377–411 [in German].

4. Zeek PM. Periarteritis nodosa and other forms of necrotizing angiitis. N Engl J Med 1953;248(18):764–72.

5. Wainwright J, Davson J. The renal appearances in the microscopic form of periarteritis nodosa. J Pathol Bacteriol 1950;62(2):189–96.

6. Savage CO, Winearls CG, Evans DJ, et al. Microscopic polyarteritis: presentation, pathology and prognosis. Q J Med 1985;56(220):467–83.

7. Jennette J, Falk RJ, Andrassy K, et al. Nomenclature of systemic vasculitides. Proposal of an international consensus conference. Arthritis Rheum 1994;37: 187–92.

8. Kussmaul A, Maier R. Ueber eine bisher nicht beschriebenen Eigenthumliche arterienerkrankung (periarteritis nodosa), die mit Morbus Brightii und rapid fortschreitender allgemeiner muskellahmung Einhergeht. Dtsch Arch Klin Med 1866;1:484–518 [in German].

9. Watts R, Lane S, Hanslik T, et al. Development and validation of a consensus methodology for the classification of the ANCA-associated vasculitides and polyarteritis nodosa for epidemiological studies. Ann Rheum Dis 2007;66(2):222–7.

10. Watts RA, Jolliffe VA, Carruthers DM, et al. Effect of classification on the incidence of polyarteritis nodosa and microscopic polyangiitis. Arthritis Rheum 1996;39(7): 1208–12.

11. Godman G, Churg J. Wegener's granulomatosis: pathology and review of the literature. Arch Pathol Lab Med 1954;58:533–53.

12. Davies D, Moran J, Niall J, et al. Segmental necrotising glomerulonephritis with antineutrophil antibody: possible arbovirus aetiology. BMJ 1982;285:606.

13. Falk R, Jennette J. Anti-neutrophil cytoplasmic autoantibodies with specificity for myeloperoxidase in patients with systemic vasculitis and idiopathic necrotizing and crescentic glomerulonephritis. N Engl J Med 1988;318:1651.

14. Guillevin L, Durand-Gasselin B, Cevallos R, et al. Microscopic polyangiitis: clinical and laboratory findings in eighty-five patients. Arthritis Rheum 1999;42(3):421–30.

15. Lane SE, Scott DG, Heaton A, et al. Primary renal vasculitis in Norfolk–increasing incidence or increasing recognition? Nephrol Dial Transplant 2000;15(1):23–7.

16. Mohammad AJ, Jacobsson LT, Mahr AD, et al. Prevalence of Wegener's granulomatosis, microscopic polyangiitis, polyarteritis nodosa and Churg Strauss syndrome within a defined population in southern Sweden. Rheumatology (Oxford) 2007;46(8):1329–37.

17. Koldingsnes W, Nossent H. Epidemiology of Wegener's granulomatosis in northern Norway. Arthritis Rheum 2000;43(11):2481–7.

18. Gonzalez-Gay MA, Garcia-Porrua C, Guerrero J, et al. The epidemiology of the primary systemic vasculitides in northwest Spain: implications of the Chapel Hill Consensus Conference definitions. Arthritis Rheum 2003;49(3):388–93.

19. Mahr A, Guillevin L, Poissonnet M, et al. Prevalences of polyarteritis nodosa, microscopic polyangiitis, Wegener's granulomatosis, and Churg-Strauss syndrome in a French urban multiethnic population in 2000: a capture-recapture estimate. Arthritis Rheum 2004;51(1):92–9.

20. Kallenberg CG, Heeringa P, Stegeman CA. Mechanisms of Disease: pathogenesis and treatment of ANCA-associated vasculitides. Nature clinical practice. Rheumatology 2006;2(12):661–70.

21. Guilpain P, Servettaz A, Goulvestre C, et al. Pathogenic effects of antimyeloperoxidase antibodies in patients with microscopic polyangiitis. Arthritis Rheum 2007;56(7):2455–63.

22. Mulder A, Heeringa P, Brouwer E, et al. Activation of granulocytes by anti-neutrophil cytoplasmic antibodies (ANCA): a FcgRII-dependent process. Clin Exp Immunol 1994;98:270.
23. Little MA, Smyth CL, Yadav R, et al. Antineutrophil cytoplasm antibodies directed against myeloperoxidase augment leukocyte-microvascular interactions in vivo. Blood 2005;106(6):2050–8.
24. Xiao H, Heeringa P, Hu P, et al. Antineutrophil cytoplasmic autoantibodies specific for myeloperoxidase cause glomerulonephritis and vasculitis in mice. J Clin Invest 2002;110(7):955–63.
25. Schlieben DJ, Korbet SM, Kimura RE, et al. Pulmonary-renal syndrome in a newborn with placental transmission of ANCAs. Am J Kidney Dis 2005;45(4): 758–61.
26. Silva F, Specks U, Sethi S, et al. Successful pregnancy and delivery of a healthy newborn despite transplacental transfer of antimyeloperoxidase antibodies from a mother with microscopic polyangiitis. Am J Kidney Dis 2009;54(3):542–5.
27. Falk RJ, Hoffman GS. Controversies in small vessel vasculitis–comparing the rheumatology and nephrology views. Curr Opin Rheumatol 2007;19(1):1–9.
28. Kain R, Exner M, Brandes R, et al. Molecular mimicry in pauci-immune focal necrotizing glomerulonephritis. Nat Med 2008;14(10):1088–96.
29. Agard C, Mouthon L, Mahr A, et al. Microscopic polyangiitis and polyarteritis nodosa: how and when do they start? Arthritis Rheum 2003;49(5):709–15.
30. Lhote F, Cohen P, Guillevin L. Polyarteritis nodosa, microscopic polyangiitis and Churg-Strauss syndrome. Lupus 1998;7(4):238–58.
31. Jennette JC, Thomas DB, Falk RJ. Microscopic polyangiitis (microscopic polyarteritis). Semin Diagn Pathol 2001;18(1):3 13.
32. Westman KW, Bygren PG, Olsson H, et al. Relapse rate, renal survival, and cancer morbidity in patients with Wegener's granulomatosis or microscopic polyangiitis with renal involvement. J Am Soc Nephrol 1998;9(5):842–52.
33. Levy JB, Hammad T, Coulthart A, et al. Clinical features and outcome of patients with both ANCA and anti-GBM antibodies. Kidney Int 2004;66(4):1535–40.
34. Lindic J, Vizjak A, Ferluga D, et al. Clinical outcome of patients with coexistent antineutrophil cytoplasmic antibodies and antibodies against glomerular basement membrane. Ther Apher Dial 2009;13(4):278–81.
35. Hellmark T, Niles JL, Collins AB, et al. Comparison of anti-GBM antibodies in sera with or without ANCA. J Am Soc Nephrol 1997;8(3):376–85.
36. Lionaki S, Jennette JC, Falk RJ. Anti-neutrophil cytoplasmic (ANCA) and anti-glomerular basement membrane (GBM) autoantibodies in necrotizing and crescentic glomerulonephritis. Semin Immunopathol 2007;29(4):459–74.
37. Lauque D, Cadranel J, Lazor R, et al. Microscopic polyangiitis with alveolar hemorrhage. A study of 29 cases and review of the literature. Groupe d'Etudes et de Recherche sur les Maladies "Orphelines" Pulmonaires (GERM"O"P). Medicine (Baltimore) 2000;79(4):222–33.
38. Gomez-Puerta JA, Espinosa G, Morla R, et al. Interstitial lung disease as a presenting manifestation of microscopic polyangiitis successfully treated with mycophenolate mofetil. Clin Exp Rheumatol 2009;27(1):166–7.
39. Collins CE, Quismorio FP Jr. Pulmonary involvement in microscopic polyangiitis. Curr Opin Pulm Med 2005;11(5):447–51.
40. Franks TJ, Koss MN. Pulmonary capillaritis. Curr Opin Pulm Med 2000;6(5): 430–5.
41. Schwarz MI, Brown KK. Small vessel vasculitis of the lung. Thorax 2000;55(6): 502–10.

42. Niles JL, Bottinger EP, Saurina GR, et al. The syndrome of lung hemorrhage and nephritis is usually an ANCA-associated condition. Arch Intern Med 1996;156(4): 440–5.

43. Eschun GM, Mink SN, Sharma S. Pulmonary interstitial fibrosis as a presenting manifestation in perinuclear antineutrophilic cytoplasmic antibody microscopic polyangiitis. Chest 2003;123(1):297–301.

44. Birnbaum J, Danoff S, Askin FB, et al. Microscopic polyangiitis presenting as a "pulmonary-muscle" syndrome: is subclinical alveolar hemorrhage the mechanism of pulmonary fibrosis? Arthritis Rheum 2007;56(6):2065–71.

45. Tzelepis GE, Kokosi M, Tzioufas A, et al. Prevalence and outcome of pulmonary fibrosis in microscopic polyangiitis. Eur Respir J 2010;36(1):116–21.

46. Foulon G, Delaval P, Valeyre D, et al. ANCA-associated lung fibrosis: analysis of 17 patients. Respir Med 2008;102(10):1392–8.

47. Ortiz-Santamaria V, Olive A, Holgado S, et al. Pulmonary aneurysms in microscopic polyangiitis. Clin Rheumatol 2003;22(6):498–9.

48. Park J, Pagnoux C, Guillevin L, et al. Microscopic polyangiitis associated with diffuse panbronchiolitis. Intern Med 2004;43(4):331–5.

49. Kluger N, et al. Comparison of cutaneous manifestations in systemic polyarteritis nodosa and microscopic polyangiitis. Br J Dermatol 2008;159(3):615–20.

50. Kawakami T, Soma Y, Saito C, et al. Cutaneous manifestations in patients with microscopic polyangiitis: two case reports and a minireview. Acta Derm Venereol 2006;86(2):144–7.

51. Seishima M, Oyama Z, Oda M. Skin eruptions associated with microscopic polyangiitis. Eur J Dermatol 2004;14(4):255–8.

52. Pagnoux C, Mahr A, Cohen P, et al. Presentation and outcome of gastrointestinal involvement in systemic necrotizing vasculitides: analysis of 62 patients with polyarteritis nodosa, microscopic polyangiitis, Wegener granulomatosis, Churg-Strauss syndrome, or rheumatoid arthritis-associated vasculitis. Medicine (Baltimore) 2005;84(2):115–28.

53. Guillevin L, Pagnoux C, Teixeira L. Microscopic polyangiitis, in vasculitis. In: Ball G, Bridges S Jr, editors. Oxford (UK): Oxford University Press; 2008. p. 355–64.

54. Ueda S, Matsumoto M, Ahn T, et al. Microscopic polyangiitis complicated with massive intestinal bleeding. J Gastroenterol 2001;36(4):264–70.

55. Spahn TW, Ullerich HJ, Lebitz P, et al. Gastrointestinal bleeding secondary to hepatic artery involvement of microscopic polyangiitis: case report and review of the literature. Dig Dis Sci 2007;52(6):1558–61.

56. Tsai CN, Chang CM, Chuang CH, et al. Extended colonic ulcerations in a patient with microscopic polyangiitis. Ann Rheum Dis 2004;63(11):1521–2.

57. Passam FH, et al. Intestinal ischemia as the first manifestation of vasculitis. Semin Arthritis Rheum 2004;34(1):431–41.

58. Ohnuma K, Hosono O, Katayose T, et al. Microscopic polyangiitis initiated with liver dysfunction, calf pain and fever of unknown origin. Rheumatol Int 2009. [Epub ahead of print].

59. Takebayashi K, Aso Y, Kitamura H, et al. Microscopic polyangiitis presenting with liver dysfunction preceding rapidly progressive necrotizing glomerulonephritis. South Med J 2004;97(9):911–4.

60. Nakamoto T, Yoshikawa M, Nakatani T, et al. Microscopic polyangiitis that presented liver dysfunction prior to noted renal manifestations. Intern Med 2000; 39(6):517–21.

61. Goritsas CP, Repanti M, Papadaki E, et al. Intrahepatic bile duct injury and nodular regenerative hyperplasia of the liver in a patient with polyarteritis nodosa. J Hepatol 1997;26(3):727–30.
62. Iannone F, Falappone P, Pannarale G, et al. Microscopic polyangiitis associated with primary biliary cirrhosis. J Rheumatol 2003;30(12):2710–2.
63. Amezcua-Guerra LM, Prieto P. Microscopic polyangiitis associated with primary biliary cirrhosis: a causal or casual association? J Rheumatol 2006;33(11): 2351–3.
64. Zhang W, Zhou G, Shi Q, et al. Clinical analysis of nervous system involvement in ANCA-associated systemic vasculitides. Clin Exp Rheumatol 2009;27(1 Suppl 52): S65–9.
65. Hattori N, Mori K, Misu K, et al. Mortality and morbidity in peripheral neuropathy associated Churg-Strauss syndrome and microscopic polyangiitis. J Rheumatol 2002;29(7):1408–14.
66. Cattaneo L, Chierici E, Pavone L, et al. Peripheral neuropathy in Wegener's granulomatosis, Churg-Strauss syndrome and microscopic polyangiitis. J Neurol Neurosurg Psychiatr 2007;78(10):1119–23.
67. Furukawa Y, Matsumoto Y, Yamada M. Hypertrophic pachymeningitis as an initial and cardinal manifestation of microscopic polyangiitis. Neurology 2004;63(9): 1722–4.
68. Ku BD, Shin HY. Multiple bilateral non-hemorrhagic cerebral infarctions associated with microscopic polyangiitis. Clin Neurol Neurosurg 2009;111(10):904–6.
69. Stone J, Talor M, Stebbing J, et al. Test characteristics of Immunofluorescence and ELISA tests in 856 consecutive patients with possible ANCA-associated conditions. Arthritis Care Res 2000;13(6):424–34.
70. Choi HK, Merkel PA, Walker AM, et al. Drug-associated antineutrophil cytoplasmic antibody-positive vasculitis: prevalence among patients with high titers of antimyeloperoxidase antibodies. Arthritis Rheum 2000;43(2):405–13.
71. Zhao MH, Jayne DR, Ardiles LG, et al. Autoantibodies against bactericidal/permeability-increasing protein in patients with cystic fibrosis. Q J Med 1996; 89(4):259–65.
72. Bauer A, Jabs WJ, Sufke S, et al. Vasculitic purpura with antineutrophil cytoplasmic antibody-positive acute renal failure in a patient with Streptococcus bovis case and Neisseria subflava bacteremia and subacute endocarditis. Clin Nephrol 2004;62(2):144–8.
73. Hermann J, Demel U, Stunzner D, et al. Clinical interpretation of antineutrophil cytoplasmic antibodies: parvovirus B19 infection as a pitfall. Ann Rheum Dis 2005;64(4):641–3.
74. Fauci A, Wolff S. Wegener's granulomatosis: studies in eighteen patients and a review of the literature. Medicine 1973;52:53–61.
75. Hoffman GS, Kerr GS, Leavitt RY, et al. Wegener's granulomatosis: an analysis of 158 Patients. Ann Intern Med 1992;116:488–98.
76. Jayne D. Randomised trial of cyclophosphamide versus azathioprine during remission in ANCA-associated systemic vasculitis (CYCAZAREM). J Am Soc Nephrol 1999;10:105A.
77. Pagnoux C, Mahr A, Hamidou MA, et al. Azathioprine or methotrexate maintenance for ANCA-associated vasculitis. N Engl J Med 2008;359(26):2790–803.
78. Jayne DR, Gaskin G, Rasmussen N, et al. Randomized trial of plasma exchange or high-dosage methylprednisolone as adjunctive therapy for severe renal vasculitis. J Am Soc Nephrol 2007;18(7):2180–8.

79. Silva F, Specks U, Kalra S, et al. Mycophenolate mofetil for induction and maintenance of remission in microscopic polyangiitis with mild to moderate renal involvement–a prospective, open-label pilot trial. Clin J Am Soc Nephrol 2010; 5(3):445–53.

80. De Groot K, Rasmussen N, Bacon PA, et al. Randomized trial of cyclophosphamide versus methotrexate for induction of remission in early systemic antineutrophil cytoplasmic antibody-associated vasculitis. Arthritis Rheum 2005;52(8): 2461–9.

81. Metzler C, Miehle N, Manger K, et al. Elevated relapse rate under oral methotrexate versus leflunomide for maintenance of remission in Wegener's granulomatosis. Rheumatology (Oxford) 2007;46(7):1087–91.

82. Stone JH, Merkel PA, Seo P, et al. Rituximab versus cyclophosphamide for induction of remission in ANCA-Associated Vasculitis: a Randomized Controlled Trial (RAVE). Arthritis Rheum 2009;60(Suppl):S204.

83. Calabrese LH, Molloy ES. Therapy: rituximab and PML risk-informed decisions needed! Nat Rev Rheumatol 2009;5(10):528–9.

Pauci-Immune Necrotizing Glomerulonephritis

Abraham Rutgers, MD, PhD[a],*, Jan S.F. Sanders, MD, PhD[b],
Coen A. Stegeman, MD, PhD[b], Cees G.M. Kallenberg, MD, PhD[a]

KEYWORDS

- ANCA • Renal-limited vasculitis
- Rapidly progressive glomerulonephritis
- Vasculitis • Myeloperoxidase • Proteinase 3

Pauci-immune necrotizing glomerulonephritis is a somewhat confusing term. Pauci originates from the Latin word paucus meaning little or few. It reflects the almost complete absence of immunoglobulin deposits (as assessed by immunofluorescence) when studying renal biopsies of a subgroup of patients with rapidly progressive glomerulonephritis.[1] Historically, pauci-immune glomerulonephritis has been described as a form of glomerulonephritis with no evidence of linear immunoglobulin deposition (type I glomerulonephritis, as in Goodpasture disease) or immune complex deposition (type II glomerulonephritis, as in lupus nephritis). However, paucity of immune deposits does not imply that the immune system is not involved in the disease process; on the contrary, pauci-immune renal disease is believed to be a typical immune-mediated disease and is treated accordingly.

Pauci-immune renal disease can be renal-limited vasculitis (RLV) or the renal manifestations of microscopic polyangiitis (MPA), Wegener's granulomatosis (WG), or Churg-Strauss syndrome (CSS). These diseases are designated as antineutrophil cytoplasmic antibodies (ANCA)-associated vasculitides (AAV). The latter 3 conditions are described in different articles in this issue (see the articles by Chung and Seo; Holle and colleagues; Baldini and colleagues elsewhere in this issue for further exploration of this topic). Renal involvement is frequent in AAV; depending on the cohort studied it varies between 71% and 88% for patients with WG and MPA.[2] In CSS, renal involvement is around 25% of cases, with higher percentages for patients with positive ANCA.[3]

Funding: no conflicting interests.
[a] Department of Rheumatology en Clinical Immunology, AA21, University Medical Center Groningen, University of Groningen, PO Box 30.001, 9700 RB Groningen, The Netherlands
[b] Department of Nephrology, University Medical Center Groningen, University of Groningen, PO Box 30.001, 9700 RB Groningen, The Netherlands
* Corresponding author.
E-mail address: a.rutgers@int.umcg.nl

Rheum Dis Clin N Am 36 (2010) 559–572
doi:10.1016/j.rdc.2010.05.002
0889-857X/10/$ – see front matter © 2010 Elsevier Inc. All rights reserved.

In this review the histopathologic changes seen in renal biopsies of patients with pauci-immune glomerulonephritis are described. This article discusses why the disease is sometimes limited to the kidneys, the clinical course of renal involvement, treatment issues, how to deal with disease relapses, and strategies to prevent disease recurrence. Furthermore, the necessity of renal biopsy and repeat biopsy, the usefulness of rapid detection of ANCA for diagnosis, the relevance of serial measurement of ANCA during follow-up, the effect of dialysis on the disease process, and the issue of renal transplantation after disease remission are also discussed.

RENAL PATHOLOGY

The glomerular lesion in patients with systemic and renal-limited ANCA-associated diseases is identical, that is, crescentic glomerulonephritis characterized by necrotizing inflammation and paucity of immune deposits.[4] The most frequently encountered histologic appearance is focal segmental glomerular fibrinoid necrosis with crescent formation and only mild hypercellularity, although neutrophils are modestly present at sites of necrosis (**Figs. 1** and **2**).[5] Periglomerular granulomatous inflammation, first described by Wegener in 1939,[6] is seen in a small number of patients (see **Fig. 1**).[7,8] Interstitial disease is present frequently, mostly characterized by a mild to severe interstitial infiltrate (**Figs. 3** and **4**). The infiltrate consists mostly of mononuclear inflammatory cells and neutrophils to a lesser extent, and in up to 22% of biopsies a small number of eosinophils are also found. In a few cases, interstitial vasculitis can be found.[9]

Chronic damage can be observed, including fibrous crescents, interstitial fibrosis, and tubular atrophy (see **Fig. 4**). Renal biopsy in RLV and in MPA shows more chronicity than in WG, even though the amount of active lesions is comparable. This could be caused by unrecognized renal disease, or because of the different nature of these 2 diseases. The renal biopsy characteristics and comparison among MPA, WG, and RLV are described by Hauer and colleagues (**Table 1**) and De Lind van Wijngaarden.[8,10]

Although pauci-immune necrotizing glomerulonephritis is characterized by a lack of immunoglobulin deposits by immunofluorescence, electron microscopy studies from renal biopsies of patients with pauci-immune crescentic glomerulonephritis can demonstrate glomerular immune complex deposits in up to 54% of patients.[11]

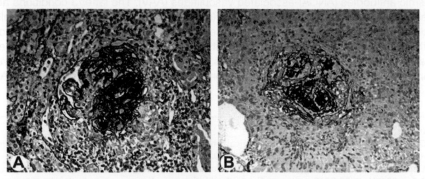

Fig. 1. (*A*) Periglomerular granulomas surrounding a sclerotic and crescentic glomerulus, with complete destruction of Bowman capsule. (*B*) A similar process, with incomplete destruction of Bowman capsule. Methenamine silver staining; original magnification: (*A*) ×400, (*B*) ×200.[7] (*Reprinted from* Rutgers A, Slot M, van Paassen P, et al. Coexistence of anti-glomerular basement membrane antibodies and myeloperoxidase-ANCAs in crescentic glomerulonephritis. Am J Kidney Dis 2005;46(2):253–62; with permission.)

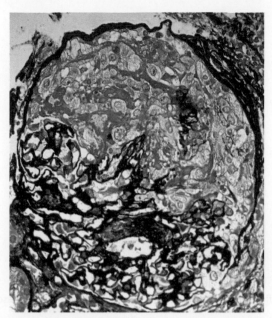

Fig. 2. Glomerulus with a crescent and fibrin interspersed with the cells of the crescent and focal disruption of Bowman capsule.

WHY IS THE DISEASE SOMETIMES LIMITED TO THE KIDNEYS?

This issue is much debated in the literature and no definite answer has emerged. Two types of reasoning exist. First, the disease process itself might specifically target a particular, organ-specific vasculature.[12] Second, the unique characteristics of certain types of vasculature could make them vulnerable to an immunologically mediated

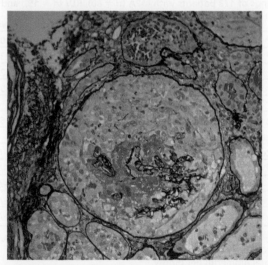

Fig. 3. Glomerulus with large circumferential cellular crescent and fibrinoid necrosis of the glomerular basement membrane. Interstitial inflammation is present; within the tubuli, erythrocytes form erythrocyte casts.

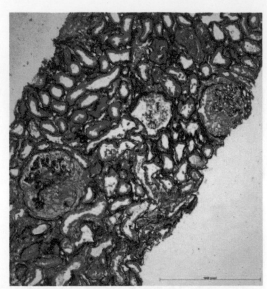

Fig. 4. Low magnification view of renal biopsy specimen containing crescentic glomeruli.

attack. The unique characteristics could be intrinsically present but not previously recognized by the immune system (eg, the noncollagenous domain of type IV collagen in Goodpasture disease), or could be acquired by the vasculature either by deposition of antigen (eg, in situ formation of immune complexes in poststreptococcal glomerulonephritis), change of a preexisting antigen (formation of neoepitopes), or change in

Table 1
Renal biopsy findings of 173 patients with MPA (n = 80), RLV (n = 19), and WG (n = 73)

Lesions	MPA	RLV	WG	All (%)
Normal glomeruli[a]	21%	27%	40%	29
Fibrinoid necrosis[a]	21	21	23	22
Crescents[a]	47	49	42	45
Cellular[a]	45	55	45	
Fibrous[a]	7	3	4	
Glomerulosclerosis[a]	30	23	16	23
Periglomerular[a] granulomatous reaction	4	2	2	
Interstitial infiltrate[b]		++	+/−	
Interstitial fibrosis[b]		++	+/−	
Tubular atrophy[b]		++	+/−	
Tubular necrosis[b]		++	+/−	
Arteriosclerosis[b]		++	+/−	70

These biopsies were derived from 2 European Vasculitis Study Group (EUVAS) trials: 98 were derived from the CYCAZAREM study[53] and 75 from the MEPEX study.[45]

[a] Percentage of total glomeruli per biopsy.

[b] Semiquantitative comparison.

Data from Hauer HA, Bajema IM, van Houwelingen HC, et al. Renal histology in ANCA-associated vasculitis: differences between diagnostic and serologic subgroups. Kidney Int 2002;61(1):80–9.

endothelial function.[13,14] Essential to the pathogenesis of pauci-immune renal disease is inflammation of blood vessels (see the article by Flint and colleagues elsewhere in this issue for further exploration of this topic). The endothelium plays a crucial role in this process. Thus, organ-specific endothelial antibodies could explain organ-specific disease manifestations,[12] although the authors and others have not been able to confirm the presence of these antibodies in most patients.[15]

The glomerulus has a unique type of fenestrated endothelium allowing for filtration of blood and the production of urine. The fenestrae are covered by a highly negatively charged glycocalyx, which is in part responsible for the glomerular filtration barrier.[16] These characteristics could facilitate capturing of ANCA antigens (especially the highly positively charged myeloperoxidase) resulting in local inflammation in the presence of ANCA. Also, local cytokine production in the kidney could induce on-site neutrophil priming, a necessary step for ANCA-induced neutrophil activation and endothelial damage.[17,18] The unique microvasculature in the glomerulus could allow local trapping of activated neutrophils and thus could be responsible for local inflammation.[19] Likely a combination of local and systemic factors determines the location and severity of active vasculitis and its disease course.

CLINICAL COURSE

Basically, 4 patterns of disease course can be discriminated in pauci-immune glomerulonephritis. First, the disease may be brought into remission and remain quiescent, with acquired damage remaining at a stable level. Second, the disease may be brought into remission, but relapses with increasing damage after each relapse. Third, the disease may not be able to be brought into remission and end-stage renal failure develops. In this situation, if there are no other extrarenal disease manifestations, the disease is quiescent and further immunosuppressive therapy provides no clinical benefit. Fourth, the disease may be brought into clinical remission, but there is persistent proteinuria, low-grade inflammation, and slowly declining renal function. The latter form is mostly seen in patients with MPA or RLV, the former 2 more in patients with WG.

Patients with renal involvement without ear, nose, and throat (ENT) involvement are at increased risk of death, and, in general, WG patients have better survival rates than patients with MPA (**Fig. 5**).[20]

TREATMENT CONTROVERSIES

Treatment involves 2 phases: induction of remission and prevention of relapse (ie, maintenance therapy).[21] The induction phase is aimed at rapid control of inflammation and the prevention of further organ dysfunction and damage. Remission should be achieved within weeks after start of treatment; otherwise therapy should be intensified (**Table 2**). After induction of remission, the maintenance phase starts and is aimed at prevention of relapse of disease, averting treatment-related damage as much as possible.

Standard induction therapy consists of 3 to 6 months of treatment with cyclophosphamide along with glucocorticoids (see **Table 2**). Glucocorticoids are tapered gradually according to various experience-based protocols. The PEXIVAS study (Plasma Exchange and Glucocorticoids for Treatment of ANCA-Associated Vasculitis) (clinicaltrials.gov identifier NCT00987389; http://clinicaltrials.gov/ct2/show/NCT00987389) is the first randomized trial designed to compare different tapering regimens; this study will soon start recruiting patients. Recently, a meta-analysis of available trials involving treatment of AAV was performed evaluating the effect of different corticosteroid dosing regimens in relapse prevention. Patients in

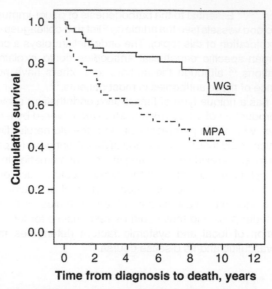

Fig. 5. Cumulative survival of patients with MPA compared with patients with WG. (*Reprinted from* Mohammad AJ, Jacobsson LT, Westman KW, et al. Incidence and survival rates in Wegener's granulomatosis, microscopic polyangiitis, Churg-Strauss syndrome and polyarteritis nodosa. Rheumatology (Oxford) 2009;48(12):1560–5; with permission.)

studies with a nonzero corticosteroid target dose at the end of the study had fewer relapses than patients in studies with a zero corticosteroid target dose (14% vs 43%, respectively).[22] Whether the benefits of a lower relapse rate outweigh the negative effects of longer corticosteroid therapy is not known.

Recent investigations have shown that intravenous (IV) pulse cyclophosphamide is equally effective as oral cyclophosphamide, with lower cumulative cyclophosphamide dose and fewer episodes of leukopenia, but no reduction in infectious complications.[23] After achieving disease remission at 9 months, however, a nonsignificant difference in disease relapse rate was noted for the IV pulse group compared with the oral cyclophosphamide group (13 of 67 vs 6 of 64, respectively; hazard ratio 2.01, 95% confidence interval 0.77–5.30). This is concordant with the data from a previously performed meta-analysis on the same subject.[24] Data on the effects of giving a lower cumulative dose of cyclophosphamide on long-term relapse rate, damage, and quality of life are not yet available.[25]

Standard maintenance therapy consists of azathioprine until 18 months after disease onset. The ongoing Prevention of Relapses in PR3-ANCA-Associated Vasculitis (REMAIN) study (clinicaltrials.gov identifier NCT00128895) is investigating the benefit of maintenance therapy continuing after 18 months. It is already known that patients positive for PR3-ANCA who remain ANCA positive after induction of stable disease remission are at increased risk for relapse of disease; therefore immunosuppression for a longer period might be considered in these patients.[26] **Table 2** summarizes the available alternative therapies applicable to patients with pauci-immune renal disease.

Controversies exist on how to treat patients with end-stage renal disease (ESRD) at the time of diagnosis. Current dogma is that patients with ESRD without any active inflammatory lesions within the kidney will not benefit from immunosuppressive therapy and will not regain independent renal function. Are there conditions in which treatment is definitely futile? This is probably only the case when there is severe tubular atrophy and 2% or fewer of glomeruli are normal. In such cases, plasma exchange treatment with concomitant standard therapy increases the risk of therapy-related death more than it raises the likelihood of attaining independence from dialysis.[27] Of course, extrarenal disease activity may necessitate therapy independent of the renal disease.

In patients with ESRD patients, maintenance immunosuppressive therapy prevents relapse of extrarenal manifestations. In 2009, Lionaki and colleagues[28] compared the clinical course of patients with ANCA-associated small vessel vasculitis with and without ESRD. They showed that relapse rates of patients on dialysis were significantly lower than in the same patients before onset of ESRD, and were lower than patients not on dialysis. Moreover, patients on maintenance immunosuppressive therapy were at increased risk for infectious complications and death.

In general, relapse should be managed similar to new-onset disease, taking into account the acquired disease- and treatment-related damage.

ROLE OF RENAL BIOPSY/REBIOPSY

Histologic findings remain the gold standard for diagnosing patients with AAV.[21] Renal biopsy in patients with WG and evidence of active renal disease (by urinary sediment) demonstrates extracapillary proliferation in more than 91.5% of patients.[29] However, ANCA positivity in the context of clinical symptoms of AAV has a high specificity for AAV and may justify the start of immunosuppressive therapy without confirmation of glomerulonephritis by biopsy.[30,31] Jennette and colleagues[30] combined the sensitivity and specificity data of ANCA testing from the study of Hagen and colleagues[32] with their own prevalence data from a cohort of 4185 patients who had undergone renal biopsy. They showed that, depending on the clinical context, the positive predictive value of ANCA for pauci-immune crescentic glomerulonephritis varies between 47% and 99% (**Tables 3** and **4**).

Repeat kidney biopsy can be helpful in differentiating patients with poor treatment response as a result of chronic damage from those who might benefit from intensified treatment.[21,31]

USEFULNESS OF MEASUREMENT OF AUTOANTIBODIES FOR DIAGNOSIS AND FOLLOW-UP

As can be concluded from **Tables 3** and **4**, ANCA measurement in the proper clinical context greatly aids in diagnosing AAV. Most patients with pauci-immune crescentic glomerulonephritis are ANCA positive; however, 10% to 30% of patients lack ANCA. Patients without ANCA might have fewer extrarenal symptoms than those who are ANCA positive.[33,34]

With the development of easy to use and rapid assays, such as the dotblot assay, any hospital can make use of rapid ANCA testing for patients with rapidly progressive renal failure.[35,36] The value of measuring ANCA during follow-up of patients is less straightforward. In a small study, it was shown that relapse could be prevented when patients were treated with cyclophosphamide after an increase in ANCA titer. Cumulative cyclophosphamide dosage was lower in patients on preemptive treatment than in a control group of patients who were untreated except in cases of clinical relapse after an increase in titer.[37] However, cyclophosphamide toxicity makes it inadvisable to preemptively treat all patients with such a regimen, as some, but not all increases in ANCA titer were followed by a disease relapse.[36] Boomsma and colleagues[38] performed a prospective study on 100 patients with AAV; ANCA were measured every 2 months. A relapse was preceded by an

Table 2
Overview of existing and accepted treatment modalities for ANCA-associated vasculitis (AAV) with pauci-immune renal involvement

	Induction	Remission	Remarks and References
Oral cyclophosphamide	Cyclophosphamide (2 mg/kg orally, max 200 mg/d)	Azathioprine (1.5–2 mg/kg)	Dose adjustments[21]: 25% lower dose if patient is >60 y old 50% lower dose if patient is >75 y old
Intravenous (IV) pulse cyclophosphamide	Cyclophosphamide (IV 15 mg/kg, max 1.2 g) every 2 weeks for the first 3 pulses, followed by infusions every 3 weeks for the next 3–6 pulses	Azathioprine (2 mg/kg)	Dose adjustment[23]: 60–70 y of age: 12.5 mg/kg/pulse >70 y of age: 10 mg/kg/pulse Creatinine 300–500 μmol/L: lower dose by 2.5 mg/kg/pulse (creatinine >500 μmol/L: see plasmapheresis)
Plasmapheresis	Added to other therapy in severe renal/pulmonary involvement or refractory disease Seven plasma exchanges within 14 days, each exchange at least 60 mg/kg, volume replacement with 5% albumin		A randomized study[45] of 70 patients receiving plasma exchange versus 67 patients receiving 3000 mg of IV methylprednisolone. At 3 months, 49% of patients treated with IV methylprednisolone compared with 69% treated with plasma exchange were alive and independent of dialysis (P = .02). Patient survival and severe adverse event rates were similar in both groups
Rituximab	Rituximab (375 mg/m² IV weekly for 4 weeks) No maintenance therapy, corticosteroids up to 6 months		RAVE study presented at the ACR 2009 (Arthritis Rheum 2009;60:S204), full length publication pending). Rituximab is not inferior for the induction of remission in severe AAV, compared with cyclophosphamide induction and azathioprine maintenance
	Rituximab (375 mg/m² IV weekly for 4 weeks) combined with 1 pulse methylprednisolone and 2 pulses cyclophosphamide Low dose corticosteroids as maintenance therapy		RITUXVAS study completed, full length publication pending. Data presented at the World Congress of Nephrology in 2009 (Abstract Sa773) show that the study's primary end point, sustained remission at 12 months, was achieved by 25 of 33 (76%) patients in the rituximab-based therapy group, and by 9 of 11 (82%) patients in the cyclophosphamide group (P = .67)

Mycophenolate mofetil (MMF)	MMF (2×1000 mg orally/d), 1–3 times 1 g of methylprednisolone followed by prednisolone 1 mg/kg/d	Open-label study[46] with 17 patients with MPO-ANCA and MPA. 13 reached the primary end point: remission at 6 months and stable renal function Currently, a randomized open-label study is being conducted
Intravenous immunoglobulin	Total 2 g/kg over 5 days	34 patients with active AAV, without rapidly progressive glomerulonephritis, after at least 2 months treatment with prednisolone and cyclophosphamide or azathioprine were randomized to IVIG or placebo. IVIG reduced disease activity, but this effect was not maintained beyond 3 months[47,48]
Methotrexate	Methotrexate (20–25 mg orally/wk)	Not suitable in pauci-immune renal disease. Only early systemic disease, serum creatinine <150 μmol/L, more relapses were observed compared with cyclophosphamide[49]
15-Deoxyspergualin	0.5 mg/kg/d subcutaneous injection for 21 days in six 28-day cycles. Cycles were stopped early for white blood count less than 4000 cells/mm³	Three open-label studies[50–52] in refractory cases. Complete remission was achieved in 32 of 75 patients (43%). Most frequent side effect was leukopenia

All protocols contain high-dose corticosteroids (1 mg/kg/d, maximum 60–80 mg) at the start of therapy. The initial high dose should be maintained for 4 weeks, after which the dose is tapered according to various tapering schedules. Corticosteroid dose should not be reduced to less than 15 mg/d for the first 3 months.

Abbreviation: IVIG, intravenous high-dose immunoglobulin.

Data from Mukhtyar C, Guillevin L, Cid MC, et al. EULAR recommendations for the management of primary small and medium vessel vasculitis. Ann Rheum Dis 2009;68(3):310–7.

Table 3
Estimated positive predictive value (PPV) and negative predictive value (NPV) of ANCA for pauci-immune renal disease in patients >18 years of age with different clinical contexts

Clinical Context		Prevalence of Pauci-Immune Renal Disease (%)	PPV (%)	NPV (%)
Rapidly progressive glomerulonephritis[a]		47	98	80
Hematuria, proteinuria, and serum creatinine (μmol/L)	>265	21	92	93
	130–265	7	77	98
	<130	2	47	99

[a] Rapidly progressive glomerulonephritis was presumed when >50% of glomeruli in a biopsy were crescentic.

From Jennette JC, Wilkman AS, Falk RJ. Diagnostic predictive value of ANCA serology. Kidney Int 1998;53(3):796–8; with permission.

increase in ANCA titer in 34 of the 37 (92%) patients who experienced a relapse during the study period. Forty-three percent of patients who showed an increase in cANCA (by indirect immunofluorescence) and 29% with an increase in PR3-ANCA (by enzyme-linked immunosorbent assay) did not subsequently experience a relapse. More recently, however, data from the WG etanercept trial (WGET) in which ANCA levels of 136 WG patients were prospectively monitored every 3 months, demonstrate that changes in ANCA levels explain less than 10% of the variation in disease activity.[39] The recently performed RITUXVAS study showed that all patients treated with rituximab became ANCA negative, compared with two-thirds of the patients in the cyclophosphamide group (data presented at World Congress of Nephrology 2009: see http://www.medscape.com/viewarticle/703732). Longer follow-up data will have to show the clinical relevance of this finding.

Thus, measuring ANCA greatly aids in the diagnosis of patients with AAV; during follow-up, increases in ANCA titer and persistent high ANCA titers might indicate a higher risk of relapse although the therapeutic implications of this association are unclear.

RENAL TRANSPLANTATION IN PAUCI-IMMUNE RENAL DISEASE

Twenty to forty percent of patients with ANCA-associated renal vasculitis develop ESRD.[40–42] Renal transplantation in these patients is a feasible option and allograft survival is comparable with other inflammatory renal diseases. Moreover, disease

Table 4
Estimated positive predictive value (PPV) and negative predictive value (NPV) of ANCA for pauci-immune renal disease in patients >50 years of age with different clinical contexts

Clinical Context		Prevalence of Pauci-Immune Renal Disease (%)	PPV (%)	NPV (%)
Rapidly progressive glomerulonephritis[a]		66	99	65
Hematuria, proteinuria, and serum creatinine (μmol/L)	>265	30	95	89
	130–265	11	85	97
	<130	4	66	99

[a] Rapidly progressive glomerulonephritis was presumed when >50% of glomeruli in a biopsy were crescentic.

From Jennette JC, Wilkman AS, Falk RJ. Diagnostic predictive value of ANCA serology. Kidney Int 1998;53(3):796–8; with permission.

relapse is lower after transplant compared with before transplant.[43] Little and colleagues[44] recently published an overview on safety issues when considering a renal transplantation in patients with ANCA-associated vasculitis. They concluded that the presence of circulating ANCA at the time of transplantation was associated with the development of vascular lesions in the graft, but was not significantly correlated with graft survival. Also, in multivariate analysis, patients were more likely to die when transplantation was performed within 12 months after reaching disease remission compared with transplantation after 12 months.

ACKNOWLEDGMENTS

Dr M.C.R.F. van Dijk, pathologist, is greatly appreciated for the commentary on the renal biopsy specimens.

REFERENCES

1. Jennette JC, Falk RJ, Andrassy K, et al. Nomenclature of systemic vasculitides. Proposal of an international consensus conference. Arthritis Rheum 1994;37(2): 187–92.
2. Pagnoux C, Hogan SL, Chin H, et al. Predictors of treatment resistance and relapse in antineutrophil cytoplasmic antibody-associated small-vessel vasculitis: comparison of two independent cohorts. Arthritis Rheum 2008;58(9):2908–18.
3. Sinico RA, Di Toma L, Maggiore U, et al. Renal involvement in Churg-Strauss syndrome. Am J Kidney Dis 2006;47(5):770–9.
4. Jennette JC, Falk RJ. Antineutrophil cytoplasmic autoantibodies and associated diseases: a review. Am J Kidney Dis 1990;15(6):517–29.
5. Jennette JC, Wilkman AS, Falk RJ. Anti-neutrophil cytoplasmic autoantibody-associated glomerulonephritis and vasculitis. Am J Pathol 1989;135(5):921–30.
6. Wegener F. Uber die eigenartige rhinogene Granulomatose mit besonderer Beteiligung des Arteriensystems unde der nieren. Beitrage zur Path Anat 1939;102: 36–68 [in German].
7. Rutgers A, Slot M, van Paassen P, et al. Coexistence of anti-glomerular basement membrane antibodies and myeloperoxidase-ANCAs in crescentic glomerulonephritis. Am J Kidney Dis 2005;46(2):253–62.
8. Hauer HA, Bajema IM, van Houwelingen HC, et al. Renal histology in ANCA-associated vasculitis: differences between diagnostic and serologic subgroups. Kidney Int 2002;61(1):80–9.
9. Hogan SL, Nachman PH, Wilkman AS, et al. Prognostic markers in patients with antineutrophil cytoplasmic autoantibody-associated microscopic polyangiitis and glomerulonephritis. J Am Soc Nephrol 1996;7(1):23–32.
10. de Lind van Wijngaarden RA, Hauer HA, Wolterbeek R, et al. Clinical and histologic determinants of renal outcome in ANCA-associated vasculitis: a prospective analysis of 100 patients with severe renal involvement. J Am Soc Nephrol 2006; 17(8):2264–74.
11. Haas M, Eustace JA. Immune complex deposits in ANCA-associated crescentic glomerulonephritis: a study of 126 cases. Kidney Int 2004;65(6):2145–52.
12. Holmen C, Christensson M, Pettersson E, et al. Wegener's granulomatosis is associated with organ-specific antiendothelial cell antibodies. Kidney Int 2004; 66(3):1049–60.
13. Hoffman GS. Disease patterns in vasculitis – still a mystery. Bull NYU Hosp Jt Dis 2008;66(3):224–7.

14. Hoffman GS. Determinants of vessel targeting in vasculitis. Clin Dev Immunol 2004;11(3–4):275–9.

15. Hu N, Westra J, Huitema MG, et al. Autoantibodies against glomerular endothelial cells in anti-neutrophil cytoplasmic autoantibody-associated systemic vasculitis. Nephrology (Carlton) 2009;14(1):11–5.

16. Jarad G, Miner JH. Update on the glomerular filtration barrier. Curr Opin Nephrol Hypertens 2009;18(3):226–32.

17. Besbas N, Ozaltin F, Catal F, et al. Monocyte chemoattractant protein-1 and interleukin-8 levels in children with acute poststreptococcal glomerulonephritis. Pediatr Nephrol 2004;19(8):864–8.

18. Tam FW, Sanders JS, George A, et al. Urinary monocyte chemoattractant protein-1 (MCP-1) is a marker of active renal vasculitis. Nephrol Dial Transplant 2004; 19(11):2761–8.

19. Tse WY, Nash GB, Hewins P, et al. ANCA-induced neutrophil F-actin polymerization: implications for microvascular inflammation. Kidney Int 2005;67(1): 130–9.

20. Mohammad AJ, Jacobsson LT, Westman KW, et al. Incidence and survival rates in Wegener's granulomatosis, microscopic polyangiitis, Churg-Strauss syndrome and polyarteritis nodosa. Rheumatology (Oxford) 2009;48(12): 1560–5.

21. Mukhtyar C, Guillevin L, Cid MC, et al. EULAR recommendations for the management of primary small and medium vessel vasculitis. Ann Rheum Dis 2009;68(3): 310–7.

22. Walsh M, Merkel PA, Mahr A, et al. The effects of duration of glucocorticoid therapy on relapse rate in anti-neutrophil cytoplasm antibody associated vasculitis: a meta-analysis. Arthritis Care Res 2010. [Epub ahead of print].

23. de Groot K, Harper L, Jayne DR, et al. Pulse versus daily oral cyclophosphamide for induction of remission in antineutrophil cytoplasmic antibody-associated vasculitis: a randomized trial. Ann Intern Med 2009;150(10):670–80.

24. de Groot K, Adu D, Savage CO. The value of pulse cyclophosphamide in ANCA-associated vasculitis: meta-analysis and critical review. Nephrol Dial Transplant 2001;16(10):2018–27.

25. Levine SM. Comment on pulse versus daily oral cyclophosphamide in ANCA-associated vasculitis. Ann Intern Med 2010;152:64–5.

26. Sanders JS, Huitma MG, Kallenberg CG, et al. Prediction of relapses in PR3-ANCA-associated vasculitis by assessing responses of ANCA titres to treatment. Rheumatology (Oxford) 2006;45(6):724–9.

27. de Lind van Wijngaarden RA, Hauer HA, Wolterbeek R, et al. Chances of renal recovery for dialysis-dependent ANCA-associated glomerulonephritis. J Am Soc Nephrol 2007;18(7):2189–97.

28. Lionaki S, Hogan SL, Jennette CE, et al. The clinical course of ANCA small-vessel vasculitis on chronic dialysis. Kidney Int 2009;76(6):644–51.

29. Aasarod K, Bostad L, Hammerstrom J, et al. Renal histopathology and clinical course in 94 patients with Wegener's granulomatosis. Nephrol Dial Transplant 2001;16(5):953–60.

30. Jennette JC, Wilkman AS, Falk RJ. Diagnostic predictive value of ANCA serology. Kidney Int 1998;53(3):796–8.

31. Klein I, Vervoort G, Steenbergen E, et al. Progressive renal disease despite immunosuppressive therapy in a patient with Wegener s granulomatosis. Neth J Med 2008;66(3):125–7.

32. Hagen EC, Daha MR, Hermans J, et al. Diagnostic value of standardized assays for anti-neutrophil cytoplasmic antibodies in idiopathic systemic vasculitis. EC/BCR Project for ANCA Assay Standardization. Kidney Int 1998;53(3): 743–53.
33. Chen M, Kallenberg CG, Zhao MH. ANCA-negative pauci-immune crescentic glomerulonephritis. Nat Rev Nephrol 2009;5(6):313–8.
34. Sable-Fourtassou R, Cohen P, Mahr A, et al. Antineutrophil cytoplasmic antibodies and the Churg-Strauss syndrome. Ann Intern Med 2005;143(9):632–8.
35. Rutgers A, Damoiseaux J, Roozendaal C, et al. ANCA-GBM dot-blot: evaluation of an assay in the differential diagnosis of patients presenting with rapidly progressive glomerulonephritis. J Clin Immunol 2004;24(4):435–40.
36. Rutgers A, Heeringa P, Damoiseaux JG. ANCA and anti-GBM antibodies in diagnosis and follow-up of vasculitic disease. Eur J Intern Med 2003;14(5):287–95.
37. Tervaert JW, Huitema MG, Hene RJ, et al. Prevention of relapses in Wegener's granulomatosis by treatment based on antineutrophil cytoplasmic antibody titre. Lancet 1990;336(8717):709–11.
38. Boomsma MM, Stegeman CA, van der Leij MJ, et al. Prediction of relapses in Wegener's granulomatosis by measurement of antineutrophil cytoplasmic antibody levels: a prospective study. Arthritis Rheum 2000;43(9):2025–33.
39. Finkielman JD, Merkel PA, Schroeder D, et al. Antiproteinase 3 antineutrophil cytoplasmic antibodies and disease activity in Wegener granulomatosis. Ann Intern Med 2007;147(9):611–9.
40. Booth AD, Almond MK, Burns A, et al. Outcome of ANCA-associated renal vasculitis: a 5-year retrospective study. Am J Kidney Dis 2003;41(4):776–84.
41. Little MA, Nazar L, Farrington K. Outcome in glomerulonephritis due to systemic small vessel vasculitis: effect of functional status and non-vasculitic co-morbidity. Nephrol Dial Transplant 2004;19(2):356–64.
42. Slot MC, Tervaert JW, Franssen CF, et al. Renal survival and prognostic factors in patients with PR3-ANCA associated vasculitis with renal involvement. Kidney Int 2003;63(2):670–7.
43. Nachman PH, Segelmark M, Westman K, et al. Recurrent ANCA-associated small vessel vasculitis after transplantation: a pooled analysis. Kidney Int 1999;56(4): 1544–50.
44. Little MA, Hassan B, Jacques S, et al. Renal transplantation in systemic vasculitis: when is it safe? Nephrol Dial Transplant 2009;24(10):3219–25.
45. Jayne DR, Gaskin G, Rasmussen N, et al. Randomized trial of plasma exchange or high-dosage methylprednisolone as adjunctive therapy for severe renal vasculitis. J Am Soc Nephrol 2007;18(7):2180–8.
46. Silva F, Specks U, Kalra S, et al. Mycophenolate mofetil for induction and maintenance of remission in microscopic polyangiitis with mild to moderate renal involvement–a prospective, open-label pilot trial. Clin J Am Soc Nephrol 2010; 5(3):445–53.
47. Jayne DR, Chapel H, Adu D, et al. Intravenous immunoglobulin for ANCA-associated systemic vasculitis with persistent disease activity. QJM 2000; 93(7):433–9.
48. Muso E, Ito-Ihara T, Ono T, et al. Intravenous immunoglobulin (IVIg) therapy in MPO-ANCA related polyangiitis with rapidly progressive glomerulonephritis in Japan. Jpn J Infect Dis 2004;57(5):S17–8.
49. de Groot K, Rasmussen N, Bacon PA, et al. Randomized trial of cyclophosphamide versus methotrexate for induction of remission in early systemic

antineutrophil cytoplasmic antibody-associated vasculitis. Arthritis Rheum 2005; 52(8):2461–9.

50. Birck R, Warnatz K, Lorenz HM, et al. 15-Deoxyspergualin in patients with refractory ANCA-associated systemic vasculitis: a six-month open-label trial to evaluate safety and efficacy. J Am Soc Nephrol 2003;14(2):440–7.

51. Flossmann O, Jayne DR. Long-term treatment of relapsing Wegener's granulomatosis with 15-deoxyspergualin. Rheumatology (Oxford) 2010;49(3):556–62.

52. Flossmann O, Baslund B, Bruchfeld A, et al. Deoxyspergualin in relapsing and refractory Wegener's granulomatosis. Ann Rheum Dis 2009;68(7):1125–30.

53. Jayne D, Rasmussen N, Andrassy K, et al. A randomized trial of maintenance therapy for vasculitis associated with antineutrophil cytoplasmic autoantibodies. N Engl J Med 2003;349(1):36–44.

Ocular Manifestations of ANCA-associated Vasculitis

Anup A. Kubal, MD[a], Victor L. Perez, MD[b],*

KEYWORDS

- Wegener's granulomatosis • Churg-Strauss syndrome
- Microscopic polyangiitis • Antineutrophil cytoplasmic antibody

Vasculitis is characterized by blood vessel inflammation and necrosis of vascular endothelium. End-organ damage is the result of the destruction and occlusion of blood vessels. The antineutrophil cytoplasmic antibody (ANCA) associated vasculitides—Wegener's granulomatosis (WG), microscopic polyangiitis (MPA), and Churg-Strauss syndrome (CSS)—are diseases in which small to medium-sized blood vessels are affected. ANCAs not only serve as a marker for disease but are also thought to play a major role in disease pathogenesis. Proteinase-3 and myeloperoxidase, the two antigens that are the targets of ANCAs observed in these diseases, are found within the neutrophil, and degranulation of these leukocytes is thought to initiate the cascade of destruction.[1-3]

Of the three ANCA-associated vasculitides, WG is the most common. In a population-based study from Norfolk, England, the incidence of WG was 8.5 cases per million. The reported incidences of MPA and CSS were 3.6 cases and 2.4 cases per million, respectively.[4] Ophthalmologic findings, with ocular blood vessels as the target of disease, can be common, particularly in WG. They can sometimes be the presenting finding. Ocular or orbital involvement has been reported to occur in 29% to 52% of patients with WG.[5-7] In one cohort of 158 patients, 15% presented with ocular manifestations at diagnosis.[8] Ocular or orbital disease occurs less frequently in MPA and CSS. In a cohort of 85 patients with MPA, confirmed in most on biopsy, only one had ocular manifestations.[9] However, ocular findings can still be the initial presenting sign in these diseases.[2]

Therefore, the ability to recognize the ocular manifestations of vasculitis and associate them with the underlying systemic disease is important so that treatment can be

a Bascom Palmer Eye Institute, Miller School of Medicine, University of Miami, 900 NW 17th Street, Miami, FL 33136, USA
b Bascom Palmer Eye Institute, Miller School of Medicine, University of Miami, 1638 NW 10th Avenue, Suite 613, Miami, FL 33136, USA
* Corresponding author.
E-mail address: Vperez4@med.miami.edu

Rheum Dis Clin N Am 36 (2010) 573–586
doi:10.1016/j.rdc.2010.05.005
0889-857X/10/$ – see front matter © 2010 Elsevier Inc. All rights reserved.

initiated promptly to prevent morbidity and mortality. The systemic findings of WG, MPA, and CSS are described in other articles within this issue (see the articles by Chung and Seo; Baldini and colleagues; Holle and colleagues elsewhere in this issue for futher exploration of this topic). This article describes ocular and orbital findings (**Table 1**). However, one must be aware that many of the findings described and illustrated here are not pathognomic for ANCA-associated vasculitis and may be seen in other vasculitic, inflammatory, or infectious processes.

CONJUNCTIVAL, EPISCLERAL, AND SCLERAL DISEASE

These manifestations can sometimes be difficult to distinguish from each other because they all can present with ocular redness and discomfort. The key to distinguishing them is recognizing the depth of tissue involvement associated with the blood vessel plexus (**Fig. 1**). For example, in episcleritis, the superficial episcleral plexus is thought to be affected by the vasculitis process (see **Fig. 1**B), in contrast to scleritis, in which the deep episcleral plexus is affected (see **Fig. 1**C).

Conjunctival disease has been reported to occur in 4% to 16% of patients with WG.[10–12] Early disease presents with conjunctival hyperemia. Granulomas can also be present and disease is often bilateral. Progressive disease is characterized by cicatrizing conjunctivitis, which may result in symblepharon, or bands of fibrovascular tissue stretching across the ocular surface to the eyelids; entropion with an inturning eyelid; and trichiasis with eyelashes directed against the globe (**Fig. 2**). The palpebral surface of the upper eyelid is most commonly involved. Ocular exposure may occur, increasing the risk of secondary infectious keratitis. Exposure is often exacerbated by a tear deficiency caused by loss of the mucin-producing conjunctival goblet cells and destruction of lacrimal glands. Symptoms of conjunctival disease often include ocular redness, foreign body sensation, blurred vision from tear dysfunction, and possibly bloody tears.

The first reported case of MPA involving the conjunctiva and eyelid was in a 23-year-old black woman with renal failure and ulcerative skin and conjunctival nodules.

Table 1
Prevalence of ophthalmic findings in the ANCA-associated vasculitides

	Wegener's Granulomatosis	Microscopic Polyangiitis	Churg-Strauss Syndrome
Conjunctivitis	4%–16%	+	+
Episcleritis	+	+	+
Scleritis	16%–38%	+	−
Peripheral ulcerative keratitis	+	+	+
Retinal vasculitis	+	+	+
Orbital disease Mass/myositis/ dacryoadenitis	+	−	+
Nasolacrimal obstruction	7%–10%	−	−
Neuroophthalmic manifestations	+	−	+

Numerical values listed are obtained from the references listed in the text. Plus signs indicate manifestations that have been documented in case reports. Minus signs indicate manifestations that have not yet been reported for the respective disease entity.

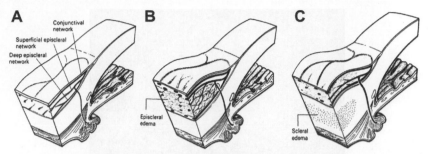

Fig. 1. Schematic illustrating depth of tissue involvement in conjunctivitis, episcleritis, and scleritis. (A) Normal anatomy. The most superficial layer, the conjunctiva is affected in conjunctivitis. (B) Episcleritis. Note the edema anterior to the sclera associated with vascular involvement of the superficial episcleralplexus (C) Scleritis. The edema is deeper than in episcleritis consistent with involvement of the deep episcleral plexus. (*From* Foster CS, de la Maza MS. The Sclera. Berlin: SpringerVerlag; 1993. p. 69; with permission.)

Laboratory testing was positive for perinuclear ANCA (p-ANCA) and the patient experienced response to treatment with cyclophosphamide.[13] Several cases of conjunctival involvement in CSS have been reported, including a 30-year-old woman with adult-onset asthma, a lung mass, peripheral eosinophilia, and a conjunctival nodule responding to oral corticosteroids.[14–17]

Conjunctival biopsy may be helpful in diagnosis because specimens may show evidence of necrosis and occlusive vasculitis. The differential diagnosis includes more common causes of conjunctivitis, such as allergies or infections, including adenovirus. More severe cicatrizing conjunctivitis can also be found in diseases such as ocular cicatricial pemphigoid and trachoma. Treatment often requires aqueous tear replacement and surgical intervention involving lysis of adhesions with removal of scar tissue, and ocular surface reconstruction with either mucous membrane or amniotic membrane grafts.

Episcleritis also presents with ocular redness. It can be unilateral or bilateral, diffuse or sectoral, or nodular in presentation. Dilated blood vessels typically appear in a radial pattern emanating from the corneoscleral limbus, and the redness blanches with application of topical 2.5% phenylephrine drops (**Fig. 3**). In addition, because the

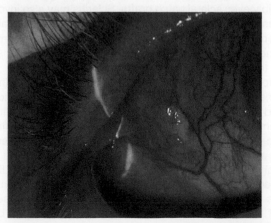

Fig. 2. Conjunctival disease. Conjunctival cicatrization with symblepharon formation in an 83-year-old woman with MPA.

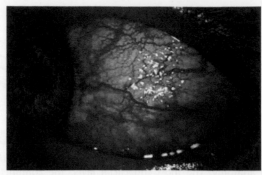

Fig. 3. Episcleritis. Note the largely radial pattern of blood vessels. This patient did not have any ocular pain and the area of inflammation is movable and blanches on installation of 2.5% phenylephrine eye drops.

lesions occur in the loose connective tissue overlying the sclera, the lesions are mobile. The ocular morbidity of episcleritis is minimal. This condition is usually idiopathic, with systemic associations such as ANCA-associated vasculitis in approximately one-third of cases.[18] In most instances these cases are associated with bilateral involvement and recurrent symptoms.

Scleritis, in contrast to episcleritis, can cause serious ocular morbidity. It often presents with deeper, boring pain and photophobia. The affected eye can be very tender to palpation. Dilated blood vessels have a crisscross or network-like appearance. The redness is not mobile and does not blanch with phenylephrine drops. Scleritis may be associated with a keratitis or iritis (as discussed later). Anterior scleritis may be diffuse, sectoral, nodular, or necrotizing, a classification scheme first described by Watson and Hayreh (**Fig. 4**).[19] In necrotizing disease, the underlying pigmented uveal tissue of the choroid and retina will appear bluish in the areas of scleromalacia.

The risk of scleral thinning and perforation can be exacerbated by secondary infection. Severe ocular complications occur in more than 90% of patients, often resulting in blindness.[20] In addition to systemic immunosuppression to treat the underlying disease, patients with necrotizing scleritis often require aggressive topical antibiotic therapy and possibly even scleral patch grafts. Scleritis may also involve the posterior sclera. In these cases, patients may present with an atypical, nonlocalizing "odd" pain with ocular movement and decreased vision from exudative retinal detachments. Choroidal folds may be seen on dilated funduscopic examination and ocular ultrasound may show thickening of the posterior globe (see **Fig. 4**D).

Scleritis is associated with an underlying systemic disorder in up to 50% of patients.[10,21,22] The differential diagnosis for scleritis is broad and includes numerous rheumatologic and inflammatory diseases, such as rheumatoid arthritis, relapsing polychondritis, systemic lupus erythematosus, Behçet's syndrome, inflammatory bowel disease, psoriatic arthritis, and sarcoidosis, and infectious processes caused by bacterial, fungal, and parasitic infection. These diseases must be considered and excluded based on history, clinical examination, and laboratory findings.

Scleritis has been reported to occur in 16% to 38% of patients with WG.[12,21] Necrotizing scleritis has a much higher association with systemic disease, and is seen in more than half of the patients with ocular WG.[23,24] Mortality has been reported to be as high as 54% in patients with necrotizing scleritis who are not undergoing immunosuppressive therapy.[25]

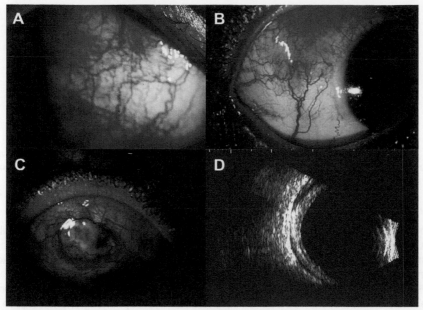

Fig. 4. Scleritis. (*A*) Diffuse anterior scleritis. Note the crisscross pattern of blood vessels. These vessels do not blanch with the application of topical phenylephrine. (*B*) Nodular scleritis. Note the elevated nature of this localized lesion. (*C*) Necrotizing scleritis. Note scleromalacia and the appearance of the underlying uveal tissue, which appears blue. (*D*) Posterior scleritis. Ocular ultrasound shows thickening of the posterior wall of the globe.

Cases of scleritis in MPA have also been reported, mostly from Japan. In one case, a 60-year-old woman presented with renal failure and bilateral scleritis, which responded to intravenous corticosteroid treatment.[26] Another report described a 79-year-old man with bilateral scleritis, fatigue, and pulmonary disease, also responsive to systemic corticosteroids.[27]

The onset of scleritis in a patient with vasculitis is a serious ophthalmic manifestation. It is either the first manifestation of the disease or a marker that systemic disease is active and aggressive therapy must be implemented to prevent not only ocular morbidity but also systemic multiorgan complications.

CORNEAL MANIFESTATIONS

Corneal findings of the ANCA-associated vasculitides are often present in concert with other anterior segment manifestations, particularly necrotizing scleritis.[12] Conjunctival scarring with resultant tear deficiency, entropion, trichiasis, and poor eyelid closure can produce an exposure keratopathy, secondary infectious ulceration, and even corneal perforation. Proptosis from orbital disease (as discussed later) can also cause exposure and its sequelae.

In addition to these secondary corneal findings, inflammatory disease may specifically target the cornea, resulting in a condition known as *peripheral ulcerative keratitis* (PUK). This condition is typically unilateral and sectoral, although bilateral disease can occur in up to 40% of patients.[28] The lesions usually are found within 2 mm of the corneoscleral limbus, and the adjacent limbal tissue and sclera show evidence of vasculitic disease (**Fig. 5**). The affected corneal stroma can be markedly thin as keratolysis

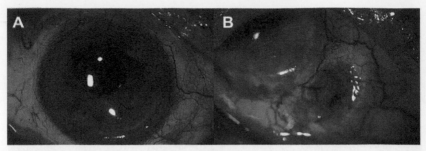

Fig. 5. (*A*) Peripheral ulcerative keratitis (PUK) in a patient with a history of prior cataract extraction and superior iridectomy. Note the inferior arc-shaped area of corneal thinning. (*B*) PUK with adjacent necrotizing scleritis.

progresses to potential corneal perforation either spontaneously or with minor ocular trauma. An epithelial defect may be present, predisposing patients to secondary infection. Patients typically present with pain, injection, photophobia, and decreased vision from corneal opacities or induced astigmatism.

PUK is typically associated with an underlying systemic disease, most commonly rheumatoid arthritis followed by WG.[29] Peripheral keratitis, although nonulcerative in appearance, was reported as a presenting sign of MPA in a 16-year-old girl who subsequently developed renal failure.[30] Recurrent PUK has also been described in a 44-year-old woman with asthma, hemorrhagic skin lesions, peripheral eosinophilia, and positive ANCA titers, confirming the diagnosis of CSS.[31] Concurrent scleritis is found in approximately one-third of patients with PUK.[32,33] Conversely, only 14% of patients with scleritis have PUK.[20] In those with both conditions, the scleritis is necrotizing in nearly 60% of cases.[28]

The differential diagnosis for PUK includes all conditions listed earlier for scleritis, in addition to localized inflammatory conditions such as rosacea. Other disease entities may resemble PUK. Mooren's ulcer has a similar appearance, but no systemic or local associations exist except for possible hepatitis C exposure. Terrien's marginal degeneration also presents with peripheral corneal thinning. However, this condition is noninflammatory and very slowly progressive. A line of lipid is present at the leading edge of the area of thinning and, unlike PUK, the epithelium remains intact. Dellen or localized corneal dehydration and thinning related to tear film irregularities can be caused by an adjacent site of tissue elevation.

Definitive treatment of PUK requires systemic immunosuppression, but adjunctive local therapies may be beneficial. Because corneal epithelial breakdown is common, topical antibiotic coverage and aggressive tear replacement should be instituted. Matrix metalloproteinases (MMPs) are believed to play a role in keratolysis, and elevated levels of these enzymes have been found in the tears and corneal tissue of patients with PUK.[34,35] Doxycycline, which has been shown to inhibit MMP activity, may therefore be helpful in limiting corneal melts.[36] Topical medroxyprogesterone acetate has also been shown to limit collagenase activity and is often used in these settings.[37]

In one series, impending or frank corneal perforation was reported to occur in one-third of patients with PUK.[28] In another series of patients with scleritis-associated PUK, 100% were in danger of perforation.[32] Imminent or overt corneal perforation can be managed by placement of cyanoacrylate glue or a contact lens as a bandage. Larger corneal defects may require the use of corneal patch grafts or therapeutic corneal transplants. The failure rate of these grafts is extremely high, because the persistence of inflammatory mediators increases the likelihood of graft rejection and may lead to progressive melting of the transplanted tissue.[38] Because the cornea is an avascular structure, and the inflammatory mediators of tissue destruction are thought to travel into the cornea from the dilated blood vessels in paralimbal tissues, conjunctival resection has been advocated in the management of PUK.[39] This procedure, however, remains controversial.

RETINOVASCULAR

Posterior segment complications are uncommon, but the blood vessels of the retinal and choroidal circulation of the eye can be affected by ANCA-associated vasculitic disease. These patients tend to present with a decline in visual acuity or loss of visual field, because vascular occlusion leads to rapid retinal ischemia and death of retinal photoreceptors (**Fig. 6**). Several cases of branch or central retinal vein occlusion (RVO) have been reported in patients with WG.[40–42] The arterial circulation of the retina and choroid also may be involved. One report described a 64-year-old man with WG and glomerulonephritis who presented with a central retinal artery occlusion (RAO) in one eye and a branch retinal artery occlusion in the other, leaving him legally blind.[43] Vitritis is usually absent.[41] RVO and RAO have been reported also in patients with CSS.[44–46] No cases have been described in patients with MPA. However, retinal cotton-wool spots, which represent nerve fiber layer infarcts and microvascular disease, have been described in MPA.[27]

Diagnosis is often confirmed through fluorescein angiography, which shows delayed or absent filling in the distribution of the involved blood vessel or patchy leakage in areas of ischemia. RVO and RAO occur more commonly in patients with other systemic inflammatory diseases such as systemic lupus erythematosus; atherosclerotic vascular disease such as hypertension and hypercholesterolemia; and hypercoagulable states than in those with ANCA-associated vasculitis. Ischemic tissues release potent stimulators of neovascularization, such as vascular endothelial growth factor (VEGF). Neovascular vessels, however, develop outside the plane of the retina. They can bleed, causing vitreous hemorrhage, and their fibrous scaffold can contract, causing retinal detachment. Neovascularization and contraction of fibrous tissue can also occur in the anterior segment, closing off the trabecular meshwork to drainage of aqueous humor and causing intraocular pressure elevation and glaucoma, which further affects the visual field. Treatment involves intraocular injections with anti-VEGF agents such as ranibizumab and bevacizumab,[47] and panretinal laser

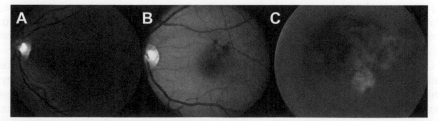

Fig. 6. Retinovascular disease. (*A*) Normal retina. Note the pink-appearing optic nerve with blood vessels (both arteries and veins) emanating from the nerve. The macula, which appears darker than the surrounding retina, is in the center of the photograph. (*B*) Retinal vasculitis affecting the superior macula of this left eye. Note the small hemorrhages and associated retinal swelling. (*C*) More extensive retinal vasculitis with profound hemorrhage.

photocoagulation because thermal destruction of the peripheral retina decreases release of VEGF from ischemic tissues.

ORBITAL

Orbital involvement is one of the most common manifestations of WG, occurring in almost half of the patients with WG and ophthalmic disease.[5,48] In a review of 29 patients with orbital and adnexal WG, signs and symptoms included proptosis in 69% of patients; sinusitis in 69%; epiphora (overflow of tears from obstruction of lacrimal duct) in 52%; diplopia in 52%; eyelid edema and erythema in 31%; orbital pain in 24%; and decreased visual acuity with evidence of optic nerve compression in 17%.[49] Although proptosis from mass effect and infiltration of orbital structures such as the lacrimal gland is a common finding, enophthalmos (recession of the eyeball within the orbit) has also been reported.[50] This condition is thought to be a late sequelae of chronic orbital inflammation as scar tissue contracts, and is therefore relatively unresponsive to immunosuppressive treatment.

Orbital disease is often contiguous with sinus disease, correlating with the high percentage of sinus complaints in this cohort of patients. Epiphora is often caused by nasolacrimal duct obstruction, but lacrimal sac mucocele is also a common cause. Diplopia has many causes, including direct mass effect on the globe, infiltration of extraocular muscles, vasculitis involving the vasa vasorum of the extraocular muscles, and involvement of cranial nerves (see later section on "Other Manifestations").

Orbital involvement has also been described in CSS presenting as dacryoadenitis or myositis.[51–54] A review of 17 cases of CSS suggests that patients with orbital disease, rather than the ocular findings described in the previous sections, have a better overall prognosis. All patients reported in the literature with only orbital disease in CSS have maintained good visual acuity.[52]

Imaging modalities such as ultrasound, CT, or MRI (**Fig. 7**) may be helpful in characterizing the size and extent of the lesion and its response to therapy. Imaging can also help rule out other diseases in the differential diagnosis (as discussed later). Moreover, imaging can also help in evaluating the risk for optic nerve compression and planning surgery if indicated.

When the diagnosis of the ANCA-associated vasculitides is in question, the orbit can also serve as source of tissue for histopathologic diagnosis. In one series of patients with WG, the classic triad of vasculitis, tissue necrosis, and granulomatous inflammation was found in 7 of 13 (54%) of biopsy specimens.[55] Other groups have reported a higher yield of 75% to 85%.[56,57] Open lung biopsies are the most diagnostic and are positive in up to 91% of cases.[8] Although the yield may not be as high for orbital specimens, it is often much easier to access the orbit for biopsy than other target organs, such as the lung or kidney. Orbital biopsy can also help diagnose CSS. Cases of infiltration of the lacrimal glands and extraocular muscles with eosinophils have been reported.[52]

Other orbital processes can present with similar signs and symptoms and must be included in the differential diagnosis. The most common is thyroid ophthalmopathy, which is typically associated with the hyperthyroidism of Graves' disease. These patients can present with unilateral or bilateral proptosis, strabismus and diplopia, and vision loss from compressive optic neuropathy. Histopathologic examination shows a lymphocytic infiltration of orbital tissues. When extraocular muscles are involved, the muscle tendons are often spared; this finding can often be detected with the imaging modalities described earlier. Patients also show a characteristic eyelid retraction. Infectious processes, such as orbital cellulitis, should also be

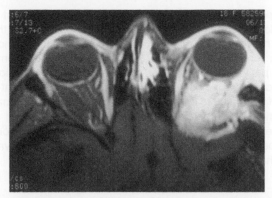

Fig. 7. T1-weighted MRI showing a diffusely infiltrating mass within the left orbit of an 18-year-old patient with WG. This patient presented with proptosis.

considered, especially because orbital infections often originate in adjacent sinuses. Orbital cellulitis may even coexist with vasculitic disease. WG that extends from a paranasal sinus can create a track for bacteria or other organisms to enter the orbit. These patients may, therefore, require systemic antibiotics in addition to systemic immunosuppression. Sarcoidosis and malignancy, such as lymphoma, can also present with orbital findings.

Orbital adnexal structures can also be affected in vasculitic disease.[58] Nasolacrimal obstruction with symptomatic epiphora has been reported in 7% to 10% of patients with WG.[5,56] Dacryocystorhinostomy, in which a fistula is created between the lacrimal sac and nasal cavity, is currently the preferred procedure to bypass this obstruction. Several authors have reported their success with this procedure in patients with WG.[59–61] In one series, long-term success was achieved in 60% of operations. Failures were related to recurrent disease activity or dacryopyocele.[60] Dacryocystectomy or removal of the lacrimal sac may be a better approach than dacryocystorhinostomy for lacrimal sac infections in patients with WG.[62]

OTHER MANIFESTATIONS

Anterior, intermediate, and posterior uveitis can also be seen in ANCA-associated disease but are uncommon. They have been reported to occur in 0% to 10% of patients with WG.[5–7] Iridocyclitis with an anterior chamber inflammatory reaction typically occurs secondary to keratitis or scleritis rather than as a primary manifestation.[21] Granulomatous anterior uveitis with large inflammatory deposits on the posterior corneal surface has been seen in patients with WG.[6,63] One report described a middle-aged French man with a 15-year history of recurrent anterior uveitis in the right eye treated with local corticosteroid therapy who presented with an acute decline in vision. He was found to have developed a granulomatous panuveitis with retinal vasculitis. Diagnosis of WG was confirmed on biopsy of a pulmonary nodule. The patient was initially treated with systemic corticosteroids and cyclophosphamide and experienced improvement in his vision.[63] Severe panuveitis has also been described in a patient with CSS who eventually underwent enucleation.[64] Hypopyoniridocyclitis with layering of inflammatory material in the anterior chamber, which is more commonly seen in conditions such as Behçet's syndrome or HLA-B27–associated disease, was reported in a patient with MPA who was successfully treated with oral and subconjunctival corticosteroids.[27]

Although diplopia or vision loss from optic neuropathy are most commonly from infiltration of orbital structures and mass effect, vasculitis affecting the blood vessels supplying cranial nerves or the optic nerve can also cause these findings. Numerous cases have been reported of ischemic optic neuropathy in patients with WG and CSS.[65–74] These patients often present with an acute, painless loss of vision; an afferent papillary defect; optic nerve edema; and visual field loss that can be sectoral. In a large series of 324 patients from the Mayo Clinic with WG, external ophthalmoplegia was documented in almost 5%.[75] Oculomotor, trochlear, and abducens nerve involvements have all been described in WG.[76,77] Palsies of the oculomotor and trochlear nerves have been reported in patients with CSS.[78,79] Horner's syndrome may also rarely occur and has been seen in WG.[80]

SUMMARY

The ANCA-associated vasculitides can affect virtually any ocular or adnexal structure. WG commonly involves the eye, whereas ophthalmic findings in CSS and particularly MPA are much rarer. These diseases can have significant visual morbidity, with some of the manifestations causing pain and blindness. More importantly, because these diseases can be fatal, physicians must recognize ocular symptoms and findings on examination as being indicators of a serious underlying systemic disease, so that the necessary systemic workup can be promptly initiated.

Localized medical and surgical therapies can be helpful in managing associated ocular disease. For example, topical and periocular depot steroids can help to quiet iridocyclitis, and dacryocystorhinostomy can bypass a tear outflow obstruction. However, the key to management is often systemic immunosuppression, even though disease activity may at first seem to be isolated to the eye. Caring for patients with WG, MPA, and CSS requires a multidisciplinary approach, because collaboration among specialists is critical for achieving the best outcomes for patients.

REFERENCES

1. Savage CO, Harper L, Holland M. New findings in pathogenesis of antineutrophil cytoplasm antibody-associated vasculitis. Curr Opin Rheumatol 2002;14:15–22.
2. Seo P, Stone JH. The anti-neutrophil cytoplasmic antibody-associated vasculitides. Am J Med 2004;117(1):39–50.
3. Ewert BH, Jennette JC, Falk RJ. Anti-myeloperoxidase antibodies stimulate neutrophils to damage human endothelial cells. Kidney Int 1992;41:373–83.
4. Watts RA, Carruthers DM, Scott DG. Epidemiology of systemic vasculitis: changing incidence or definition? Semin Arthritis Rheum 1995;25:28–34.
5. Bullen CL, Liesegang TJ, McDonald TJ, et al. Ocular complications of Wegener's granulomatosis. Ophthalmology 1983;90:279–90.
6. Haynes BF, Fishman ML, Fauci AS, et al. The ocular manifestations of Wegener's granulomatosis. Fifteen years experience and review of the literature. Am J Med 1977;63:131–41.
7. Straatsma BR. Ocular manifestations of Wegener's granulomatosis. Am J Ophthalmol 1957;44:789–99.
8. Hoffman GS, Kerr GS, Leavitt RY, et al. Wegener granulomatosis: an analysis of 158 patients. Ann Intern Med 1992;116:488–98.
9. Guillevin L, Durand-Gasselin B, Cevallos R, et al. Microscopic polyangiitis: clinical and laboratory findings in eighty-five patients. Arthritis Rheum 1999;42(3):421–3.

10. Pakrou N, Selva D, Leibovitch I. Wegener's granulomatosis: ophthalmic manifestations and management. Semin Arthritis Rheum 2006;35:284–92.
11. Robinson MR, Lee SS, Sneller MC, et al. Tarsal-conjunctival disease associated with Wegener's granulomatosis. Ophthalmology 2003;110:1770–80.
12. Fauci AS, Haynes BF, Katz P, et al. Wegener's granulomatosis: prospective clinical and therapeutic experience with 85 patients for 21 years. Ann Intern Med 1983;98:76–85, 198.
13. Caster JC, Shetlar DJ, Pappolla MA, et al. Microscopic polyangiitis with ocular involvement. Arch Ophthalmol 1996;114(3):346–8.
14. Meisler DM, Stock EL, Wertz RD, et al. Conjunctival inflammation and amyloidosis in allergic granulomatosis and angiitis (Churg-Strauss syndrome). Am J Ophthalmol 1981;91:216–9.
15. Margolis R, Kosmorsky GS, Lowder CY, et al. Conjunctival involvement in Churg-Strauss syndrome. Ocul Immunol Inflamm 2007;15(2):113–5.
16. Shields CL, Shields JA, Rozanski TI. Conjunctival involvement in Churg-Strauss syndrome. Am J Ophthalmol 1986;102(5):601–5.
17. Nissim F, Von derValde J, Czernobilsky B. A limited form of Churg-Strauss syndrome: ocular and cutaneous manifestations. Arch Pathol Lab Med 1982; 106(6):305–7.
18. Akpek EK, Uy HS, Christen W, et al. Severity of episcleritis and systemic disease association. Ophthalmology 1999;106:729–31.
19. Watson PG, Hayreh SS. Scleritis and episcleritis. Br J Ophthalmol 1976;60: 163–91.
20. Sainz de la Maza M, Jabbur NS, Foster CS. Severity of scleritis and episcleritis. Ophthalmology 1994;101:389–96.
21. Thorne JE, Jabs DA. Ocular manifestations of vasculitis. Rheum Dis Clin North Am 2001;27:761–9.
22. Watson PG, Hyreh SS. Episcleritis and scleritis. Br J Ophthalmol 1976;98:467–71.
23. Sainz de la Maza M, Foster CS, Jabbur NS. Scleritis associated with systemic vasculitis diseases. Ophthalmology 1995;102:687–92.
24. Harper SL, Letko E, Samson CM, et al. Wegener's granulomatosis: the relationship between ocular and systemic disease. J Rheumatol 2001;28(5):1025–32.
25. Foster CS, Forstot SL, Wilson LA. Mortality rate in rheumatoid arthritis patients developing necrotizing scleritis or peripheral ulcerative keratitis. Effects of systemic immunosuppression. Ophthalmology 1984;91(10):1253–6.
26. Hara A, Ohta S, Takata M, et al. Microscopic polyangiitis with ocular manifestations as the initial presenting sign. Am J Med Sci 2007;334(4):308–10.
27. Mihara M, Hayasaka S, Watanabe K, et al. Ocular manifestations in patients with microscopic polyangiitis. Eur J Ophthalmol 2005;15(1):138–42.
28. Sainz de la Maza M, Foster CS, Jabbur NS, et al. Ocular characteristics and disease associations in scleritis-associated peripheral keratopathy. Arch Ophthalmol 2002;120:15–9.
29. Ladas JB, Mondino BJ. Systemic disorders associated with peripheral corneal ulceration. Curr Opin Ophthalmol 2000;11:468–71.
30. Darlington JK, Mannis MJ, Segal WA, et al. Peripheral nonulcerative keratitis as a presenting sign of microscopic polyangiitis. Cornea 2001;20:522–4.
31. Bawazeer AM, Jackson WB. Marginal infiltrative ulcerative keratitis secondary to Churg-Strauss syndrome: a case report. Cornea 2000;19(3):402–4.
32. Tauber J, Sainz de la Maza M, Hoang-Xuan T, et al. An analysis of therapeutic decision making regarding immunosuppressive chemotherapy for peripheral ulcerative keratitis. Cornea 1990;9(1):66–73.

33. Galor A, Thorne JE. Scleritis and peripheral ulcerative keratitis. Rheum Dis Clin North Am 2007;33(4):835–54.
34. Geerling G, Joussen AM, Daniels JT, et al. Matrix metalloproteinases in sterile corneal melts. Ann N Y Acad Sci 1999;878:571–4.
35. Smith VA, Hoh HB, Easty DL. Role of ocular metalloproteinases in peripheral ulcerative keratitis. Br J Ophthalmol 1999;83:1376–83.
36. Smith VA, Cook SD. Doxycycline-a role in ocular surface repair. Br J Ophthalmol 2004;88:619–25.
37. Newsome NA, Gross J. Prevention by medroxyprogesterone of perforation in the alkali-burned rabbit cornea: inhibition of collagenolytic activity. Invest Ophthalmol Vis Sci 1977;16:21–31.
38. Maeno A, Naor J, Lee HM, et al. Three decades of corneal transplantation:indications and patient characteristics. Cornea 2000;19:7–11.
39. Feder RS, Krachmer JH. Conjunctival resection for the treatment of the rheumatoid corneal ulceration. Ophthalmology 1984;91:111–5.
40. Greenberger MH. Central retinal artery closure in Wegener's granulomatosis. Am J Ophthalmol 1967;63:515–6.
41. Wang M, Khurana RN, Sadda SR. Central retinal vein occlusion in Wegener's granulomatosis without retinal vasculitis. Br J Ophthalmol 2006;90:1435–6.
42. Venkatesh P, Chawla R, Tewari HK. Hemiretinal vein occlusion in Wegener's granulomatosis. Eur J Ophthalmol 2003;13:722–5.
43. Iida T, Spaide RF, Kantor J. Retinal and choroidal arterial occlusion in Wegener's granulomatosis. Am J Ophthalmol 2002;133:151–2.
44. Dagi LR, Currie J. Branch retinal artery occlusion in the Churg-Strauss syndrome. J Clin Neuroophthalmol 1985;5:229–37.
45. De Salvo G, Li Calzi C, Anastasi M, et al. Branch retinal vein occlusion followed by central retinal artery occlusion in Churg-Strauss syndrome: unusual ocular manifestations in allergic granulomatous angiitis. Eur J Ophthalmol 2009;19(2):314–7.
46. Partal A, Moshfeghi DM, Alcorn D. Churg-Strauss syndrome in a child: retina and optic nerve findings. Br J Ophthalmol 2004;88:971–2.
47. Ciulla TA, Rosenfeld PJ. Antivascular endothelial growth factor therapy for neovascular age-related macular degeneration. Curr Opin Ophthalmol 2009;30(3): 166–74.
48. Perry SR, Rootman J, White VA. The clinical and pathologic constellation of Wegener granulomatosis of the orbit. Ophthalmology 1997;104:683–94.
49. Woo TL, Francis IC, Wilcsek GA, et al. Australasian orbital and adnexal Wegener's granulomatosis. Ophthalmology 2001;108:1535–43.
50. Talar-Williams C, Sneller MC, Langford CA, et al. Orbital socket contracture: a complication of inflammatory orbital disease in patients with Wegener's granulomatosis. Br J Ophthalmol 2005;89:493–7.
51. Billing K, Malhotra R, Selva D, et al. Orbital myositis in Churg-Strauss syndrome. Arch Ophthalmol 2004;122(3):393–6.
52. Takanashi T, Uchida S, Arita M, et al. Orbital inflammatory pseudotumor and ischemic vasculitis in Churg-Strauss syndrome: report of two cases and review of the literature. Ophthalmology 2001;108(6):1129–33.
53. McNab AA. Orbital inflammation in Churg-Strauss syndrome. Orbit 1998;17(3): 203–5.
54. Bosch-Gil JA, Falga-Tirado C, Simeon-Aznar CP, et al. Churg-Strauss syndrome with inflammatory orbital pseudotumor. Br J Rheumatol 1995;34:485–6.
55. Kalina PH, Lie JT, Campbell RJ, et al. Diagnostic value and limitations of orbital biopsy in Wegener's granulomatosis. Ophthalmology 1992;99:120–4.

56. Sadiq SA, Jenning CR, Jones NS, et al. Wegener's granulomatosis: the ocular manifestations revisited. Orbit 2000;19:153–61.
57. Fechner FP, Faquin WC, Pilch BZ. Wegener's granulomatosis of the orbit: a clinicopathological study of 15 patients. Laryngoscope 2002;112:1945–50.
58. Ghanem RC, Chang N, Aoki L, et al. Vasculitis of the lacrimal sac wall in Wegener granulomatosis. Ophthal Plast Reconstr Surg 2004;20:254–7.
59. Eloy P, Leruth E, Bertrand B, et al. Successful endonasal dacryocystorhinostomy in a patient with Wegener's granulomatosis. Clin Ophthalmol 2009;3:651–6.
60. Hardwig PW, Bartley GB, Garrity JA. Surgical management of nasolacrimal duct obstruction in patients with Wegener's granulomatosis. Ophthalmology 1992;99: 133–9.
61. Glatt HJ, Putterman AM. Dacryocystorhinostomy in Wegener's granulomatosis. Ophthal Plast Reconstr Surg 1990;6:207–10.
62. Holds JB, Anderson RL, Wolin MJ. Dacryocystectomy for the treatment of dacryocystitis patients with Wegener's granulomatosis. Ophthalmic Surg 1989;20: 443–4.
63. Huong du LT, Tran TH, Piette JC. Granulomatous uveitis revealing Wegener's granulomatosis. J Rheumatol 2006;33:1209–10.
64. Cury B, Breakey AS, Payne BF. Allergic granulomatous angiitis associated with uveoscleritis and papilledema. Arch Ophthalmol 1966;55:261–6.
65. Belden CJ, Hamed LM, Macuso AA. Bilateral isolated retrobulbar optic neuropathy in limited Wegener's granulomatosis. J Clin Neuroophthalmol 1993;13: 119–23.
66. Niskopoulou M, Du Toit N. Optic neuritis as a feature of Wegener's granulomatosis. Eye 2002;16:320–1.
67. Duran E, Merkel PA, Sweet S, et al. ANCA-associated small vessel vasculitis presenting with ischemic optic neuropathy. Neurology 2004;13(62):152–3.
68. Howe L, D'Cruz D, Chopdar A, et al. Anterior ischaemic optic neuropathy in Wegener's granulomatosis. Eur J Ophthalmol 1995;5:277–9.
69. Rosenblatt BJ, Foroozan R, Savino PJ. Asymptomatic optic neuropathy associated with Churg-Strauss syndrome. Ophthalmology 2003;110:1650–2.
70. Kattah JC, Chrousos GA, Katz PA, et al. Anterior ischemic optic neuropathy in Churg-Strauss syndrome. Neurology 1994;44:2200–2.
71. Androudi S, Iaccheri B, Brazitikos P, et al. Bilateral chronic anterior uveitis & neuro-ophthalmologic manifestations in a patient with Churg-Strauss syndrome: an unusual ocular presentation. Ocul Immunol Inflamm 2004;12:59–63.
72. Vitali C, Genovesi-Ebert F, Romani A, et al. Ophthalmological and neuro-ophthalmological involvement in Churg-Strauss syndrome: a case report. Graefes Arch Clin Exp Ophthalmol 1996;234:404–8.
73. Acheson JF, Cockerell OC, Bentley CR, et al. Churg-Strauss vasculitis presenting with severe visual loss due to bilateral sequential optic neuropathy. Br J Ophthalmol 1993;77:118–9.
74. Weinstein JM, Chui H, Lane S, et al. Churg-Strauss syndrome (allergic granulomatous angiitis). Neuro-ophthalmologic manifestations. Arch Ophthalmol 1983; 101:1217–20.
75. Nishino H, Rubino FA, DeRemee RA, et al. Neurological involvement in Wegener's granulomatosis: an analysis of 324 consecutive patients at the Mayo Clinic. Ann Neurol 1993;33:4–9.
76. Nowack R, Wachtler P, Kunz J, et al. Cranial nerve palsy in Wegener's granulomatosis–lessons from clinical cases. J Neurol 2009;256:299–304.

77. Kamimura T, Shimazaki H, Morita M, et al. Limited Wegener's granulomatosis manifested by abducens nerve palsy resulting from pachymeningitis. J Clin Rheumatol 2006;12:259–60.
78. Tsuda H, Ishikawa H, Majima T, et al. Isolated oculomotor nerve palsy in Churg-Strauss syndrome. Intern Med 2005;44:638–40.
79. Borruat FX. Neuro-ophthalmologic manifestations of rheumatologic and associated disorders. Curr Opin Ophthalmol 1996;7:10–8.
80. Weijtens O, Mooy N, Paridaens D. Horner's syndrome as manifestation of Wegener's granulomatosis. Eye 2004;18:846–8.

Outcome Measures in ANCA-associated Vasculitis

Ravi Suppiah, BHB, MBChB, PGDipSM, Joanna Robson, MBBS, PhD, MRCP,
Raashid Luqmani, DM, FRCP, FRCP(E)*

KEYWORDS

- Vasculitis • Outcome measures
- Birmingham Vasculitis Activity Score
- Vasculitis Damage Index
- Combined Damage Assessment Index
- Patient-reported outcome measures

The antineutrophil cytoplasm antibody (ANCA)–associated group of vasculitides encompass Wegener's granulomatosis (WG), microscopic polyangiitis (MPA), and Churg-Strauss syndrome (CSS) but also includes some patients with syndromes that do not neatly fit into these disease categories. The ANCA-associated vasculitides are multisystem diseases that predominantly affect small vessels (including the renal glomeruli and lung capillaries) and, if left untreated, have a uniformly high mortality.[1–4] Modern therapy has improved outcome,[5] but early death and chronic morbidity (eg, dialysis dependence) remains a feature of these diseases.[6–12]

With advances in acute therapy for vasculitis, other long-term consequences such as cardiovascular events, thromboembolic events, and malignancy become increasingly important. End-stage organ failure such as kidney failure or respiratory failure can make life difficult for survivors. This morbidity coupled with the effects of drug toxicity can significantly reduce quality of life, which is a crucial end point for patients.[13,14] In addition, relapse, and low-grade persistent disease manifestations are common and require ongoing immunosuppression that may result in poor long-term outcomes.[15–18] Clinical trials in the past decade have attempted to determine the optimal therapeutic strategy for induction and maintenance therapy.[10–12,19–21] Outcomes can be judged in terms of life, death, and defined organ failure, but for chronic low-grade morbidity, it is useful to quantify this in a systematic way for clinical trials and for practical use when evaluating the accrual of morbidity in daily practice. To accurately quantify disease morbidity, make appropriate treatment decisions (ie, only use immunosuppression

RS is funded by the Rose Hellaby Medical Scholarship, New Zealand.
Department of Rheumatology, Nuffield Orthopaedic Centre, Windmill Road, Oxford, OX3 7LD, UK
* Corresponding author.
E-mail address: raashid.luqmani@noc.nhs.uk

Rheum Dis Clin N Am 36 (2010) 587–607
doi:10.1016/j.rdc.2010.04.001
0889-857X/10/$ – see front matter © 2010 Elsevier Inc. All rights reserved.

for active disease rather than chronic scarring), and to serve as appropriate outcome measures in clinical trials, several clinical tools have been developed to specifically measure disease activity and disease damage. In addition to reporting the incidence of death and renal failure, these tools can be used to define the main outcome being measured in trials of ANCA-associated vasculitis.

This article provides an overview of the outcomes measured in clinical trials of ANCA-associated vasculitis and describes the main clinical tools that are used to quantify these concepts. **Table 1** provides a summary of definitions and outcome measures, some of which are more comprehensively validated than others. The current focus is on disease activity and damage, but future attention will be on patient-reported outcome measures and functional status (eg, ability to work or participate in normal activities).

MORTALITY

Death is an important and valid outcome measure when assessing the balance of efficacy and safety of treatment regimens. Most early deaths in ANCA vasculitis are attributable to infection or active vasculitis,[6,22] whereas late deaths may relate to increased cardiovascular disease and malignancy.[23–25] Severity and distribution of organ involvement are currently the best predictors of short- and medium-term survival.[16,26,27] Predictors of mortality in ANCA-associated vasculitis are shown in **Table 1**.[6,27–29] As a result of routine treatment with immunosuppressive therapy, mortalities have fallen dramatically for patients with ANCA-associated vasculitis (**Table 2**).[30] Mortality is now too insensitive to use as a primary end point in clinical trials, which, as a consequence, has driven the development and adoption of clinical tools that can better differentiate between treatments in terms of disease activity and organ damage.

DISEASE ACTIVITY

Disease activity is a well-recognized concept for most chronic inflammatory diseases, and there has been a move away from subjective physician assessments to objective measures of activity. In the context of vasculitis, determining disease activity is complex because of the heterogeneous and multisystem nature of disease. There is no single clinical, serologic, or radiological marker that informs us about disease activity. Inflammatory markers such as serum C-reactive protein (CRP) and erythrocyte sedimentation rate (ESR) provide some information about disease activity but are not specific because they can be high, due to infection or other disease processes, or low as a result of recent glucocorticoid therapy. In addition, CRP and ESR do not correlate well with our current best clinical measures of disease activity.[31] An increase in ANCA titers using new capture and anchor enzyme-linked immunosorbent assay techniques has been proposed as a potential method of predicting an imminent relapse (ie, an increase in disease activity), but currently this assay is not able to adequately perform this role.[32] Therefore, in the absence of any single measure, a comprehensive clinical tool that incorporates the multiorgan nature of vasculitis has been required to adequately measure disease activity.

ANCA Titers to Measure Disease Activity and Relapse

From the first descriptions of ANCA directed against proteinase-3 (PR3) and myeloperoxidase (MPO) in the small-vessel vasculitides, measurement of ANCA has been proposed as a tool to measure disease activity.[33,34] The measurement of increasing MPO- and PR3-ANCA titers has been shown to predict clinical relapse in patients with WG, CSS, and MPA.[35–40] A meta-analysis of 8 studies evaluating the increase of ANCA titers showed a positive likelihood ratio of 3.39 (95% confidence interval [CI]: 1.69–6.82) for a future flare with the absence of an increase in ANCA having a negative likelihood ratio of 0.45 (95% CI: 0.23–0.87).[41] In addition, patients in clinical remission but with rising titers of ANCA who are then randomized to increased immunosuppression have a lower rate of clinical relapse than those with positive titers who are randomized to no increase in immunosuppression.[42,43] However, there is controversy about the use of ANCA as a sole marker of disease activity because discordance between ANCA levels and relapse has also been shown.[32,44–46] In clinical practice, rising ANCA titers must be used in conjunction with evidence of other clinical disease activity when determining the presence of relapse, especially before an increase in immunosuppression is considered!

Early Clinical Tools

Early measures of disease activity include the Groningen Index for WG.[47] This tool used a combination of clinical features and laboratory results but required biopsy evidence of active vasculitis for each time disease activity was measured. Biopsy findings are appropriate at diagnosis, but are not practical for follow-up of patients. An alternative called the Vasculitis Activity Index (VAI) was developed by the Baltimore group.[48] The VAI consists of 9 organ systems that are graded 0 to 4 depending on the impressions of the physician regarding overall activity in that organ system. The main problem with this scale is observer bias; hence, it is not widely used.[49]

Birmingham Vasculitis Activity Score

The current standard, and the tool recommended by the European League Against Rheumatism (EULAR) for assessing disease activity in clinical trials is the Birmingham Vasculitis Activity Score (BVAS).[50] The original version of the BVAS was developed and validated in 1994.[51] It was constructed by a consensus group of physicians interested in vasculitis and comprised 59 individual items, organized into 9 organ systems (systemic; cutaneous; mucous membranes/eyes; ear, nose, and throat [ENT]; chest; cardiovascular; abdominal; renal; and neurologic). Most of the symptoms and signs were easily ascertainable by history and clinical examination but a few items, such as hematuria and serum creatinine, required additional investigations. Positive findings were only recorded if directly attributed to active vasculitis and other potential causes had been excluded; this distinction was made because several features in this tool, such as fever or hematuria, could easily relate to infection, malignancy, drug toxicity, or some other cause. The symptoms and signs were recorded if present at time of assessment or during the preceding 4 weeks. The individual items were given a weight (between 1 and 9) based on the relative importance placed on them by the consensus group (objective items, and items involving the renal, gastrointestinal (GI), and neurologic systems were rated the highest), with a maximum score applied to each organ system. The overall range of possible scores for the BVAS is 0 to 63, with the higher the score the more active the disease. The original BVAS was validated in a sample of 213 patients with mixed primary and secondary vasculitis, and evaluated against a physician global assessment, VAI, Groningen Index and assessed for feasibility, sensitivity to change, and inter observer reliability. In addition, the expert observers agreed that BVAS made biologic sense (construct validity).[51]

Table 1
Important outcome measures and definitions

Term or Outcome Measure	Definition	How is it Measured or Expressed?	Comment About Use as an Outcome Measure	Recognized Predictors of Outcome	References
Mortality	Death	Straightforward to measure. Patients who died or survived can be expressed as a proportion of the overall group for a specific timeframe	Mortality depends on the type and severity of ANCA vasculitis and can range from 0% to 27.4% in 1 y. It can be a useful end point for clinical studies of very severe vasculitis, but, in milder forms for which mortality is low, it is not a useful end point. It is an important outcome for long-term studies	Older age Dialysis dependence at baseline Renal involvement Five Factor Score (FFS): >0, increased risk; >1, highest risk Higher Birmingham Vasculitis Activity Score (BVAS) Vasculitis Damage Index (VDI) score ≥1 Albumin ≤30 g/L at baseline Lung involvement Upper respiratory tract involvement reduces risk of mortality	Koldingsnes and Nossent, 2002[27] Reinhold-Keller et al, 2002[70] Aasarod et al, 2000[28] Bligny et al, 2004[6] Guillevin et al, 1996[16] and 2008[26]

Remission	The complete absence of disease activity attributable to vasculitis, including other inflammatory features like granulomatous inflammation in WG or tissue eosinophilia in CSS. The minimum duration of remission should be stated. Proposed that remission should only be defined as occurring if patient is on prednisolone/prednisone ≤7.5 mg/d for a defined period	Usually measured by the BVAS (BVAS1 = 0 and BVAS2 ≤1). Remission should be qualified by type, duration, and maximum dosage of immunosuppressive therapy	The rates of remission achieved by modern therapy are typically ≥90%. Therefore remission is a realistic primary end point for studies of induction therapy	Type of induction therapy used will determine time to remission. Maintenance therapy will determine whether a patient stays in remission. Severe disease (defined as BVAS >23) was predictive of higher rate of remission. A higher VDI at baseline predicts lower rate of remission	Aasarod et al, 2000[28] de Groot et al, 2005[10] and 2009 Koldingsnes and Nossent, 2003[20] Stegeman et al 1996 Jayne et al, 2003[11] and 2007[12]
Response	A quantifiable measure of improvement from baseline disease activity	A percentage improvement in a measurable disease activity score. A reduction in the BVAS of ≥50% is the recommended measure	In patients refractory to conventional induction therapy, remission is only achieved in 35%–83% of those given second-line treatment. In this difficult-to-treat group, detecting partial improvement may be clinically important	Each 1-point increase in the VDI increases treatment resistance (odds ratio [OR] 1.53)	Hellmich et al, 2007[50] Koldingsnes and Nossent, 2003[20]

(continued on next page)

Table 1
(continued)

Term or Outcome Measure	Definition	How is it Measured or Expressed?	Comment About Use as an Outcome Measure	Recognized Predictors of Outcome	References
Relapse	Recurrence or new onset of disease activity attributable to active inflammation	Major relapse is defined as the Recurrence or new onset of potentially organ- or life-threatening disease activity that cannot be treated with increased glucocorticoids alone (ie, requires cyclophosphamide) All other relapses are considered minor	Rate of relapse is used as an end point in studies comparing strategies for maintenance therapy	Predictors of higher rate of relapse include positive ANCA at baseline, fourfold increase in ANCA titer, chronic nasal carriage of *Staphylococcus aureus*, cardiac involvement at baseline, CrCl>60 mL/min, cumulative cyclophosphamide dose <10 g in 6 mo and prednisone dose ≥ 20 mg for <2.75 mo Adjunctive cotrimoxazole to normal maintenance therapy reduces rate of relapse	Boomsma et al, 2000[35] Stegman et al, 1994 and 1996[18,21] Koldingsnes and Nossent, 2003[20]
Refractory disease	Patients who fail to achieve remission following induction with standard therapy are termed refractory. (ie, do not achieve remission following cyclophosphamide and glucocorticoids for generalized/severe ANCA-associated vasculitis [AAV])	Unchanged or increased disease activity in acute AAV after 4 wk of standard therapy or lack of response (≤50% reduction in BVAS) after 6 wk or 1 major or 3 minor items present on BVAS after 12 wk of treatment	Can be used as the entry criteria for studies evaluating new or second-line induction treatments	Each 1 point increase in the VDI increases treatment resistance (OR 1.53)	Hellmich et al, 2007[50] Koldingsnes and Nossent, 2003[20]

Grumbling (low-grade persistent) disease	Arthralgia, fatigue, or low-grade nasal crusting may continue in patients who are otherwise considered to be in remission	BVAS versions 2 or 3 can be used to score persistent disease. This low-grade disease state does not usually require change in immunosuppressive treatment	Not currently used as an outcome measure in clinical trials but may become relevant in long-term follow-up studies	Hellmich et al, 2007[50]
Damage or organ-specific damage	Irreversible end organ damage as a result of previously active vasculitis	Damage can be recorded globally using an instrument such as the VDI or Combined Damage Assessment (CDA) index or can be focused on a single organ system such as renal failure. Reporting of proportion of patients who are dialysis independent is recommended	End-stage renal failure is clinically important for AAV and used as the primary end point in trials involving patients with severe renal presentations. Global damage assessment is important in long-term follow-up studies but, to date, this has not been used as the primary end point in therapeutic trials	Seo et al, 2007[66]; Hellmich et al, 2007[50]; Koldingsnes and Nossent, 2002[27]
Adverse events	Adverse change in health status or a side effect that occurs in a person during or after receiving specific therapy. This therapy can be a medication, or procedure (eg, plasma exchange in the context of ANCA vasculitis)	Usually reported as the cumulative frequency of each event. Normally grouped into serious (resulting in death, life-threatening adverse event, or requiring hospital admission) and mild/moderate severity. In ANCA vasculitis the common serious adverse events are infection and malignancy	Potential end point for noninferiority studies. This is when a new therapy is assumed to be as effective as conventional therapy and the perceived benefit is a reduction in side effects	Type and intensity of immunosuppressive therapy	de Groot et al, 2005[10] and 2009[9]; Jayne et al, 2003[11] and 2007[12]

(continued on next page)

Table 1
(continued)

Term or Outcome Measure	Definition	How is it Measured or Expressed?	Comment About Use as an Outcome Measure	Recognized Predictors of Outcome	References
Patient-reported outcomes	Outcomes that patients regard as important. These outcomes usually encompass the ability to function at home and work, and quality of life	There are currently no vasculitis-specific patient-reported outcome measures. Generic tools such as the Short Form 36 (SF-36) questionnaire, Health Assessment Questionnaire (HAQ), and the Hospital Anxiety and Depression Score (HADS) are currently used	Vasculitis-specific patient-reported outcome measures are needed	We are not sure what factors will ultimately predict patient-reported outcomes but we suspect that they will be different from physician-based assessments	McHorney et al, 1992[71] Fries et al, 1982[72] Zigmond and Snaith, 1983[73]

Table 2 Five-year survival in the ANCA vasculitides	
Diagnosis	Five-Year Survival (%)
WG	75
MPA	45–75
CSS	68–100

Data from Phillip R, Luqmani R. Mortality in systemic vasculitis: a systematic review. Clin Exp Rheumatol 2008;26(5 Suppl 51):S94–104.

The BVAS was adopted by the European Vasculitis Study Group (EUVAS) for its clinical trials in ANCA-associated vasculitis, and as a result underwent further refinement.[9–12] Adjustments were made to the items, including the addition of smoldering disease; that is, not new or worse activity but grumbling (low-grade persistent disease) activity was recorded in a separate column that could have a maximum score of 36. Four of the original items that were believed to occur very rarely were removed and 7 new items, including features available after subspecialist opinion, were added (total of 64 items); however, the overall range of scores for the BVAS remained the same. This tool is now called BVAS version 2, but is scored as 2 separate components; BVAS1 (new/worse disease) and BVAS2 (persistent disease). For the EUVAS trials, the BVAS scores were used to determine remission when assessing induction therapy, and to define relapse when assessing maintenance therapy. Remission was defined as the absence of new or worse clinical disease activity (BVAS1 = 0), but allowed persistent activity (BVAS2) in 1 item scoring less than 2 points. Major relapse was defined by the recurrence or first appearance of at least 1 item on the BVAS1 involving a vital organ (kidney, lung, brain, eye, motor nerve, or gut), and minor relapse by the recurrence or first appearance of at least 3 other items on the BVAS1.[9–12] In the last decade, the BVAS has been used in numerous clinical trials in ANCA-associated vasculitis,[9–12,52–55] with some trials incorporating the BVAS score as part of the primary end point (see **Table 1**).[10,11,52,56]

The latest iteration of the BVAS is version 3, which was published and validated in 2009 (**Table 3**).[31] The changes were made by consensus expert opinion and include reduction in the total number of items to 56 by omission or merging, and the persistent boxes for each variable were replaced by a single persistent box for the whole form that is only checked if all the items are considered persistent disease. The weighting of items was unchanged. The new version was validated in 313 patients with primary and secondary vasculitis (although most had ANCA-associated vasculitis) for convergent validity against the previous BVAS versions, treatment decisions, physician global assessment, CRP, and VAI, and was shown to be reliable, reproducible, and sensitive to change.[31]

A modified version of the BVAS called the BVAS/WG has been adapted by North American investigators for trials involving patients with WG.[55] Features unlikely to occur in WG (such as loss of pulses) were omitted and new items specific for WG, such as endobronchial lesions, were introduced. The weighting of the BVAS was changed, assigning 1 point to any item judged to be of minor importance, and 3 points to major items (which typically require aggressive therapy with cyclophosphamide). A physician global assessment (as a 10-cm visual analog scale) is incorporated into the BVAS/WG and allows for the assignment of remission, minor flare, or major flare.[55] The BVAS/WG has only been validated in patients with WG, but has been shown to correlate with the BVAS (old and new) in cases of WG and MPA in the literature.[57] However, it has not been validated in current patients with MPA, other ANCA

Table 3
Comparison of the range of BVAS observed in 2 different cohorts of mixed primary and secondary vasculitis

	Original BVAS (Luqmani et al, 1994[51]) N = 213	BVAS v3 (Suppiah et al, 2010) N = 285
CSS	Not available	0–24
MPA	Not available	0–25
Wegener's granulomatosis	11–25	0–37
Nonrenal Wegener's	1–19	0–25
Behcet disease	4–19	0–19
Giant cell arteritis	1–9	Not available
Polyarteritis nodosa	10–29	0–6
Rheumatoid vasculitis	1–16	0–12
Takayasu arteritis	7–14	0–5

Online BVAS v3 calculator: http://www.epsnetwork.co.uk/BVAS/bvas_flow.html.
Downloadable BVAS v3 Microsoft Excel calculator: http://www.ndorms.ox.ac.uk/profiles.php?profile=rluqmani.

vasculitis, or any other types of vasculitis; caution is therefore advised if considering the use of BVAS/WG for assessment in diseases other than WG.

As with any biologic tool, the BVAS will benefit from continual review and improvement, ideally through a data-driven process. We anticipate that this process will be facilitated in the future through the Outcome Measures in Rheumatoid Arthritis Clinical Trials (OMERACT) initiative.[58] The main target for future improvements should be to rationalize the weighting system (which is currently based on expert opinion) to one that is based on hard outcomes from prospective studies.

Other Disease Assessment Tools

The Disease Extent Index (DEI) measures the number of organ systems (out of a possible 10) involved, each given a score of 2, and the presence of constitutional symptoms are given a score of 1 (maximum score = 21). The DEI can be calculated from the individual components of the BVAS, and therefore also correlates with the BVAS score.[56,57,59] The DEI can complement the BVAS by showing whether a high BVAS score is due to multiorgan involvement or severe involvement of 1 organ.

The French Vasculitis Study Group (FVSG) developed a prognostic tool called the Five Factor Score (FFS).[16] The original version was created from a cohort of patients with polyarteritis nodosa (PAN) and CSS. Renal failure, proteinuria, cardiomyopathy, GI tract involvement, and central nervous system (CNS) signs are scored as being present or absent, with a higher total score being predictive of higher 5-year mortality (**Table 4**).[16] This score has been revised to include patients with WG and MPA, and incorporates ENT involvement, which is associated with a reduced risk of death (see **Table 4**).[26]

DISEASE DAMAGE

Chronic scarring from vasculitis or its treatment is termed disease damage and is distinct from active inflammation, with further immunosuppression given only to patients with the latter. Current immunosuppressive therapy for acute

Table 4
A comparison of the original and revised FFS as a prognostic tool for mortality

	Original FFS (Guillevin et al, 1996[16]) Includes PAN, MPA, CSS	Revised FFS (Guillevin et al, 2008[26]) Includes PAN, MPA, CSS, WG
Criteria and how to score	Each of the following have a score of +1: • Proteinuria >1 g/24 h • Serum creatinine >1.58 mg/dL • GI involvement • Cardiomyopathy • CNS signs	Each of the following have a score of +1: • Age >65 y • Cardiac symptoms • GI involvement • Renal insufficiency (>1.7 mg/dL) The following has a score of −1: • ENT involvement
5-y mortality risk (%)	FFS of 0 = 11.9 FFS of 1 = 26 FFS of ≥2 = 46	FFS of 0 = 7.5 FFS of 1 = 20 FFS of ≥2 = 47

ANCA-associated vasculitis achieves remission in more than 90% of cases, but long-term sequelae from vasculitis or treatment are a problem for most patients.[15,60,61] Therefore, accurate quantification of this damage is now an important long-term measure of outcome in ANCA vasculitis.

Impairment of renal function is probably the most important organ-specific damage in ANCA-associated vasculitis; however, outcomes such as respiratory failure and peripheral neuropathy are other examples of important end organ damage. In the Methyl Prednisolone Versus Plasma Exchange (MEPEX) trial (**Table 5**), the primary end point was renal survival as measured by dialysis independence at 3 months.[12] Plasma exchange significantly improved this end point, compared with standard therapy. Improvements in renal function by increase in creatinine clearance or achievement of target creatinine are also recognized end points for trials in ANCA-associated vasculitis. Changes in estimated glomerular filtration rate (GFR) as well as end-stage renal disease or requirement for temporary dialysis were secondary end points in the CYCLOPS and Cyclophosphamide Versus Azathioprine for Early Remission (CYCAZAREM) studies (see **Table 5**).[9,10] However, this approach does not encompass all the damage that can occur in these multisystem diseases; nevertheless, renal function is an important and easy-to-measure end point and should be considered for all studies in which the kidney is likely to be involved.

Vasculitis Damage Index

The Vasculitis Damage Index (VDI) has been used as the formal assessment tool of damage in most of the major clinical trials of the ANCA-associated vasculitides conducted in the last decade.[9–12,52] The VDI was first developed by the Birmingham Vasculitis Group in the United Kingdom.[63] They identified that a tool was needed to separate damage, as an irreversible process or scarring, from active inflammation or grumbling (persistent) disease.[63] The decision was made to exclude any damage accrued before the onset of vasculitis and to have an arbitrary cutoff of at least 3 months before disease manifestations can be scored as damage rather than ongoing activity.[63] The VDI records damage as present or absent with no weighting attached to specific items. The score is cumulative and all previously scored items are carried over to the next assessment. Items of damage are scored irrespective of whether they are later attributed to effect of treatment or other comorbidities, provided

Table 5
Major therapeutic trials in ANCA-associated vasculitis which used the BVAS to determine the primary end point

Trial Name/Author	Trial Description	Primary Outcome	Version of BVAS
CYCAZAREM trial Jayne et al, 2003[11]	Comparison of azathioprine with cyclophosphamide for maintenance therapy in 155 patients with newly diagnosed ANCA-associated vasculitis and a renal manifestation (Cr<500 mmol/L) or with generalized life-threatening disease	Relapse rate (major relapse defined as ≥1/24 items on the BVAS1 that indicate threatened function of a vital organ (kidney, lung, brain, eye, motor nerve, or gut) and minor relapse defined as ≥3 other items in the BVAS1)	BVAS version 2
Wegener's Granulomatosis Etanercept Trial (WGET) WGET research group, 2005[52]	180 patients with Wegener's granulomatosis randomized to receive etanercept or placebo as an adjunct to standard maintenance therapy	Sustained remission (BVAS = 0 for at least 6 mo)	BVAS/WG
NORAM trial de Groot et al, 2005[10]	A comparison of methotrexate with cyclophosphamide for induction therapy in 100 patients with newly diagnosed ANCA vasculitis and Cr<150 mmol/L and without critical organ-threatening disease	Remission rate at 6 mo (remission defined as BVAS1 = 0 and BVAS2 ≤1)	BVAS version 2
CYCLOPS trial de Groot et al, 2009[9]	149 patients who had newly diagnosed generalized ANCA-associated vasculitis with renal involvement but not immediately life-threatening disease. Randomized to continuous oral vs pulsed intravenous cyclophosphamide for induction therapy	Time to remission (remission defined as BVAS1 = 0 and BVAS2 ≤1)	BVAS version 2
RITUXVAS Jones et al, 2009[62]	44 patients with ANCA-associated vasculitis and renal involvement randomized 3:1 to induction therapy with a rituximab-based regimen vs standard intravenous pulse cyclophosphamide	Sustained remission (BVAS = 0 at 6 mo and sustained for 6 mo)	BVAS version 3

they occur after the onset of vasculitis.[63] Items to be scored were reached by consensus between physicians from different specialties in the Birmingham Vasculitis Group, and further refined through discussion with the EUVAS group.[64] There are 64 items grouped into 11 systems: musculoskeletal, skin/mucous membranes, ocular, ENT, pulmonary, cardiovascular, peripheral vascular disease, GI, renal, neuropsychiatric, and other (including malignancy and gonadal failure). The VDI has been validated for use in patients with a range of systemic vasculitides and is a sensitive and comprehensive tool to assess damage, with good inter- and intraobserver repeatability.[63] The VDI correlates well with the only other index of activity specific for vasculitis, the Systemic Necrotizing Vasculitis (SNV) Damage Index, which had been used previously to assess damage in a cohort of patients with PAN and CSS.[63,65] The SNV is shown in **Table 6** but is not discussed further because it has been superseded by the VDI. In addition to acting as a tool to assess damage in individual patients and as an outcome measure in clinical trials, the VDI has also been used to study the natural history of the ANCA-associated vasculitides. An example is the use of the VDI in outcome studies that have proven that most damage occurs in the first 6 months, which gives weight to the use of early aggressive immunosuppressive therapy in organ-threatening disease.[27,66] The VDI can also be used as a prognostic score; at baseline VDI greater than or equal to 1 predicts decreased survival by 42 months (HR 6.10 [95%CI 1.7–22.1]),[27] and at 6 months a VDI greater than or equal to 5 predicts decreased survival by 2 years (HR 12.3 [95%CI 4.2–36.9]).[66]

Combined Damage Assessment Index

Using the VDI in many clinical trials has created a realization in Europe and North America that item selection and weighting could be optimized further. The ANCA-associated Vasculitis Instrument of Damage (AVID) is an American tool that has yet to be validated but is currently being compared with the VDI in the Rituximab for ANCA-associated Vasculitis (RAVE) trial. A more collaborative approach through the OMERACT initiative is a joint project between the Vasculitis Clinical Research Consortium (VCRC; http://www.RareDiseasesNetwork.org/vcrc) and EUVAS

Table 6 Summary of the damage assessment tools		
Assessment Tool	**Description**	**Comments**
SNV Damage Index Abu-Shakra et al, 1994[65]	34 items, some items have double weighting, no ENT damage items included	Replaced by VDI
VDI Exley et al, 1997[63,66]	64 items in 11 systems. No weighting in current version. For use in all types of vasculitis	Validated and widely used
ANCA Vasculitis Index of Damage (AVID) Seo et al, 2007[67]	Left and right sides scored separately for damage for eyes and ears. Specific for AAVs	Awaiting validation through use in Rituximab for ANCA-associated Vasculitis (RAVE) trial
Combined Damage Assessment Index (CDA) Seo et al, 2007[67]	135 items in 17 systems, left and right both scored for damage to eyes and ears Specific for AAVs	Collaborative development, weighting of items planned for future, awaiting validation

The VDI form, glossary, and training sheets are available online at the EUVAS Web site (http://www.vasculitis.org/.)

(http://www.Vasculitis.org), supported by grants from the US National Institutes of Health and EULAR. The agenda for this international project was published in 2007 and details the development of a new tool: the Combined Damage Assessment Index (CDA).[67] Information recorded in the Other category of the VDI on patients in the Wegener's Granulomatosis Etanercept Trial (WGET) has been used as the basis for expanding the items included in the CDA.[61] The CDA now includes 17 categories with a total of 135 items, with a gradation of severity for 8 items.[67] In contrast to the VDI, it has been suggested that all items should be attributed to vasculitis or treatment, and that there should be a change in the time cutoff from 3 to 6 months.[67] An exercise to reach a consensus between experts in vasculitis about weighting of individual items suggests that renal failure, cardiovascular and respiratory failure, blindness, and malignancy are deemed the most important, whereas features such as mouth ulcers, bruising, striae, and alopecia are less so.[68] However, this is still an expert opinion–based approach to weighting that needs validation in prospective long-term studies. A comparison between the use of the VDI and the CDA (with a 3-month cutoff and items attributed to any cause), in a cohort of patients with primary and secondary vasculitis found the CDA to be more sensitive at detecting damage, but also more complex to complete, leading to decreased inter- and intraobserver reliability.[69]

An unresolved issue is the concept of damage as a finite measurement. If damage has occurred at a specific time point, but later resolves (eg, corticosteroid-induced diabetes), should the damage score still include this item? At present, the VDI and CDA measure damage as a cumulative score, but adaptations may be made in the future to capture the changing clinical picture.

ADVERSE EVENTS

Although the term adverse event encompasses all outcomes during the course of a clinical trial or study, the focus is usually on drug toxicity, commonly seen with the use of immunosuppression and glucocorticoids. Adverse events range from acute allergic reactions, leukopenia, and infection to long-term problems such as diabetes, osteoporosis, and malignancy. Infection, which is likely related to aggressive immunosuppressive therapy, is the most common cause of death early in the disease course.[7,22] In therapeutic trials in which noninferiority of a new medication is being tested, the advantage of the new drug is usually a reduction in adverse events. For example, when methotrexate was evaluated for induction therapy in nonrenal ANCA-associated vasculitis against cyclophosphamide in the Non-renal Vasculitis Alternative Treatment with Methotrexate (NORAM) trial, one of the main outcomes evaluated was the difference in adverse events compared with cyclophosphamide.[10] In this example, methotrexate was equally effective at inducing remission, but had lower rates of leukopenia (although major adverse events were similar between the groups.)[10] Similarly, in the RAVE trial, which is a noninferiority trial of rituximab versus cyclophosphamide for induction therapy in ANCA vasculitis (in progress), the perceived benefit of rituximab compared with cyclophosphamide is fewer therapy-related adverse events (such as infection in the acute setting, and malignancy in the long term), highlighting that safety and reducing adverse events are important outcomes when assessing new therapies. One of the main findings of the etanercept versus placebo study on WG (WGET) was the increased risk of solid-organ malignancy in those patients treated with etanercept.[52] Even though patients treated with etanercept had also previously been exposed to cyclophosphamide, as a result of this study, it is likely that etanercept will never be used in ANCA-associated vasculitis. In a Danish cohort of 293 patients with WG, cyclophosphamide at cumulative doses greater than

36 g was associated with markedly increased rates of acute myeloid leukemia (standardized incidence ratios [SIR] 59.0, 95%CI 12–172) and bladder cancer (SIR 9.5, 95%CI 2.6–24).[25] In this cohort, leukemia and bladder cancer were diagnosed many years after receiving therapy (6.9–18.5 years after first dose of cyclophosphamide).[25] In addition, the risk of nonmelanoma skin cancers was also raised (SIR 4.7, 95% CI 2.8–7.3) with any exposure to cyclophosphamide.[25] Therefore, the long-term risk of developing a serious adverse event (eg, malignancy) needs to be considered in the context of the potential short-term benefit of controlling current disease activity with greater immunosuppression. It will ultimately be up to patients and their treating physician whether they are willing to take greater risks in the short term (eg, avoiding cyclophosphamide in induction therapy) to prevent long-term harm, or whether the acute benefits of treatment outweigh the future risk of serious adverse events.

PATIENT-REPORTED OUTCOMES

Patients with ANCA-associated vasculitis are now living longer, but the effect of the diagnosis on ability to function at home and work, on quality of life, and on interpersonal relationships is significant.[13,70] In patients aged less than 40 years with WG, more than a quarter of those employed at diagnosis were unemployed by 39 months.[71] Unemployed patients with WG have significantly lower levels of physical and social functioning and patient-perceived health status than patients who are employed.[71] The generic Medical Outcomes Survey Short Form 36 questionnaire (SF-36),[72] Health Assessment Questionnaire (HAQ),[73] and the Hospital Anxiety and Depression Score (HADS)[74] have been used to show significantly reduced quality of life and functioning, and increased levels of disability and symptoms of depression and anxiety in patients with systemic vasculitides.[14,65]

The OMERACT Vasculitis Working Group is a collaboration between international investigators working toward optimal outcome measures for use in clinical trials. The report from OMERACT 9 highlights the need to develop vasculitis-specific patient-reported outcome measures, because of concern than generic questionnaires developed for use in other chronic disease may be less responsive in this group of patients with multisystem disease.[58] One possibility is the development of specific tools for the symptoms or organ systems involved.[58] Hoffman and colleagues[13] designed a tool to assess the social, health, and economic

Table 7 Current tools available to assess function	
Assessment Tool	Description
Medical Outcomes Survey SF-36	Generic measure of health status and quality of life widely used for chronic diseases. Dimensions include physical function, role limitation due to physical or emotional difficulties, social functioning, mental health, energy levels, pain, and perceptions of general health
HAQ	Widely used in clinical trials to measure physical function and disability
Hospital Anxiety and Depression Scale (HADS)	Developed to determine levels of anxiety and depression in patients with chronic physical disease
Hoffman et al[5,13] developed questionnaire specific for WG	Developed with focus group comprising patients and their partners; separate questionnaire for partners

effects of WG, which was refined through discussion with a focus group of patients, their spouses, and clinicians. Most questions were multiple choice and divided into categories of health, function, income, and interpersonal relationships, with a separate questionnaire to capture responses from spouses or life partners.[13] With minor adjustments, this questionnaire has also been applied to patients with systemic lupus erythematosus, showing a broadly similar effect on patients' lives to that found in WG.[70] The current tools for measuring patient-reported outcomes are detailed in **Table 7**; efforts to refine these measures are ongoing.

SUMMARY

The goal for treatment of ANCA-associated vasculitis has changed from preventing death to improving the quality of survival. Survival in ANCA vasculitis is often characterized by disease activity, drug toxicity, and permanent long-term damage. Patient well-being may remain unsatisfactory, with poor function and quality of life. The use of outcome measures to define and quantify these problems is the basis for improvement, in terms of clinical studies and therapeutic trials but also in everyday practice. Currently, their main use is in scientific research but, with the advent of expensive potentially useful biologic interventions, it will be increasingly necessary to quantify response to therapy in a way that can be readily compared between patients. This requirement may be driven primarily through a need to justify costly therapy, as has occurred following the introduction of biologic therapy in the treatment of inflammatory arthritis and spondyloarthropathy.[75–78] Current outcome measures in ANCA-associated vasculitis were designed for clinical studies but are practical and effective and are recommended for use in clinical practice. More widespread use of these instruments will promote their improvement while the search continues for more effective, reliable biomarkers.

REFERENCES

1. Davson J, Ball J, Platt R. The kidney in periarteritis nodosa. Q J Med 1948;17(67): 175–202.
2. Fahey JL, Leonard E, Churg J, et al. Wegener's granulomatosis. Am J Med 1954; 17(2):168–79.
3. Godman GC, Churg J. Wegener's granulomatosis: pathology and review of the literature. AMA Arch Pathol 1954;58(6):533–53.
4. Hollander D, Manning RT. The use of alkylating agents in the treatment of Wegener's granulomatosis. Ann Intern Med 1967;67(2):393–8.
5. Hoffman GS, Kerr GS, Leavitt RY, et al. Wegener's granulomatosis: an analysis of 158 patients. Ann Intern Med 1992;116(6):488–98.
6. Bligny D, Mahr A, Toumelin PL, et al. Predicting mortality in systemic Wegener's granulomatosis: a survival analysis based on 93 patients. Arthritis Rheum 2004; 51(1):83–91.
7. Bourgarit A, Le Toumelin P, Pagnoux C, et al. Deaths occurring during the first year after treatment onset for polyarteritis nodosa, microscopic polyangiitis, and Churg-Strauss syndrome: a retrospective analysis of causes and factors predictive of mortality based on 595 patients. Medicine (Baltimore) 2005; 84(5):323–30.

8. Burkhardt O, Kohnlein T, Wrenger E, et al. Predicting outcome and survival in patients with Wegener's granulomatosis treated on the intensive care unit. Scand J Rheumatol 2007;36(2):119–24.
9. de Groot K, Harper L, Jayne DR, et al. Pulse versus daily oral cyclophosphamide for induction of remission in antineutrophil cytoplasmic antibody-associated vasculitis: a randomized trial. Ann Intern Med 2009;150(10): 670–80.
10. de Groot K, Rasmussen N, Bacon PA, et al. Randomized trial of cyclophosphamide versus methotrexate for induction of remission in early systemic antineutrophil cytoplasmic antibody-associated vasculitis. Arthritis Rheum 2005; 52(8):2461–9.
11. Jayne D, Rasmussen N, Andrassy K, et al. A randomized trial of maintenance therapy for vasculitis associated with antineutrophil cytoplasmic autoantibodies. N Engl J Med 2003;349(1):36–44.
12. Jayne DR, Gaskin G, Rasmussen N, et al. Randomized trial of plasma exchange or high-dosage methylprednisolone as adjunctive therapy for severe renal vasculitis. J Am Soc Nephrol 2007;18(7):2180–8.
13. Hoffman GS, Drucker Y, Cotch MF, et al. Wegener's granulomatosis: patient-reported effects of disease on health, function, and income. Arthritis Rheum 1998;41(12):2257–62.
14. Koutantji M, Harrold E, Lane SE, et al. Investigation of quality of life, mood, pain, disability, and disease status in primary systemic vasculitis. Arthritis Rheum 2003; 49(6):826–37.
15. Guillevin L, Jarrousse B, Lok C, et al. Longterm followup after treatment of polyarteritis nodosa and Churg-Strauss angiitis with comparison of steroids, plasma exchange and cyclophosphamide to steroids and plasma exchange. A prospective randomized trial of 71 patients. The Cooperative Study Group for Polyarteritis Nodosa. J Rheumatol 1991;18(4):567–74.
16. Guillevin L, Lhote F, Gayraud M, et al. Prognostic factors in polyarteritis nodosa and Churg-Strauss syndrome. A prospective study in 342 patients. Medicine (Baltimore) 1996;75(1):17–28.
17. Metzler C, Hellmich B, Gause A, et al. Churg Strauss syndrome–successful induction of remission with methotrexate and unexpected high cardiac and pulmonary relapse ratio during maintenance treatment. Clin Exp Rheumatol 2004;22(6 Suppl 36):S52–61.
18. Stegeman CA, Tervaert JW, Sluiter WJ, et al. Association of chronic nasal carriage of Staphylococcus aureus and higher relapse rates in Wegener's granulomatosis. Ann Intern Med 1994;120(1):12–7.
19. de Groot K, Muhler M, Reinhold-Keller E, et al. Induction of remission in Wegener's granulomatosis with low dose methotrexate. J Rheumatol 1998;25(3): 492–5.
20. Koldingsnes W, Nossent JC. Baseline features and initial treatment as predictors of remission and relapse in Wegener's granulomatosis. J Rheumatol 2003;30(1):80–8.
21. Stegeman CA, Tervaert JW, de Jong PE, et al. Trimethoprim-sulfamethoxazole (co-trimoxazole) for the prevention of relapses of Wegener's granulomatosis. Dutch Co-Trimoxazole Wegener's Study Group. N Engl J Med 1996; 335(1):16–20.
22. Mahr A, Girard T, Agher R, et al. Analysis of factors predictive of survival based on 49 patients with systemic Wegener's granulomatosis and prospective followup. Rheumatology (Oxford) 2001;40(5):492–8.

23. Fain O, Hamidou M, Cacoub P, et al. Vasculitides associated with malignancies: analysis of sixty patients. Arthritis Rheum 2007;57(8):1473–80.

24. Faurschou M, Mellemkjaer L, Sorensen IJ, et al. Increased morbidity from ischemic heart disease in patients with Wegener's granulomatosis. Arthritis Rheum 2009;60(4):1187–92.

25. Faurschou M, Sorensen IJ, Mellemkjaer L, et al. Malignancies in Wegener's granulomatosis: incidence and relation to cyclophosphamide therapy in a cohort of 293 patients. J Rheumatol 2008;35(1):100–5.

26. Guillevin L, Pagnoux C, Mahr A, et al. The five factor score (FFS) revisited: a tool to assess the prognoses of polyarteritis nodosa (PAN), microscopic polyangiitis (MPA), Churg-Strauss syndrome (CSS) and Wegener's granulomatosis (WG) based on 1108 patients from the French Vasculitis Study Group [abstract]. American College of Rheumatology Annual Scientific Conference 2008. Available at: http://acr.confex.com/acr/2008/webprogram/Paper2220.html. Accessed December 9, 2009.

27. Koldingsnes W, Nossent H. Predictors of survival and organ damage in Wegener's granulomatosis. Rheumatology (Oxford) 2002;41(5):572–81.

28. Aasarod K, Iversen BM, Hammerstrom J, et al. Wegener's granulomatosis: clinical course in 108 patients with renal involvement. Nephrol Dial Transplant 2000;15(12):2069.

29. Reinhold-Keller E, Beuge N, Latza U, et al. An interdisciplinary approach to the care of patients with Wegener's granulomatosis: long-term outcome in 155 patients. Arthritis Rheum 2000;43(5):1021–32.

30. Phillip R, Luqmani R. Mortality in systemic vasculitis: a systematic review. Clin Exp Rheumatol 2008;26(5 Suppl 51):S94–104.

31. Mukhtyar C, Lee R, Brown D, et al. Modification and validation of the Birmingham vasculitis activity score (version 3). Ann Rheum Dis 2009;68(12):1827–32.

32. Finkielman JD, Merkel PA, Schroeder D, et al. Antiproteinase 3 antineutrophil cytoplasmic antibodies and disease activity in Wegener's granulomatosis. Ann Intern Med 2007;147(9):611–9.

33. Falk RJ, Jennette JC. Anti-neutrophil cytoplasmic autoantibodies with specificity for myeloperoxidase in patients with systemic vasculitis and idiopathic necrotizing and crescentic glomerulonephritis. N Engl J Med 1988;318(25):1651–7.

34. van der Woude FJ, Rasmussen N, Lobatto S, et al. Autoantibodies against neutrophils and monocytes: tool for diagnosis and marker of disease activity in Wegener's granulomatosis. Lancet 1985;1(8426):425–9.

35. Boomsma MM, Stegeman CA, van der Leij MJ, et al. Prediction of relapses in Wegener's granulomatosis by measurement of antineutrophil cytoplasmic antibody levels: a prospective study. Arthritis Rheum 2000;43(9):2025–33.

36. Gaskin G, Savage CO, Ryan JJ, et al. Anti-neutrophil cytoplasmic antibodies and disease activity during long-term follow-up of 70 patients with systemic vasculitis. Nephrol Dial Transplant 1991;6(10):689–94.

37. Hogan SL, Falk RJ, Chin H, et al. Predictors of relapse and treatment resistance in antineutrophil cytoplasmic antibody-associated small-vessel vasculitis. Ann Intern Med 2005;143(9):621–31.

38. Sanders JS, Huitma MG, Kallenberg CG, et al. Prediction of relapses in PR3-ANCA-associated vasculitis by assessing responses of ANCA titres to treatment. Rheumatology (Oxford) 2006;45(6):724–9.

39. Slot MC, Tervaert JW, Boomsma MM, et al. Positive classic antineutrophil cytoplasmic antibody (C-ANCA) titer at switch to azathioprine therapy associated with relapse in proteinase 3-related vasculitis. Arthritis Rheum 2004;51(2): 269–73.
40. Terrier B, Saadoun D, Sene D, et al. Antimyeloperoxidase antibodies are a useful marker of disease activity in antineutrophil cytoplasmic antibody-associated vasculitides. Ann Rheum Dis 2009;68(10):1564–71.
41. Tomasson G, Grayson P, Mahr A, et al. The value of rise in anti-neutrophil cytoplasmic antibody (ANCA) measurements for predicting relapse among patients with ANCA-associated vasculitis - a meta-analysis [abstract]. Arthritis Rheum 2009;60(Suppl 10):648.
42. Han WK, Choi HK, Roth RM, et al. Serial ANCA titers: useful tool for prevention of relapses in ANCA-associated vasculitis. Kidney Int 2003;63(3): 1079–85.
43. Tervaert JW, Huitema MG, Hene RJ, et al. Prevention of relapses in Wegener's granulomatosis by treatment based on antineutrophil cytoplasmic antibody titre. Lancet 1990;336(8717):709–11.
44. De'Oliviera J, Gaskin G, Dash A, et al. Relationship between disease activity and anti-neutrophil cytoplasmic antibody concentration in long-term management of systemic vasculitis. Am J Kidney Dis 1995;25(3):380–9.
45. Girard T, Mahr A, Noel LH, et al. Are antineutrophil cytoplasmic antibodies a marker predictive of relapse in Wegener's granulomatosis? A prospective study. Rheumatology (Oxford) 2001;40(2):147–51.
46. Kerr GS, Fleisher TA, Hallahan CW, et al. Limited prognostic value of changes in antineutrophil cytoplasmic antibody titer in patients with Wegener's granulomatosis. Arthritis Rheum 1993;36(3):365–71.
47. Kallenberg CG, Tervaert JW, Stegeman CA. Criteria for disease activity in Wegener's granulomatosis: a requirement for longitudinal clinical studies. APMIS Suppl 1990;19:37–9.
48. Whiting-O'Keefe QE, Stone JH, Hellmann DB. Validity of a vasculitis activity index for systemic necrotizing vasculitis. Arthritis Rheum 1999;42(11):2365–71.
49. Flossmann O, Bacon P, de Groot K, et al. Development of comprehensive disease assessment in systemic vasculitis. Ann Rheum Dis 2007;66(3): 283–92.
50. Hellmich B, Flossmann O, Gross WL, et al. EULAR recommendations for conducting clinical studies and/or clinical trials in systemic vasculitis: focus on anti-neutrophil cytoplasm antibody-associated vasculitis. Ann Rheum Dis 2007; 66(5):605–17.
51. Luqmani RA, Bacon PA, Moots RJ, et al. Birmingham vasculitis activity score (BVAS) in systemic necrotizing vasculitis. QJM 1994;87(11):671–8.
52. WGET Study Group. Etanercept plus standard therapy for Wegener's granulomatosis. N Engl J Med 2005;352(4):351–61.
53. Booth A, Harper L, Hammad T, et al. Prospective study of TNFalpha blockade with infliximab in anti-neutrophil cytoplasmic antibody-associated systemic vasculitis. J Am Soc Nephrol 2004;15(3):717–21.
54. Metzler C, Miehle N, Manger K, et al. Elevated relapse rate under oral methotrexate versus leflunomide for maintenance of remission in Wegener's granulomatosis. Rheumatology (Oxford) 2007;46(7):1087–91.
55. Stone JH, Hoffman GS, Merkel PA, et al. A disease-specific activity index for Wegener's granulomatosis: modification of the Birmingham vasculitis activity

score. International Network for the Study of the Systemic Vasculitides (INSSYS). Arthritis Rheum 2001;44(4):912–20.

56. de Groot K, Adu D, Savage CO. The value of pulse cyclophosphamide in ANCA-associated vasculitis: meta-analysis and critical review. Nephrol Dial Transplant 2001;16(10):2018–27.

57. Merkel PA, Cuthbertson DD, Hellmich B, et al. Comparison of disease activity measures for anti-neutrophil cytoplasmic autoantibody (ANCA)-associated vasculitis. Ann Rheum Dis 2009;68(1):103–6.

58. Merkel PA, Herlyn K, Mahr AD, et al. Progress towards a core set of outcome measures in small-vessel vasculitis. Report from OMERACT 9. J Rheumatol 2009;36(10):2362–8.

59. Mukhtyar C, Lee R, Brown D, et al. Modification and validation of the Birmingham vasculitis activity score (version 3). Ann Rheum Dis 2009;68(12):1827–32.

60. Gayraud M, Guillevin L, le Toumelin P, et al. Long-term followup of polyarteritis nodosa, microscopic polyangiitis, and Churg-Strauss syndrome: analysis of four prospective trials including 278 patients. Arthritis Rheum 2001;44(3): 666–75.

61. Seo P, Min YI, Holbrook JT, et al. Damage caused by Wegener's granulomatosis and its treatment: prospective data from the Wegener's granulomatosis etanercept trial (WGET). Arthritis Rheum 2005;52(7):2168–78.

62. Jones R, Cohen Tevaert J, Hauser T, et al. Randomized trial of rituximab vs cyclophosphamide for ANCA-associated renal vasculitis: RITUXVAS [abstract]. APMIS 2009;117(Suppl 127):78.

63. Exley AR, Bacon PA, Luqmani RA, et al. Development and initial validation of the vasculitis damage index for the standardized clinical assessment of damage in the systemic vasculitides. Arthritis Rheum 1997;40(2):371–80.

64. Bacon PA, Moots RJ, Exley A, et al. VITAL (vasculitis integrated assessment log) assessment of vasculitis. Clin Exp Rheumatol 1995;13(2):275–8.

65. Abu-Shakra M, Smythe H, Lewtas J, et al. Outcome of polyarteritis nodosa and Churg-Strauss syndrome. An analysis of twenty-five patients. Arthritis Rheum 1994;37(12):1798–803.

66. Exley AR, Carruthers DM, Luqmani RA, et al. Damage occurs early in systemic vasculitis and is an index of outcome. QJM 1997;90(6):391–9.

67. Seo P, Luqmani RA, Flossmann O, et al. The future of damage assessment in vasculitis. J Rheumatol 2007;34(6):1357–71.

68. Seo P, Jayne D, Luqmani R, et al. Assessment of damage in vasculitis: expert ratings of damage. Rheumatology (Oxford) 2009;48(7):823–7.

69. Suppiah R, Flossmann O, Mukhtyar C, et al. A cross sectional study comparing the CDA to the VDI for the assessment of damage in vasculitis [abstract]. Arthritis Rheum 2009;60(Suppl 10):644.

70. Boomsma MM, Bijl M, Stegeman CA, et al. Patients' perceptions of the effects of systemic lupus erythematosus on health, function, income, and interpersonal relationships: a comparison with Wegener's granulomatosis. Arthritis Rheum 2002;47(2):196–201.

71. Reinhold-Keller E, Herlyn K, Wagner-Bastmeyer R, et al. Effect of Wegener's granulomatosis on work disability, need for medical care, and quality of life in patients younger than 40 years at diagnosis. Arthritis Rheum 2002;47(3):320–5.

72. McHorney CA, Ware JE Jr, Rogers W, et al. The validity and relative precision of MOS short- and long-form health status scales and Dartmouth COOP charts. Results from the medical outcomes study. Med Care 1992;30(Suppl 5): MS253–65.

73. Fries JF, Spitz PW, Young DY. The dimensions of health outcomes: the health assessment questionnaire, disability and pain scales. J Rheumatol 1982;9(5): 789–93.
74. Zigmond AS, Snaith RP. The hospital anxiety and depression scale. Acta Psychiatr Scand 1983;67(6):361–70.
75. Botteman MF, Hay JW, Luo MP, et al. Cost effectiveness of adalimumab for the treatment of ankylosing spondylitis in the United Kingdom. Rheumatology (Oxford) 2007;46(8):1320–8.
76. McLeod C, Bagust A, Boland A, et al. Adalimumab, etanercept and infliximab for the treatment of ankylosing spondylitis: a systematic review and economic evaluation. Health Technol Assess 2007;11(28):1–158, iii–iv.
77. Smith N, Ding T, Butt S, et al. The importance of the baseline disease activity score 28 in determining responders and non-responders to anti-TNF in UK clinical practice. Rheumatology (Oxford) 2008;47(9):1389–91.
78. Smith N, Gadsby K, Butt S, et al. Is pre-assessment for anti-TNF therapy in RA necessary in the UK? Analysis of DAS28 in six centres. Rheumatology (Oxford) 2007;46(10):1557–9.

The Future of ANCA-associated Vasculitis

Julia U. Holle, MD[a,*], Stefan Wieczorek, MD[b],
Wolfgang L. Gross, MD, PhD[a]

KEYWORDS

- ANCA-associated vasculitis • Wegener's granulomatosis
- Clinical manifestations • Treatment

In the 1950s, the vasculitides associated with antineutrophil cytoplasmic antibodies (ANCA) (Wegener's granulomatosis [WG], microscopic polyangiitis [MPA], and Churg-Strauss syndrome [CSS]) were characterized by fatal outcome with a mortality of 80% within 1 year. A median patient survival of 5 months was described for WG because no effective treatments for WG and other ANCA-associated vasculitis (AAV) were available.[1] In the 1970s, the introduction of the Fauci regimen, namely treatment with cyclophosphamide (Cyc) and glucocorticoids, represented a milestone in the improvement of patients survival.[2] Since then, several important advances have been made in the pathophysiology and treatment of AAV. The detection of ANCA as a serologic marker in the 1980s facilitated the diagnosis of AAV.[3] Subsequently, it was shown by in vitro studies and animal models that ANCA plays an important role in the pathogenesis of small-vessel vasculitis.[4–6] In the 1990s, the establishment of classification criteria[7] and disease definitions[8] led to major progress in categorizing disease entities. The European Vasculitis Study Group (EUVAS) defined disease stages for AAV (such as localized and generalized)[9,10] and initiated the first controlled trials to provide evidence for efficacy of therapy based on disease stage and disease activity.[11] Validated scores were introduced to assess disease activity (Birmingham Vasculitis Activity Score [BVAS]), disease extent (Disease Extent Index [DEI]), and damage caused by AAV (Vasculitis Damage Index [VDI]).[12–14]

Today, we have a good understanding of the pathophysiology of ANCA-induced vasculitis, but the pathophysiologic role of granulomatous lesions in WG and CSS and the role of eosinophils in CSS remain largely unknown. The authors follow a stage- and activity-based treatment regimen[11] that helps to further improve outcome and

[a] Department of Rheumatology and Clinical Immunology, Vasculitis Center, University Hospital Schleswig-Holstein, Bad Bramstedt, Oskar-Alexander-Straße 26, 24576 Bad Bramstedt, Germany
[b] Department of Human Genetics, Ruhr University MA 5/39, 44780 Bochum, Germany
* Corresponding author.
E-mail address: Holle@klinikumbb.de

Rheum Dis Clin N Am 36 (2010) 609–621
doi:10.1016/j.rdc.2010.05.007
0889-857X/10/$ – see front matter © 2010 Elsevier Inc. All rights reserved.

curtail toxic treatment regimens.[15,16] Nevertheless, there is an ongoing need for less toxic treatment strategies. Furthermore, the diagnosis of vasculitis is often made using classification criteria or disease definitions, because diagnostic criteria for the primary vasculitides are still lacking.

Future milestones in the understanding of the pathophysiology of AAV will be to elucidate the role of granulomatous lesions in WG and CSS. Understanding the genetic background of AAV (eg, by genome-wide association and subsequent fine-mapping studies) will probably offer valuable information to fully understand questions surrounding the pathogenesis of AAV and its different phenotypes. A strict classification of disease entities and phenotypes is needed, and diagnostic criteria need to be established. Regarding treatment strategies, the substitution of a less toxic treatment option instead of Cyc would be a major milestone. Rituximab is a good candidate, but long-term studies are needed to evaluate its side effects and toxicity. Moreover, answers need to be found to the questions regarding the duration of maintenance therapy required in AAV and delineation of the doses of glucocorticoids needed to control the disease during remission induction and maintenance.

ISSUES TO RESOLVE IN THE PATHOPHYSIOLOGY OF AAV
Genetics

The limited knowledge to date on the genetic background of AAV has been gained from candidate-gene approaches. The most remarkable genetic associations in WG, which have been replicated by several studies, are those with the deficiency allele PI∗Z and PI∗S of the protease-inhibitor 1 (also referred to as alpha1-antitrypsin) gene (odds ratio [OR] for ZZ/SS/SZ compared with MM, 14.62)[17,18]; for the HLA-DPB1∗0401 allele (OR 3.38–3.91)[19,20] and the 620 W allele of PTPN22 (OR 1.76).[21] Deficiency of alpha1-antitrypsin may lead to an increased presence of the autoantigen PR3 in the circulation, which may be one factor for the induction of autoimmunity against PR3. However, not all homozygous PI∗Z carriers develop WG, so additional factors must be required for the development of WG. HLA genes contribute to the risk of almost all autoimmune diseases, although the exact mechanism is not well understood. Certain HLA alleles induce a specific structure of the major histocompatibility complex peptide and/or its binding cleft, which facilitates the presentation of self-antigens to autoreactive lymphocytes. Outside the HLA region, PTPN22 is a susceptibility gene for many autoimmune diseases.[22,23] PTPN22 encodes lymphoid tyrosine kinase (LYP), a protein tyrosine phosphatase that decreases IL-2 production and inhibits T-cell receptor signaling. As a result of a single nucleotide polymorphism inducing a change in the encoded protein from arginine to tryptophan at position 620, the T cell receptor signaling is reduced. The exact pathogenic mechanism of reduced T-cell receptor signaling predisposing to autoimmunity is not fully understood, but may be related to impaired negative selection of T cells in the thymus or a reduction of regulatory T cells.[23] HLA-DPB1∗0401 and the PTPN22 R620 W allele have been linked to ANCA-positive WG with the latter also being associated with vasculitic manifestations such as glomerulonephritis.[19,20] Moreover, PTPN22 R620 W is a genetic risk factor for MPA,[24] including association with positive ANCA status. In contrast, among AAV, HLA-DPB∗0401 seems to be a specific risk factor for WG, as no associations with this allele have been found in MPA (unpublished observation) or CSS.[25] Other HLA genes have been implicated as risk factors for CSS (such as HLA-DRB1, -DRB3, -DRB4).[26] Recently, a protective haplotype of IRF5 has been identified for WG (OR 0.73) in a large study population (n>600), implicating that the interferon (IFN) type I system (IFNα and IFNβ) is involved in the pathogenesis of WG.[27] Compared with controls, the protective effect was stronger in patients with systemic disease than in those with localized disease (OR 0.68, P = .0000641 vs OR 0.8, P = not significant). In another recent study, a certain haplotype of the *IL-10* gene (IL-10.2 haplotype) has been associated with CSS, in particular with ANCA-negative CSS, but not with WG[28]; this finding may be linked to the increased serum levels of IL-10 observed in CSS. Although the results of the latter two studies need replication, they are important because they have been performed in a large study population and point to the differences in genetic background of the different diseases, and to different phenotypes within one disease.

In summary, the evidence from genetic studies in AAV suggests that the genetic background consists of risk factors that are common to several autoimmune diseases, including AAV (such as *PTPN22 R620 W*). There are also unique genetic risk factors characteristic of one AAV (such as HLA-*DPB1∗0401* for WG) or even for a phenotype within one AAV (such as the *IL10.2* haplotype being associated mainly with ANCA-negative CSS). Therefore, disease groups and phenotypes need to be considered carefully for genetic association studies to dissect the underlying pathogenetic disease mechanisms.

In the future, the genome-wide association studies will be a powerful tool to identify further genetic risk factors. It will then be important to link identified genetic risk factors to functional studies to fully understand the genetic basis for AAV and their subgroups or phenotypes.

INDUCTION OF AN ADAPTIVE IMMUNE RESPONSE IN WG
Target Antigens in AAV

Whereas there is at least some evidence from in vitro studies and from animal models for the pathophysiologic role of circulating ANCA,[4–6,29,30] far less is known about the induction or generation of ANCA. Proteinase 3 (PR3) and myeloperoxidase (MPO) are currently recognized as the main target antigens in AAV. This view has recently been challenged, however, by the detection of human lysosomal membrane protein-2 (LAMP-2) antibodies in the serum of patients with pauci-immune glomerulonephritis, 50% of whom also display antibodies against PR3 or MPO.[30] It is not certain therefore whether all relevant target antigens have been identified and whether the possible disease mechanisms elucidated in vitro or in animal models based on the assumption that PR3 and MPO are indeed the main target antigens reflect the true basis for the pathogenesis of AAV. Furthermore, it is not known why immunity against PR3 is more likely to induce the phenotype of WG characterized by formation of granulomatous lesions and vasculitic manifestations, whereas immunity against MPO seems to convey the phenotype of more or less purely vasculitic MPA.

Factors that May Contribute to the Induction of an Adaptive Immune Response

Assuming that PR3 is the main target antigen in WG, there is some evidence of how an adaptive immune response in WG is induced. Factors that may contribute to the induction of an adaptive immune response include increased presence of the autoantigen itself. In addition, cofactors may help to induce the activation of autoreactive immune cells. These cofactors may include bacterial stimuli that provide a proinflammatory environment or function as molecular mimics; or drugs that may modify the autoantigen to render it immunogenic. In WG there is an increased presence of the autoantigen PR3 in the circulation: Polymorphonuclear cells of patients with WG patients have increased percentages of membrane PR3 expression[31] and a higher percentage of mPR3 expression has been detected in relapsing patients.[32]

Furthermore, there is good evidence to assume that infectious agents function as triggers of autoimmunity. First, localized or systemic infections have been shown to increase the presence of PR3 or MPO.[33] Second, nasal carriage of *Staphyloccous aureus* is associated with increased relapse.[34] Third, the occurrence of ANCA (mainly PR3-ANCA) and of vasculitic manifestations during infections such as endocarditis, parvovirus B 19 infection–associated arthritis, and chronic hepatitis C infection have been described.[35,36] ANCA and clinical vasculitic manifestations typically disappear after adequate antibiotic therapy in endocarditis[36] and other infections. Recently, the breaking of tolerance to another potential ANCA target antigen (LAMP-2) by the bacterial antigen FimH was described for the first time in a rat model,[30] suggesting that bacterial agents may indeed function as molecular mimics for ANCA antigens and may therefore play an important role in the generation of an adaptive immune response in AAV.

Drugs are other candidates that have been associated with induction of ANCA and vasculitis. Most frequently, propylthiouracil (PTU) has been implicated in the induction of MPO-ANCA, and hydralazine, sulfasalazine, and cocaine have been associated with the induction of ANCA.[37–39] Several cross-sectional and prospective studies showed a prevalence of 20% to 64% of PTU-induced ANCA, however few patients suffered from PTU-induced vasculitic manifestations.[39] The mechanism of ANCA induction by drugs remains unclear. It has been suggested that modification of ANCA target antigen by the drug and/or its metabolites may render the target antigen immunogenic, as suggested for PTU.[39] Antibodies to citrullinated peptides in rheumatoid arthritis are a good example of peptide modification that induces an autoimmune response.[40] The concept of a target antigen requiring modification to become immunogenic is intriguing and may be a prerequisite for AAV. Nevertheless, it is not understood why the exposure to certain drugs leads to the induction of ANCA in only some of the exposed individuals; moreover, it remains to be elucidated why some individuals develop drug-induced ANCA only and some develop drug-induced ANCA with vasculitis.

In Vitro and in Vivo Models for the Induction of an Adaptive Immune Response

So far, the most convincing evidence of how an immune response is raised against ANCA target antigens comes from 2 studies. An in vitro study showed that PR3 induces maturation of GM-CSF/IL-4 dendritic cells (DC) derived from monocytes in vitro via protease receptor-2 (PAR-2)[41]; these DC can activate PR3-specific CD4+ T cells.[41] Furthermore, Kain and colleagues[30] showed that immunization of rats with the bacterial protein FimH induced antibodies cross-reactive to LAMP-2 that are expressed on the surface of neutrophils; these antibodies to LAMP-2 cause pauci-immune focal necrotizing glomerulonephritis when injected into rats. As mentioned earlier, antibodies to human LAMP-2 were detected with a high prevalence (93%) in a cohort of patients with pauci-immune glomerulonephritis who were positive for PR3- or MPO-ANCA in only 50% of cases. Another study suggests a link between infection and AAV by showing that ANCA production could be induced solely by CpG stimulation of B cells isolated from the circulation of AAV patients[42]; further studies are needed to clarify the mechanism involved in this finding.

The focus of most other studies of animal models was to prove pathogenicity of ANCA rather than to elucidate the mechanisms of ANCA induction (see later discussion).

In the future, it will be essential to identify the exact conditions that are required to induce autoimmunity against ANCA antigens. The search for other potential target antigens and the revelation of how an autoantigen relates to a certain disease or disease phenotype will be central issues to elucidate the pathophysiology of AAV. The understanding of ANCA induction will offer new targets for therapeutic interventions that interfere with the inception of the disease, even before ANCA is induced.

ANIMAL MODELS TO PROVE THE CONCEPT OF SMALL-VESSEL VASCULITIS INDUCED BY ANCA

To date, an animal model supporting the pathogenicity of ANCA has been successfully developed for MPO-ANCA, but not for PR3-ANCA. Xiao and colleagues[6] provided the first convincing model of immunity against MPO in which necrotizing vasculitis could be induced. Immunization of MPO-deficient mice with mouse MPO led to the induction of MPO-ANCA. Injection of MPO-ANCA into immunodeficient or wild-type mice generated pauci-immune focal necrotizing glomerulonephritis. A relatively small proportion of glomeruli were affected, which may be a consequence of the passive transfer of antibodies. When splenocytes from MPO-injected MPO-deficient mice were transferred into Rag2$^{-/-}$ mice, they developed necrotizing crescentic glomerulonephritis that was more severe than that induced by the passive transfer of the antibody. In a second model, the passive transfer of MPO-ANCA was circumvented by immunizing MPO$^{-/-}$ mice with MPO followed by irradiation and transplantation of bone marrow from MPO$^{+/+}$ mice. Engraftment resulted in pauci-immune necrotizing glomerulonephritis in all mice and pulmonary capillaritis in some mice.[29] Furthermore, it was shown that neutrophil localization to the glomeruli is dependent on the C5a receptor.[29] Murine models show that immunity to MPO can cause small-vessel vasculitis; it remains to be elucidated whether this occurs with or without cofactors.

PR3-ANCA–associated small-vessel vasculitis has yet to be induced in rodents, for unclear reasons (see Ref.[43] for a review). Establishing models of immunity against PR3 are further complicated because human and murine PR3 are different in structure and their antibodies do not cross-react.[44] Immunization of rats and mice with chimeric human/mouse proteinase 3 has been shown to induce autoantibodies to mouse PR3 and rat granulocytes, but did not cause vasculitis.[45] In another model, the injection of PR3 into PR3-deficient mice induced antibodies to mouse PR3, but passive transfer of anti-mouse PR3 antibodies did not induce vasculitis. After injection of tumor necrosis factor (TNF) into the skin of PR3-immunized mice, a local infiltrate of inflammatory cells could be detected.[46]

Additional studies need to dissect the pathophysiologic pathways of vasculitis induced by MPO/MPO-ANCA. Whether a model for PR3-mediated immunity will be successfully established remains unknown.

THE ROLE OF GRANULOMATOUS LESIONS IN WG

WG is not only characterized by ANCA-associated small-vessel vasculitis but also by mass formation (eg, pulmonary granuloma or orbital masses). In biopsy specimens of such masses, granuloma formation can be detected in addition to vasculitis and geographic necrosis. It has been hypothesized that WG starts with inflammation in the upper and lower respiratory tract characterized by granulomatous lesions and progresses to ANCA-associated small-vessel vasculitis in subsequent stages.[47] According to this hypothesis, an aberrant immune response may be triggered by an unknown bacterial antigen (eg, *S aureus*) leading to formation of granulomatous lesions and a subsequent adaptive immune response against PR3 (PR3-ANCA production). Consistent with this, PR3-ANCA is detected in almost all patients with generalized disease, but is less frequent in localized disease.[48,49] Likewise, anti-LAMP-2 antibodies were detected in almost all patients with focal necrotizing glomerulonephritis, but patients with localized nonrenal disease were almost uniformly negative for anti-LAMP-2 antibodies.[30]

WG granulomas may contain PR3+ cell clusters of neutrophils and monocytes[50] and lymphoid follicle-like aggregates of B cells expressing an immunoglobulin gene repertoire with potential affinity to PR3.[51] These B cells are surrounded by antigen-presenting cells and Th1-type CD4+ CD28- T cells, which are expanded and represent a major source of Th1-type cytokines (such as TNF and interferon-γ) that may function as an essential driving force in granuloma formation.[52] Whether WG granulomatous lesions are indeed the site of ANCA production remains to be clarified.

In the future, the potential role of granulomatous lesions in the pathogenesis of WG needs to be elucidated: What causes granulomatous lesions in WG? Is there a unique feature of WG granulomatous lesions and what is their function? Does autoantibody production take place in granulomatous lesions? What is the mechanism of the formation of masses (granuloma in the clinical sense) and what is the mechanism of tissue destruction induced by granulomatous masses (eg, bone erosion)?

BIOMARKERS

ANCA are a useful diagnostic tool in the diagnosis of AAV but have limitations as a biomarker. Their correlation with disease activity is controversial.[53,54] Furthermore, a substantial proportion of patients in the localized stage of WG are ANCA-negative.[48] Consequently, there is need for the identification of other biomarkers. Potential new biomarkers include circulating endothelial cells (CEC) as a marker of endothelial cell damage,[55] circulating angiopoietin-2,[56] and microparticles derived from platelets and leukocytes.[57] Levels of CECs and microparticles are increased in ANCA-associated vasculitis and correlate with disease activity.[55,57]

Other newly identified markers may also be useful in differentiating between the AAV entities or between disease subgroups. HMGB-1, a nonhistone nuclear protein released during cell necrosis and late apoptosis, is increased in WG characterized by vasculitis and granulomatous necrotic inflammation, but is not increased in MPA (Wibisono and colleagues, personal communication, 2010). Woywodt and colleagues[58] found that the level of CEC can help to distinguish between granulomatous (ie, nonvasculitic) disease and vasculitis disease in WG. Granulomatous WG is characterized by only slightly increased CEC numbers, whereas vasculitic WG is associated with high CEC numbers during active disease and relapse. Nevertheless, CEC, microparticles, and HMGB-1 are not specific for AAV and therefore cannot be used as diagnostic markers.[59–61]

In the future, biomarkers that are diagnostic of AAV and correlate well with disease activity are needed. Ideally, biomarkers should also predict relapse. Furthermore, biomarker assays should be performed quickly and reproducibly and should be simple enough to become widely available.

CLINICAL ISSUES TO RESOLVE IN AAV
Need for Diagnostic Criteria

Today, classification criteria and disease definitions[7,8] facilitate the classification of vasculitis patients into certain subgroups once vasculitis is diagnosed. These criteria are often applied as diagnostic criteria, but they were not developed for diagnostic purposes. Testing for ANCA is a useful tool to identify AAV if suspected, yet ANCA are not included in current classification criteria. A positive ANCA is absent in a substantial proportion of patients with CSS and WG, suggesting the presence of subphenotypes within these diseases.[48,62] This refuels the debate of whether AAV represent one disease entity with several subgroups or whether the individual AAVs represent single disease entities.

In the future, there is a need to establish diagnostic criteria for AAV. Common and different pathogenic features including the genetic background and the clinical phenotype need to be considered.

FUTURE TREATMENT OPTIONS IN WG
Alternatives to Cyclophosphamide for Remission Induction of Generalized AAV

In remission induction of generalized AAV, cyclophosphamide (Cyc) in conjunction with glucocorticoids is the mainstay of therapy, but preliminary results of 2 trials suggest that rituximab may be an alternative treatment option. The RAVE trial[63] compared oral Cyc (2 mg/kg body weight/d for 3–6 months) for remission induction in AAV (around 80% with WG, 20% with MPA, serum creatinine <4 mg/dL) to 4 weekly infusions of 375 mg/m^2 of rituximab. In both arms, patients received 3 pulses of 1 g methylprednisolone initially, were tapered off glucocorticoids after 6 months, and received azathioprine for remission maintenance for 18 months. Of 197 patients in the trial, 84 patients on rituximab and 81 patients on Cyc completed 6 months. After 6 months, there was no difference in the induction of remission (defined as BVAS/WG = 0 while on no glucocorticoids); 64% of patients in the rituximab group and 55% of the Cyc group achieved this primary end point. Furthermore, there was no difference in the response (defined as BVAS/WG = 0 on <10 mg prednisone/d) in the rate of flares by 6 months and of serious adverse events including infections. The rate of primary end point achievement was significantly higher in patients who received rituximab for a severe disease flare, whereas there was no significant difference in the rate of complete remissions of patients who were treated for new disease. In conclusion, the RAVE trial shows that rituximab is not inferior to oral Cyc for the induction of remission in severe AAV. Similar results were observed in the RITUXVAS trial,[64] assessing the efficacy of rituximab (375 mg/m^2 intravenously once a week for 4 weeks) plus 2 Cyc pulses compared with Cyc pulses for 3 to 6 months (44 patients, 3:1 randomization). Patients in both treatment arms received concomitant glucocorticoids, which were discontinued after 12 months; furthermore, patients on Cyc pulse therapy were switched to remission maintenance with azathioprine after 3 to 6 months. In this trial, there were no differences in the primary end point of remission at 12 months (76% vs 82%); deaths (18% in both arms); the rate of serious adverse events; the recovery of renal function; or the cumulative glucocorticoid dose. From this trial it was concluded that the combined cyclophosphamide-rituximab regimen is not inferior to a Cyc alone regimen and that rituximab was efficient in sparing Cyc pulses.

In the future, long-term data will be required to further support the role of rituximab as an alternative treatment of cyclophosphamide. Nevertheless, the data from the RAVE and RITUXVAS studies provide preliminary evidence for an alternative, noninferior treatment to Cyc in remission induction of generalized AAV. Other B-cell–depleting therapies (other than rituximab) such as ocrelizumab (humanized anti-CD20), ofatumumab (human anti-CD20), epratuzumab (humanized anti-CD22), and belimumab (humanized anti-BAFF) may also be promising options.[65,66]

Small-molecule inhibitors are yet another treatment approach, although their development is less advanced than the investigational new therapies mentioned earlier.[67] Inhibitors of kinases such as mitogen-activated protein (MAP) kinases, tyrosine kinases, and lipid kinases are currently in development and are under investigation for other rheumatic diseases. Kinases have key roles in regulation of cytokine production and responses in various rheumatic diseases. Among the MAP kinase inhibitors, p38 inhibitors have been studied in preclinical arthritis models.[68] MAP kinases (eg, JNK and ERK) and tyrosine kinases (eg, Janus kinases [JAKs] or spleen tyrosine kinase [Syk]) are potential targets to treat autoimmune disease including vasculitis. Syk is involved in the mediation of ANCA-induced neutrophil activation and neutrophil adhesion[69,70] and therefore a potential target in AAV.

Inhibition of proteasomes may be a promising therapeutic option in WG. Proteasomes are multicatalytic proteinase complexes that regulate the intracellular breakdown of various proteins, including those involved in the activation of proinflammatory signaling pathways (eg, NFkB), cell proliferation, and survival. Ex vivo, the proteasome inhibitor bortezomib inhibited the release of NFkB-inducible cytokines (such as TNF) and induced apoptosis in activated T cells from patients with rheumatoid arthritis.[71] In mice with lupus-like disease, bortezomib induces depletion of plasma cells and protects from lupus nephritis.[72] The principle of inhibiting signaling pathways (NFkB) to suppress cytokine production, especially of cytokines such as TNF, renders the drug a promising therapeutic option in WG.

ISSUES TO RESOLVE IN MAINTENANCE TREATMENT

Today it is still unclear how long maintenance therapy is required. Furthermore, it is not known whether some patients are more prone to relapse than others or which factors may be associated with relapse. A current EUVAS study addresses the duration of maintenance therapy. In the REMAIN trial, newly diagnosed patients with generalized MPA or WG receive Cyc for remission induction, and are switched to maintenance therapy with azathioprine after successful induction of remission. Patients are then randomized to receive azathioprine for 24 months or for 48 months and evaluated for the duration of remission. No preliminary data are available from this study. Similarly, there is no evidence from controlled trials as to whether glucocorticoid treatment should be continued long-term or tapered and discontinued early in the disease course. According to EULAR/EUVAS recommendations, less than 10 mg prednisone/d is recommended; glucocorticoids are to be further tapered and discontinued after 6 to 18 months in remission.[11] In contrast, in a recent study in the United States (WGET), glucocorticoids were discontinued only 6 months after the initiation of treatment.[73]

Currently, there are 4 conventional treatment options for maintenance: methotrexate (MTX), azathioprine (Aza), leflunomide (Lef), and mycophenolate mofetil (MMF). These 4 options have never been tested for efficacy in a head-to-head trial. In the WEGENT study comparing MTX and Aza, there was no significant difference between medications with regard to relapse-free survival or toxicity.[74] The IMPROVE trial reported significantly higher relapse rates with MMF (55%) compared with Aza (38%).[75] A head-to-head study comparing all 4 drugs would be desirable to determine which drug is most efficacious. Apart from conventional immunosuppressants, biologics such as rituximab may also present an option for maintenance therapy. A controlled trial (MAINRITSAN) by the French Vasculitis Study Group is currently assessing the efficacy of rituximab infusions (500 mg every 6 months) versus Aza for the maintenance of remission in AAV.

SUMMARY

Great progress is being made toward understanding the pathogenesis of AAV and improving outcomes by alternate treatment strategies with new drugs. A major problem in dealing with vasculitis is the lack of diagnostic criteria; a consensus needs to be reached on the debate whether AAV represents 1 entity or multiple individual diseases. There is further research to be done to understand the genetic background of AAV and to understand the pathophysiologic role of granulomatous lesions and mass formation in WG; so far there has been no convincing animal model demonstrating autoimmunity against PR3. Regarding treatment options, long-term data on the efficacy of rituximab are required to evaluate whether rituximab may be a substitute for cyclophosphamide for remission induction and whether it is also efficacious for maintenance therapy. Controlled data regarding the treatment of refractory disease and addressing the duration of maintenance therapy are also needed.

REFERENCES

1. Walton EW. Giant cell granuloma of the respiratory tract (Wegener's granulomatosis). Br Med J 1958;2:265–70.
2. Fauci AS, Katz P, Haynes BF, et al. Cyclophosphamide therapy of severe systemic necrotizing vasculitis. N Engl J Med 1979;301:235–8.
3. Lüdemann G, Gross WL. Autoantibodies against cytoplasmic structures of neutrophil granulocytes in Wegener's granulomatosis. Clin Exp Immunol 1987; 69:350–7.
4. Falk RJ, Terrell RS, Charles LA, et al. Anti-neutrophil cytoplasmatic autoantibodies induce neutrophils to degranulate and produce oxygen radicals in vitro. Proc Natl Acad Sci U S A 1990;87:4115–9.
5. Calderwood JM, Williams JM, Morgan MD, et al. ANCA induces beta2 integrin and CXC chemokine-dependent neutrophil-endothelial cell interactions that mimic those of highly cytokine-activated endothelium. J Leukoc Biol 2005;77: 33–43.
6. Xiao H, Heeringa P, Hu P, et al. Antineutrophil cytoplasmatic antibodies specific for myeloperoxidase cause glomerulonephritis and vasculitis in mice. J Clin Invest 2002;110:955–63.
7. Jennette JC, Falk RJ, Andrassy K, et al. Nomenclature of systemic vasculitides. Proposal of an international consensus conference. Arthritis Rheum 1994;37(2): 187–92.
8. Fries JF, Hunder GG, Bloch DA, et al. The American College of Rheumatology 1990 criteria for the classification of vasculitis. Summary. Arthritis Rheum 1990; 33:1135–6.
9. Rasmussen N, Jayne RWD, Abramowicz D, et al. European therapeutic trials in ANCA-associated systemic vasculitis: disease scoring, consensus regimens and proposed clinical trials. Clin Exp Immunol 1995;101(Suppl 1):29–34.
10. Hellmich B, Flossman O, Gross WL, et al. EULAR recommendations for conducting clinical studies and/or clinical trials in systemic vasculitis: focus on antineutrophil cytoplasm antibody-associated vasculitis. Ann Rheum Dis 2007;66: 605–17.
11. Mukhtyar C, Guillevin L, Cid MC, et al. EULAR recommendations for the management of primary small vessel vasculitis. Ann Rheum Dis 2009;68:310–7.
12. Luqmani RA, Bacon PA, Moots RJ, et al. Birmingham Vasculitis Activity Score (BVAS) in systemic necrotizing vasculitis. QJM 1994;87:671–81.
13. De Groot K, Gross WL, Herlyn K, et al. Development and validation of a Disease Extent Index for Wegener's granulomatosis. Clin Nephrol 2001;55:31–8.
14. Exley AR, Bacon PA, Luqmani RA, et al. Development and initial validation of the Vasculitis Damage Index for the standardized clinical assessment of damage in the systemic vasculitides. Arthritis Rheum 1997;40:371–80.

15. Eriksson P, Jacobsson L, Lindell A, et al. Improved outcome in Wegener's granulomatosis and microscopic polyangiitis? A retrospective analysis of 95 cases in two cohorts. J Intern Med 2009;265:496–506.

16. Stratta P, Marcuccio C, Campo A, et al. Improvement in relative survival of patients with vasculitis: study of 101 cases compared to the general population. Int J Immunopathol Pharmacol 2008;21:631–42.

17. Esnault VL, Testa A, Audrian M, et al. Alpha 1-antitrypsin genetic polymorphism in ANCA-positive systemic vasculitis. Kidney Int 1993;43:1329–32.

18. Mahr AD, Edberg J, Stone J, et al. Alpha 1-antitrypsin deficiency and the risk for Wegener's granulomatosis. In: Proceedings of the 14th International Vasculitis and ANCA Workshop [abstract N1]. APMIS 2009;117(Suppl 127):157.

19. Jagiello P, Gencik M, Arning L, et al. New genomic region for Wegener's granulomatosis as revealed by an extended association screen with 202 apoptosis-related genes. Hum Genet 2004;114:468–77.

20. Heckmann M, Holle JU, Arning L, et al. The Wegener's granulomatosis quantitative trait locus on chromosome 6p21.3 as characterized by tagSNP genotyping. Ann Rheum Dis 2008;67:972–9.

21. Jagiello P, Aries P, Arning L, et al. The PTPN22 620W allele is a risk factor for Wegener's granulomatosis. Arthritis Rheum 2005;12:4039–43.

22. Gregersen PK, Olsson LM. Recent advances in the genetics of autoimmune disease. Annu Rev Immunol 2009;27:363–91.

23. Arechiga AF, Habib T, He Y, et al. Cutting edge: the PTPN22 allelic variant associated with autoimmunity impairs B cell signaling. J Immunol 2009;182:3343–7.

24. Carr EJ, Niederer HA, Williams J, et al. Confirmation of the genetic association of CTLA4 and PTPN22 with ANCA-associated vasculitis. BMC Med Genet 2009;10:121.

25. Wieczorek S, Hellmich B, Gross WL, et al. Associations of the Churg-Strauss syndrome with the HLA-DRB1 locus, and relationship to the genetics of antineutrophil cytoplasmic antibody-associated vasculitides: comment on the article by Vaglio et al. Arthritis Rheum 2007;58:329–30.

26. Vaglio A, Martorana D, Maggiore U, et al. HLA-DRB4 as a genetic risk factor for Churg-Strauss syndrome. Arthritis Rheum 2007;56:3159–66.

27. Wieczorek S, Holle JU, Müller S, et al. A functionally relevant IRF5 haplotype is associated with reduced risk to Wegener's granulomatosis. J Mol Med 2010;88:413–21.

28. Wieczorek S, Hellmich B, Arning L, et al. Functionally relevant variations of the interleukin-10 gene associated with antineutrophil cytoplasmic antibody-negative Churg-Strauss syndrome. Arthritis Rheum 2008;58:1839–48.

29. Xiao H, Schreiber A, Heeringa P, et al. Alternative complement pathway in the pathogenesis of disease mediated by antineutrophil cytoplasmic autoantibodies. Am J Pathol 2007;170:52–64.

30. Kain R, Exner M, Brandes R, et al. Molecular mimicry in pauci-immune focal necrotizing glomerulonephritis. Nat Med 2008;14:1088–96.

31. Witko-Sarsat V, Lesavre P, Lopez S, et al. A large subset of neutrophils expressing membrane proteinase 3 is a risk factor for vasculitis and rheumatoid arthritis. J Am Soc Nephrol 1999;10:1224–33.

32. Rarok AA, Stegeman CA, Limburg PC, et al. Neutrophil membrane expression of proteinase 3 (PR3) is related to relapse in PR3-ANCA-associated vasculitis. J Am Soc Nephrol 2002;13:2232–8.

33. Matsumoto T, Kaneko T, Wada H, et al. Proteinase 3 expression on neutrophil membranes from patients with infectious disease. Shock 2006;26(2):128–33.
34. Stegeman CA, Taervert JW, Sluiter JW, et al. Association of chronic nasal carriage of *Staphylococcus aureus* and higher relapse rates in Wegener granulomatosis. Ann Intern Med 1994;120:12–7.
35. Belizna CC, Hamidou MA, Levesque H, et al. Infection and vasculitis. Rheumatology 2009;48:475–82.
36. Choi HK, Lamprecht P, Niles JL, et al. Subacute bacterial endocarditis with positive cytoplasmatic antineutrophil cytoplasmatic antibodies and anti-proteinase 3 antibodies. Arthritis Rheum 2000;43:226–31.
37. Gao Y, Zhao MH. Drug-induced antineutrophil cytoplasmic antibody-associated vasculitis. Nephrology (Carlton) 2009;14:33–41.
38. Wiik A. Drug-induced vasculitis. Curr Opin Rheumatol 2008;20:35–9.
39. Otsuka S, Kinebuchi A, Tabata H, et al. Myeloperoxidase-antineutrophil cytoplasmic antibody-associated vasculitis following propylthiouracil therapy. Br J Dermatol 2000;142:828–30.
40. Rantapää-Dahlqvist S, de Jong BA, Berglin E, et al. Antibodies against cyclic citrullinated peptide and IgA rheumatoid factor predict the development of rheumatoid arthritis. Arthritis Rheum 2003;48:2741–9.
41. Csernok E, Ai M, Gross WL, et al. Wegener autoantigen induces maturation of dendritic cells and licenses them for Th1 priming via protease-activated receptor-2 pathway. Blood 2006;107:4440–8.
42. Hurtado RR, Jeffs L, Nitschke J, et al. CpG oligodeoxynucleotide stimulates production of antineutrophil cytoplasmic antibodies in ANCA associated vasculitis. BMC Immunol 2008;9:34.
43. Kain R, Firmin DA, Rees AJ. Pathogenesis of small-vessel vasculitis associated with autoantibodies to neutrophil cytoplasmic antigens: new insights from animal models. Curr Opin Rheumatol 2010;22:15–20.
44. Wiesner O, Litwiller RD, Hummel AM, et al. Differences between human proteinase 3 and neutrophil elastase and their murine homologues are relevant for murine model experiments. FEBS Lett 2005;579:5305–12.
45. Van der Geld YM, Hellmark T, Selga D, et al. Rats and mice immunised with chimeric human/mouse proteinase 3 produce autoantibodies to mouse PR3 and rat granulocytes. Ann Rheum Dis 2007;66:1679–82.
46. Pfister H, Ollert M, Fröhlich LF, et al. Antineutrophil cytoplasmic autoantibodies against the murine homolog of proteinase 3 (Wegener autoantigen) are pathogenic in vivo. Blood 2004;104:1411–8.
47. Fienberg R. The protracted superficial phenomenon in pathergic (Wegener's) granulomatosis. Hum Pathol 1981;12:458–67.
48. Reinhold-Keller E, de Groot K, Rudert H, et al. Response to trimethoprim/sulfamethoxazole in Wegener's granulomatosis depends on the phase of disease. QJM 1996;89:15–23.
49. Reinhold-Keller E, Beuge N, Latza U, et al. An interdisciplinary approach to the care of patients with Wegener's granulomatosis: long-term outcome in 155 patients. Arthritis Rheum 2000;43(5):1021–32.
50. Voswinkel J, Mueller A, Lamprecht P. Is PR3-ANCA formation initiated in Wegener's granulomatosis lesions? Granulomas as potential lymphoid tissue maintaining antibody production. Ann N Y Acad Sci 2005;1051:12–9.
51. Voswinkel J, Mueller A, Kraemer JA, et al. B lymphocyte maturation in Wegener's granulomatosis: a comparative analysis of VH genes from endonasal lesions. Ann Rheum Dis 2006;65:859–64.

52. Csernok E, Trabandt A, Müller A, et al. Cytokine profiles in Wegener's granulomatosis: predominance of type 1 (Th1) in the granulomatous inflammation. Arthritis Rheum 1999;42:742–50.
53. Cohen Taervert JW, van der Woude FJ, Fauci AS, et al. Association between active Wegener's granulomatosis and anticytoplasmatic antibodies. Arch Intern Med 1989;149:2461–5.
54. Finkielman JD, Merkel PA, Schroeder D, et al, WGET Research Group. Antiproteinase 3 antineutrophil cytoplasmatic antibodies and disease activity in Wegener granulomatosis. Ann Intern Med 2007;147:611–9.
55. Woywodt A, Streiber F, de Groot K, et al. Circulating endothelial cells as markers for ANCA-associated small vessel vasculitis. Lancet 2003;361:206–10.
56. Kümpers P, Hellpap J, David S, et al. Circulating angiopoietin-2 is a marker and potential mediator of endothelial cell detachment in ANCA-associated vasculitis with renal involvement. Nephrol Dial Transplant 2009;24:1845–50.
57. Erdbrügger U, Grossheim M, Hertel B, et al. Diagnostic role of endothelial microparticles in vasculitis. Rheumatology 2008;57:1820–5.
58. Woywodt A, Goldberg C, Kirsch T, et al. Circulating endothelial cells in relapse and limited granulomatous disease due to ANCA-associated vasculitis. Ann Rheum Dis 2006;65:164–8.
59. Grundmann M, Woywodt A, Kirsch T, et al. Circulating endothelial cells: a marker of vascular damage in patients with preeclampsia. Am J Obstet Gynecol 2008;198:317, e1–5.
60. Kniff-Dutmer EA, Koerts J, Nieuwland R, et al. Elevated levels of platelet microparticles are associated with disease activity in rheumatoid arthritis. Arthritis Rheum 2002;46:1498–503.
61. Ek M, Popovic K, Harris HE, et al. Increased extracellular levels of the novel proinflammatory cytokine high mobility group box chromosomal protein 1 in minor salivary glands of patients with Sjögren's syndrome. Arthritis Rheum 2006;54:2289–94.
62. Pagnoux C, Guillevin L. Churg-Strauss syndrome: evidence for disease subtypes? Curr Opin Rheumatol 2010;22:21–8.
63. Stone JH, Merkel PA, Seo P, et al. Rituximab versus cyclophosphamide for the induction of remission in ANCA-associated vasculitis: a randomized controlled trial (RAVE) [abstract 550]. Arthritis Rheum 2009;60(Suppl 10):S204.
64. Jones R, Cohen-Tervaert JW, Hauser T, et al. Randomized trial of rituximab vs. cyclophosphamide for ANCA-associated renal vasculitis: RITUXVAS [abstract A24]. APMIS 2009;117(Suppl 127):78.
65. Levesque MC. Translational mini-review series on B cell-directed therapies: recent advances in B-cell-directed biological therapies for autoimmune disorders. Clin Exp Immunol 2009;157:198–208.
66. Krumbholz M, Specks U, Wick M, et al. BAFF is elevated in serum of patients with Wegener's granulomatosis. J Autoimmun 2005;25:298–302.
67. Goeb V, Bunch MH, Vital EM, et al. Costimulation blockade in rheumatic diseases: where we are? Curr Opin Rheumatol 2009;21:244–50.
68. Badger AM, Griswold DE, Kapadia R, et al. Disease-modifying activity of SB 242235, a selective inhibitor of p38 mitogen-activated protein kinase, in rat adjuvant-induced arthritis. Arthritis Rheum 2000;43:175–83.
69. Zarbock A, Lowell CA, Lay K. Spleen tyrosine kinase Syk is necessary for E-selection-induced alpha(L)beta2 integrin-mediated rolling on intercellular adhesion molecule-1. Immunity 2007;26:773–83.

70. Hewins P, Williams JM, Wakelam MJ, et al. Activation of Syk in neutrophils by anti-neutrophil cytoplasm antibodies occurs via Fcgamma receptors and CD18. J Am Soc Nephrol 2004;15:796–808.
71. van der Heijden JW, Oelremans R, Lems WF, et al. The proteasome inhibitor bortezomib inhibits the release of NFKappaB-inducible cytokines and induces apoptosis of activated T-cells from rheumatoid arthritis patients. Clin Exp Rheumatol 2009;27:92–8.
72. Neubert K, Meister S, Moser K, et al. The proteasome inhibitor bortezomib depletes plasma cells and protects mice with lupus-like disease from nephritis. Nat Med 2008;14:748–55.
73. Wegener's Granulomatosis Etanercept Trial (WGET) Research Group. Etanercept plus standard therapy for Wegener's granulomatosis. N Engl J Med 2005;352(4): 351–61.
74. Pagnoux C, Mahr A, Hamidou MA, et al. Azathioprine of methotrexate maintenance for ANCA-associated vasculitis. N Engl J Med 2008;359:2790–803.
75. Hiemstra T, Walsh M, de Groot K, et al. Randomized trial of mycophenolate mofetil vs. azathioprine for maintenance therapy in ANCA-associated vasculitides (AAV) [abstract A23]. APMIS 2009;117(Suppl 127):77.

Index

Note: Page numbers of article titles are in **boldface** type.

A

Abdominal pain
  in Churg-Strauss syndrome, 531
  in microscopic polyangiitis, 550–551
Adverse events, as outcome measure, 593, 600–601
Age factors, in Wegener's granulomatosis, 448–449
Allergic rhinitis, in Churg-Strauss syndrome, 529
Alveolar hemorrhage
  diffuse, diagnosis of. *See* ANCA-associated vasculitis, diagnosis of.
  in microscopic polyangiitis, 549
ANCA-associated vasculitis. *See also specific diseases.*
  autoantibodies in, **479–489**
  Churg-Strauss syndrome, **527–543**
  clinical presentations in, 491–494
  diagnosis of, **491–506,** 527
    clinical presentations in, 491–494
    criteria for, 614–615
    general approach to, 491–496
    histopathological, 500
    in multisystem involvement, 499–500
    in specific organ systems, 496–499
    laboratory testing in, 494–496, 532–533
    recurrent, 500
    research needs in, 614–615
  epidemiology of, **447–461**
  future of, **609–621**
  histopathology of, 500
  history of, **439–446**
  laboratory testing in, 494–496, 532–533
  microscopic polyangiitis, **545–558**
  ocular manifestations of, **573–586**
  outcome measures of, **587–607**
  pathogenesis of, **463–477**
    ANCA in, 464
    animal models of, 466–467
    antiendothelial cell antibodies in, 468–469
    etiology theories in, 470–471
    issues to resolve in, 610–611
    lymphocytes in, 469–470
    lysosomal membrane protein 2 in, 468
    neutrophils in, 464–467
  pauci-immune necrotizing glomerulonephritis, **559–572**

Rheum Dis Clin N Am 36 (2010) 623–636
doi:10.1016/S0889-857X(10)00062-1
0889-857X/10/$ – see front matter © 2010 Elsevier Inc. All rights reserved.

rheumatic.theclinics.com

Moving?

Make sure your subscription moves with you!

To notify us of your new address, find your **Clinics Account Number** (located on your mailing label above your name), and contact customer service at:

Email: journalscustomerservice-usa@elsevier.com

800-654-2452 (subscribers in the U.S. & Canada)
314-447-8871 (subscribers outside of the U.S. & Canada)

Fax number: 314-447-8029

Elsevier Health Sciences Division
Subscription Customer Service
3251 Riverport Lane
Maryland Heights, MO 63043

*To ensure uninterrupted delivery of your subscription, please notify us at least 4 weeks in advance of move.